Human Health and Physiology Essentials: Vitamin C

Human Health and Physiology Essentials: Vitamin C

Editor: Mavis Keller

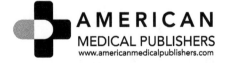

AMERICAN
MEDICAL PUBLISHERS
www.americanmedicalpublishers.com

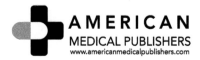

AMERICAN
MEDICAL PUBLISHERS
www.americanmedicalpublishers.com

Cataloging-in-Publication Data

Human health and physiology essentials : vitamin C / edited by Mavis Keller.
    p. cm.
Includes bibliographical references and index.
ISBN 978-1-63927-693-6
1. Vitamin C. 2. Vitamin C--Physiological effect. 3. Vitamin C--Metabolism.
4. Vitamin C--Therapeutic use. 5. Vitamin C--Health aspects. 6. Vitamin C deficiency.
I. Keller, Mavis.
QP772.A8 H86 2023
612.399--dc23

American Medical Publishers,
41 Flatbush Avenue,
1st Floor, New York,
NY 11217, USA

ISBN 978-1-63927-693-6 (Hardback)

Contents

Preface

Every book is a source of knowledge and this one is no exception. The idea that led to the conceptualization of this book was the fact that the world is advancing rapidly; which makes it crucial to document the progress in every field. I am aware that a lot of data is already available, yet, there is a lot more to learn. Hence, I accepted the responsibility of editing this book and contributing my knowledge to the community.

Vitamin C is a vital water-soluble vitamin, which is needed by a human body for a variety of metabolic functions. It is one of the most important nutrients required for treating common cold and cough. It is synthesized naturally in many animals but humans must consume vitamin C-rich meals to derive the vitamin-C. It is also utilized in repairing damaged tissues and for the production of crucial neurotransmitters. It plays a major role in appropriate functioning of the immune system. It is also utilized in the form of a cofactor for enzymes essential in the hydroxylation of lysine and proline to produce collagen. The lack of vitamin C can lead to decreased production of collagen that eventually results in the breakdown of body tissues, scaly skin, gingivitis, decreased wound healing, nosebleed, and decreased ability of the body to prevent infections. This book provides significant information to help develop a good understanding of vitamin C and its impact on human health. The topics included herein on vitamin C are of utmost significance and bound to provide incredible insights to readers. The extensive content of this book provides the readers with a thorough understanding of the subject.

While editing this book, I had multiple visions for it. Then I finally narrowed down to make every chapter a sole standing text explaining a particular topic, so that they can be used independently. However, the umbrella subject sinews them into a common theme. This makes the book a unique platform of knowledge.

I would like to give the major credit of this book to the experts from every corner of the world, who took the time to share their expertise with us. Also, I owe the completion of this book to the never-ending support of my family, who supported me throughout the project.

Editor

Vitamin C Transporters and their Implications in Carcinogenesis

Kinga Linowiecka [1,*], **Marek Foksinski** [2,*] **and Anna A. Brożyna** [1,*]

1   Department of Human Biology, Faculty of Biological and Veterinary Sciences,
     Nicolaus Copernicus University, 87-100 Toruń, Poland
2   Department of Clinical Biochemistry, Faculty of Pharmacy, Collegium Medicum,
     Nicolaus Copernicus University, 85-092 Bydgoszcz, Poland
*   Correspondence: klinowiecka@umk.pl (K.L.); marekf@cm.umk.pl (M.F.); anna.brozyna@umk.pl (A.A.B.)

Abstract: Vitamin C is implicated in various bodily functions due to its unique properties in redox homeostasis. Moreover, vitamin C also plays a great role in restoring the activity of 2-oxoglutarate and Fe^{2+} dependent dioxygenases (2-OGDD), which are involved in active DNA demethylation (TET proteins), the demethylation of histones, and hypoxia processes. Therefore, vitamin C may be engaged in the regulation of gene expression or in a hypoxic state. Hence, vitamin C has acquired great interest for its plausible effects on cancer treatment. Since its conceptualization, the role of vitamin C in cancer therapy has been a controversial and disputed issue. Vitamin C is transferred to the cells with sodium dependent transporters (SVCTs) and glucose transporters (GLUT). However, it is unknown whether the impaired function of these transporters may lead to carcinogenesis and tumor progression. Notably, previous studies have identified SVCTs' polymorphisms or their altered expression in some types of cancer. This review discusses the potential effects of vitamin C and the impaired SVCT function in cancers. The variations in vitamin C transporter genes may regulate the active transport of vitamin C, and therefore have an impact on cancer risk, but further studies are needed to thoroughly elucidate their involvement in cancer biology.

Keywords: vitamin C; SVCT polymorphisms; carcinogenesis

1. Vitamin C Properties and Redox Homeostasis

Vitamin C, a common name for l-ascorbic acid or l-ascorbate, is a six-carbon lactone. It can be synthesized from glucose by enzyme l-gulono-1,4-lactone oxidase, which can be found in almost every mammal's liver, with the exception of humans, other primates, bats, and guinea pigs [1,2]. Consequently, these species must provide their organisms with l-ascorbate exogenously. Since l-ascorbate is a key factor in intensifying the activity of numerous enzymes located throughout the human body, the external intake of vitamin C is particularly important. Its unique properties are connected with its structure and biochemistry: ascorbic acid can be transformed into ascorbate monoanion or ascorbate dianion via the dissociation of one or two hydrogen ions from hydroxyl groups located at carbon 2 and carbon 3. In physiological pH ascorbate functions as a monoanion, which is its primary form. Ascorbic acid is known to be a significant reducing factor, easily subject to the compilations of two one-electron oxidations. The first one is accomplished via ascorbate radical generation [3], providing a specific chemical structure (resonance stabilization) with a stable yet not highly reactive form [4]. The ascorbate radical can then undergo the second one-electron oxidation to form dehydroascorbic acid (DHA) (Figure 1) [3]. This ability makes ascorbate a particularly good defender against other free radicals by substituting them with more stable and less reactive compounds [4]. Furthermore, in vitro studies demonstrated that an increased level of ascorbate can act as a stimulus to cooperate with superoxide dismutase in the removal of superoxides [5]. DHA and ascorbate radicals can also be reduced to ascorbate in a reversible manner [3].

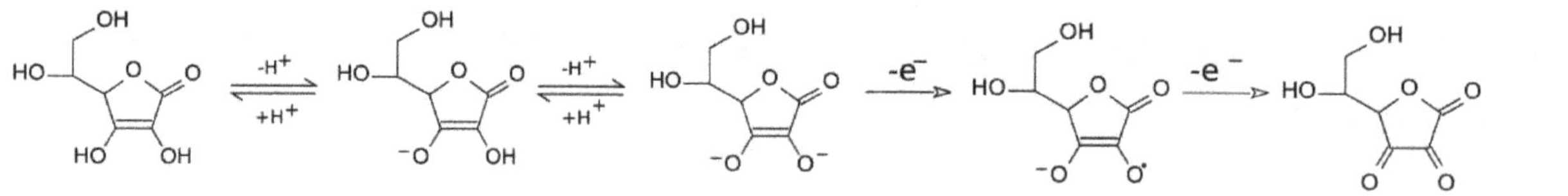

Figure 1. Vitamin C redox states. Ascorbic acid undergoes two reversible hydrogen dissociations to form ascorbate monoanions and ascorbate dianions, respectively. Then, ascorbate dianons can be subsequently subjected to one-electron oxidation to create ascorbate radicals. These are not highly reactive components; however, they can undergo another one-electron oxidation to form dehydroascorbic acid.

Despite its ability to act as a reducing agent, ascorbate can also perform a key role as an oxidative factor. Although the oxidation process of ascorbate occurs mainly in the presence of catalytic metals, the process can be performed by ascorbate itself (autooxidation) but at a significantly slower rate in neutral pH [6]. The effect of vitamin C oxidation is hydrogen peroxide formation, which can affect cellular metabolism, by changing intracellular redox stability [6,7]. Moreover, vitamin C can act as a prodrug through its ability to serve as a reducing and oxidizing factor [7]. The privileged form of vitamin C is determined by the vitamin C concentration in plasma. In physiological concentrations, ascorbic acid preferentially exerts its antioxidant functions, which help restore cellular 2-oxoglutarate and Fe^{2+} dependent dioxygenase activity (2-OGDDs) [8]. On the other hand, a higher level of ascorbic acid is linked to pro-oxidative functions [7].

2. Vitamin C and Its Role in 2-OGDD Enzymes Activity

Due to its antioxidant potential, vitamin C can also serve as an enzyme cofactor. 2-OGDD enzymes require 2-oxoglutarate (2-OG) and Fe^{2+} to maintain their catalytic activity. However, most 2-OGGDs also require ascorbate as a cofactor [9]. The family of 2-OGDDs consists of more than 60 enzymes that contain specific double-stranded β-helix (DSBH) motifs with Fe^{2+} ions in their cores. Their catalytic functions relate to the hydroxylation of particular substrates with the decarboxylation of 2-OG to succinate in the presence of oxygen [10]. Ascorbic acid crucially increases the rate of the reaction catalyzed by 2-OGGD by targeting its catalytic domain and regenerating iron ions from Fe^{3+} to Fe^{2+} (Figure 2) [11].

Research over the past decade has highlighted that vitamin C has a crucial function in epigenetics. In 2009, Tahiliani et al. shed new light on the epigenetic field. The authors discovered that ten-eleven-translocation enzymes (TET: TET1, TET2, TET3), originally considered as chromosomal translocations of the genes MLL and LCX (t(10;11)(q22;q23)) in acute myeloid leukemia patients [12,13], are actually responsible for changing the DNA methylation pattern [14]. Their research indicated that TETs have the ability to induce the hydroxylation of 5-methylcytosine (5-mC) to 5-hydroxymethylcytosine (5-hmC), which leads to DNA demethylation [14]. Later developments in this field revealed that TETs are also involved in the further hydroxylation of 5-hmC to the other cytosine derivatives, which can be subsequently excised by DNA glycosylases [15]. A number of studies have found that ascorbate is an important compound for TET protein activity, since these proteins belong to the 2-OGDD superfamily. It has been proven that ascorbic acid enhances 5-hmC generation by promoting the hydroxylation of 5-mC provided by TET proteins [16]. Additionally, it was conclusively demonstrated that ascorbic acid's impact on TET proteins is not only due to its reducing ability, as other strong oxidizing agents do not present a similar activity [17]. In line with this finding, vitamin C was proposed to be an agent that promotes DNA demethylation [16,17]. DNA methylation and demethylation are not only linked with cytosine modifications, but also with chromatin reorganization through changes in the amino acids in histones. The enzymes responsible for histone demethylation are Jumonji C-domain-containing histone demethylases (JHDMs), which also belong to the 2-OGDD superfamily [18]. As mentioned in the literature review, more than 20 JHDMs are capable of eliminating the methyl groups of lysines, which are located in histones [9,19]. Previous studies identified that the methylation of lysines can induce or inhibit transcription depending on their location in the histones. Methylation located at lysine 9 in histone H3 and at lysine 20 in histone H4 provides gene silencing, whereas the methylation of lysine 4, lysine 36, and lysine 79 in histone H3 is linked with enhancing transcription [20,21]. A large and growing body of evidence has investigated the essential role of the impaired balance between methylation and demethylation during cancer initiation and progression [22–25]. In recent years, there has been an increasing interest in TET or JHDM mutations in different cancers, especially hematological ones [26–28]. Therefore, the plausible effects of vitamin C in cancer therapy have been the central aim of numerous works of research.

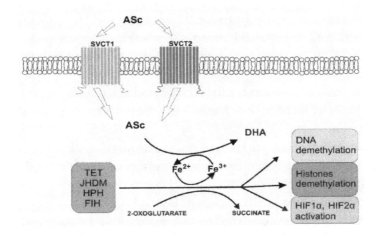

Figure 2. Vitamin C's role in 2-oxoglutarate and Fe^{2+} dependent dioxygenase (2-OGDD) activity. Legend abbreviations: ASc—ascorbate; SCVT1—sodium dependent vitamin C transporter 1; SCVT2—sodium dependent vitamin C transporter 2; DHA—dehydroascorbic acid, TET—ten–eleven translocation proteins; JHDM—Jumonji C-domain-containing histone demethylases; HPH—hypoxia-inducible factor prolyl hydroxylases; FIH—factor-inhibiting hypoxia-inducible factor; HIF1α—subunit α of the hypoxia inducible factor 1; HIF2 α—subunit α of the hypoxia inducible factor 2. Ascorbate can be engaged in restoring the activity of 2-OGDD enzymes by reducing Fe^{3+} to Fe^{2+}, which can be found in the catalytic center of those enzymes. 2-OGDD enzymes also require 2-oxoglutarate to maintain their catalytic activity. TET, JHDM, HPH and FIH are members of the 2-OGDD family, and their main roles in cell biochemistry are based on DNA demethylation (TET proteins), histone demethylation (JHDM proteins) and HIF1α and HIF2 α activation (HPH and FIH proteins). A more detailed description is given in the text.

Other members of the 2-OGDD family are the hypoxia-inducible factors prolyl hydroxylases (HPHs) and the factor-inhibiting hypoxia-inducible factor (FIH), which are arranged during the initiation of the degradation of subunit α of the hypoxia inducible factors HIF1 and HIF2. HIFs take part in cellular adaptation to an anaerobic state, which frequently occurs in tumors [29]. The tumor microenvironment is distinct from that observed in healthy tissues. Tumor cells have the ability to divide very quickly and frequently. Thus, boosting the tumor mass generates separation from blood vessels. Although angiogenesis is common in cancer development, the newly formed vessels are distinct from healthy ones in terms of their structures and functions [30]. Taken together, there is a decrease in the partial pressure of oxygen in tumor masses compared to the pressure observed in corresponding healthy tissue [31,32]. A hypoxic state in tumors can increase the tumor's invasiveness and ability to metastasize [33]. HIFs are composed of two constitutively expressed subunits, α and β. In normoxic conditions, subunit α is hydroxylated by HPH and FIH; after a multistage post-translational process, subunit α is degraded by proteasomes [29]. However, in a hypoxic state, subunit α is stabilized, followed by bonding with the β subunit, which eventually facilitates the transcription of specific genes.

HIF1-α and HIF2-α differ from each other via transcription regulation: HIF1-α is responsible mainly for the regulation of genes involved in cellular metabolic changes, and HIF2-α is responsible for the control of genes involved in cellular signaling and extracellular matrix remodeling factors [34–36]. Moreover, both factors exhibit different expressions during hypoxia: in an acute hypoxic state, HIF1-α is highly expressed, whereas long-termed hypoxia results in HIF2-α accumulation [37]. Given that subunit α stabilization is crucial for the expression of HIFs, HPHs and FIH are major factors contributing to cell adaptation under an anaerobic state. Hence, any dysregulation of these enzymes may itself be a trigger of cancer initiation.

3. Vitamin C Transporters: Their Function and Distribution in the Human Body

In the late 1970s, Cameron et al. published a study featuring the significant recovery of cancer patients who ingested vitamin C (10 g orally and 10 g intravenously) [38]. Several years later, two independent randomized controlled studies demonstrated that a daily oral intake of 10 g of ascorbate by patients with cancer resulted in no significant differences from those treated with a placebo [39,40]. However, all these studies suffer from some serious limitations. The main omissions in the above-mentioned research are the routes of administration for vitamin C and the vitamin's pharmacokinetics in the human body. Preliminary comprehensive work on the relationship between doses of ascorbic acid intake and its concentration in plasma and tissues, as well as bioavailability and urinary excretion, was undertaken by Levine et al. [41]. Based on the results from seven healthy volunteers, the authors determined that the daily recommended dietary allowance for vitamin C is 200 mg/day, but the dose that induces urinary excretion of ascorbic acid is lower (100 mg/day). Moreover, doses higher than 500 mg/day seemed to be ineffective, resulting in nearly complete urinary excretion. Furthermore, 100 mg of vitamin C administered daily was responsible for approximately 60 μM plasma ascorbic acid concentration, and, more importantly, higher oral intake produced plasma concentrations up to 75–90 μM [41]. This finding highlights the unambiguous relationship between the oral administration of ascorbic acid and the upper saturation of the plasma ascorbate concentration. These outcomes further support the tight control of ascorbic acid plasma concentration driven by renal reabsorption and excretion [42,43]. Furthermore, the foregoing studies clearly illustrated that the route of vitamin C administration is a crucial factor for plasma concentration. It was thoroughly demonstrated that the intravenous intake of ascorbic acid can contribute to a 30–60-fold increase in plasma concentration compared to the upper level of its oral doses [41–43].

Since vitamin C exhibits a complicated pharmacokinetic range from its absorption to its elimination, its metabolism should be conducted by specialized transporters that regulate it through active or passive transport mechanisms.

Ascorbic acid administration is followed by its absorption in the digestive tract, accumulation in tissues, and reabsorption and excretion by the kidneys. This can be achieved through active transport across cell membranes via the sodium-dependent vitamin C transporters SVCT1 and SVCT2 which were cloned for the first time from rats [44]. SVCTs can actively transport ascorbic acid against the gradient by coupling its entry with sodium inflow to the cell, thus maintaining the sodium gradient throughout the plasma membrane, which is provided by Na/K- ATPase [44–46]. However, SVCT2, unlike SVCT1, requires specific ions (Ca^{2+}/Mg^{2+}) to fully maintain its biological efficiency [46]. Both SVCT1 and SVCT2 display a high affinity to the non-transformed form of ascorbic acid, whereas no other form of vitamin C can be used as a substrate [44,47]. Each transporter is a product of a different gene, either *SLC23A1* or *SLC23A2*. *SLC23A1* is located in chromosome 5 (locus 5q31.2–31.3), whereas *SLC23A2* is mapped to chromosome 20 (locus 20p12.2–12.3). Although both enzymes exhibit 66% amino acid sequence identity, they feature distinctive tissue distributions [48,49]. Interestingly, a review by Bürzle et al. identified a third transporter, SVTC3, which is an orphan transporter whose functions remain unclear. However, this transporter exhibits approximately 30% sequence identity with SVCT1 and SVCT2 [50]. Further work is required to establish SVCT3's function. Thus far, many studies have been published on SVCT1 and SVCT2. SVCT1 is highly expressed in the epithelium of the small intestine, liver, pancreas, kidneys, reproductive organs, lungs, and skin [44,51]. Both SVCT1 and SVCT2 are found in the intestines. However, the expression of SVCT1 is greater than that of SVCT2 [44]. The most crucial location of SVCT1 is the brush-border membrane of the proximal tubule in renal tissue, which is involved in the renal reabsorption of ascorbic acid. Consequently, SVCT1 is primarily involved in maintaining the vitamin C level in the human body [52,53]. Therefore, a knockout of the *Slc23a1* gene in mice provides almost complete vitamin C urinary elimination, thereby losing approximately 70% of ascorbate tissue supplies [52]. Consequently, the loss of SVCT1 expression in primates may lead to more serious consequences, as they cannot synthetize ascorbic acid by themselves. Moreover, research concerning ascorbic acid transport affinity and capacity underline the key role of SVCT1 in ascorbate reabsorption in the kidneys: SVCT1's affinity to ascorbic acid is low, but SVCT1 can transport this compound with a high capacity [44,47]. By contrast, the other vitamin C transporter, SVCT2, transports vitamin C with high affinity but with a relatively low capacity [47]. SVCT2 is expressed in almost every cell in the human body, particularly in cells that accumulate vitamin C, such as those in the eyes, adrenal glands, and brain [44,51]. Sotiriou et al. conducted a study in which the authors applied a genetic knockout of the *Slc23a2* gene in a murine model. Prenatal supplementation of ascorbic acid in mice lacking an SVCT2 analog did not have any effect, and the mice died within several minutes after birth due to brain hemorrhage [54]. Thus, it is believed that SCVT2 is essential for brain development. In line with this research, Parker et al. indicated that the pericytes found in brain microvessels are enriched with SVCT2 transporters, which allows such microvessels to collect ascorbate [55].

Since vitamin C easily oxidizes and transforms into DHA upon a pH change, such a change does not inhibit vitamin C transport. DHA transport can be mediated via facilitated diffusion lead by glucose transporters (GLUTs), which is a sodium-independent process. Moreover, the reduced form of vitamin C (AA) is not transferred via GLUT transporters [56–58]. Following diffusion, DHA is rapidly reduced into its AA form with the simultaneous oxidation of glutathione and NADPH [59], which is called ascorbate recycling in the literature [60]. As mentioned in the literature review, the GLUT family consists of 14 members that have been identified in most tissues in the human body. Primarily, these members are responsible for glucose transport between the extracellular space and the cells [61]. Nonetheless, previous studies demonstrated that members of the GLUT family can also transport DHA via GLUT1, GLUT3, and GLUT4 [56,57], but none of these transporters is expressed in enterocytes, where vitamin C is absorbed [58]. GLUT2 and GLUT8 are expressed in the intestines, and these two transporters are putatively involved in DHA transfer [58]. However, according to Corpe et al., the DHA transport by GLUTs may be interrupted by dietary factors, which in turn lead to decreased vitamin C bioavailability [58]. Furthermore, a few GLUTs have a considerably weaker affinity for glucose than for DHA. In line with these observations, several cell culture studies suggest that DHA transport is an alternate, or even principal pathway of vitamin C accumulation [62,63]. However, later research on the murine model indicated that SVCT2 knockout in mice led to their demise, despite normally functioning GLUTs [54]. An important question is whether the same pathways of DHA transport are present in human and mice (or other animal) models. As far as we know, GLUT transporters are diverse in human and murine red blood cells [64], and humans and rats show different expressions of GLUT in the intestines [65].

On the other hand, there are several studies concerning the key role of vitamin C transport provided by GLUT in cancer cells [66,67]. A recent paper by Pena et al. suggested that the vast majority of vitamin C transferred from the extracellular space into cancer cells assumes the form of DHA [66]. The authors reported that cancer cells were able to acquire vitamin C, even if they expressed an abnormal form of SVCT2, by using GLUT transporters and converting DHA to AA inside the cells [66]. This phenomenon is called the bystander effect and was previously thoroughly described [63].

4. Effects of Vitamin C on Cancer Cells

Due to the pleiotropic functions of vitamin C, the idea of using this compound as a potential anti-cancer drug is not new. However, the past decade has seen increasingly rapid advances in novel approaches to cancer therapy. There is a general agreement that cancer patients exhibit significantly lower level of vitamin C in their plasma compared to healthy subjects [8,68,69]. Moreover, previous studies conclusively demonstrated that ascorbate deficiency can improve the invasiveness of cancer cells [70,71]. One plausible explanation of vitamin C depletion is oxidative stress in cells and reactive oxygen species (ROS) formation over the course of carcinogenesis. It is widely known that cancer cells exhibit different metabolic processes as a result of the dysfunction of the cellular organelles (mainly the mitochondria). This eventually leads to excessive ROS generation, followed by chronic inflammation [72,73]. Vitamin C acts as a radical scavenger due to its antioxidant ability and plays a pivotal role in ROS elimination, so vitamin C levels may eventually decline when free radicals are excessively generated [74]. Therefore, it was suggested that vitamin C may have great value in cancer therapy. In line with this hypothesis, a considerable amount of literature has been published on vitamin C's ability to destroy cancer cells in vitro and in vivo, even under pharmacological concentrations [7,75,76]. Moreover, it was also indicated that ascorbate has the ability to inhibit cancer growth [77]. There are several possible ways that vitamin C can exert anti-cancer action. One of them is vitamin C's pro-oxidant ability, which is revealed mainly at high doses and can be accessed only via intravenous intake. Several studies provided by Chen et al. showed that vitamin C may produce hydrogen peroxide (H_2O_2) as an intermediate of ascorbate radical generation in cancer cells [7,75,77]. H_2O_2, as one of ROS, plays a key role in maintaining the cellular redox state, it may have an impact on disrupting cancer cells' metabolism [78]. According to Uetaki et al., the main target for vitamin C's anti-cancer action is the inhibition of glycolysis via a decrease in NAD [78]. Interestingly, vitamin C cytotoxicity is observed only in tumor cells while omitting normal ones [75]. This difference may be the result of an altered mode of ATP generation in cancer cells: instead of oxidative proliferation, such cells preferentially undergo glycolysis, even in an aerobic state. This process is commonly known as the Warburg effect [79]. Hence, vitamin C is targeted in the process and is mainly responsible for energy production in the tumor cells. Furthermore, some cancer-specific mutations are actually associated with the Warburg effect, as previously demonstrated [80,81]. KRAS or BRAF mutations that occur in colorectal cancer may also contribute to glucose uptake and GLUT1 overexpression [82]. As mentioned, GLUT1 transports DHA, which is reduced to ascorbic acid directly after transferring to the cell [59]. A great amount of GLUT1 in KRAS and BRAF mutant cells can be a target for high doses of vitamin C, which can ultimately lead to ROS generation and cancer cell death [81].

However, abnormal cell functions during carcinogenesis are predisposed to reduced oxygen availability [83], and a hypoxic state in cancer cells may restrain the cytotoxic effect of vitamin C [84]. Therefore, there is a second explanation for the selective attack of vitamin C on cancer cells based on vitamin C's potential to react with iron ions, which can be found in the catalytic centers of multiple enzymes [3]. According to the hypothesis proposed by Ngo et al., there is an abundance of Fe^{2+} ions in specific cancer microenvironments, which can generate H_2O_2 and •OH through a reaction with vitamin C [85]. Moreover, the enrichment of Fe^{2+} inside cancer cells may stimulate the diffusion of H_2O_2 from extracellular space, which is an intermediate for vitamin C autooxidation [85]. In both cases, an excessive amount of H_2O_2 may lead to cytotoxicity in cancer cells.

A large and growing body of studies have demonstrated that the balance between methylation and demethylation is disturbed in many types of cancers [23,86–88]. It was found that 5-mC changes involve 5-hmC reductions in tumors [23,24]. Such alterations are proven to have an impact on the transcription of key genes in the human body, including oncogenes and tumor suppressor genes, which may provoke carcinogenesis [89]. Moreover, it was recently detected that the vitamin C level correlates with 5-hmC [90] and, since 5-hmC is potentially involved in the regulation of gene expression [25], ascorbate may also be involved in this process. Ascorbate is a co-factor of TET proteins, which are members of the 2-OGGD family. Several in vitro [16,91–93] and in vivo [94] studies have established that ascorbate has the ability to increase 5-hmC. It is also noteworthy that vitamin C removal in vitro correlates with a remarkable decrease in the 5-hmC level with a parallel increase in the 5-mC level [91]. Furthermore, TET2 mutations often occur in hematological malignancies, with approximately 10%

in acute myeloid leukemia, 30% in myelodysplastic syndrome, and 50% in chronic myelomonocytic leukemia [95]. Notably, in the case of TET2 mutations, application of vitamin C has the ability to restore TET2 deficiency and promote DNA demethylation [96]. The relationship between TET2 enzymes and ascorbate therapy in leukemic cells was also detected in a study by Zhao et al. [97], who found that vitamin C administration increased TET2 activity. However, in terms of TET2 expression, a similar effect was not detected [97]. Vitamin C in cancer therapy has other beneficial effects on the suppression of tumor growth and metastasis (discussed below) [92,98–100], which may be associated with changes in the transcription and expression of genes caused by changes in DNA methylation. As mentioned above, other enzymes regulating the epigenome that depend upon vitamin C are JHDMs connected with chromatin changes [18]. Several studies have identified vitamin C as a crucial agent contributing to the JHDM-dependent chromatin demethylation that occurs during hematopoiesis and somatic cell reprogramming [101–104]. Given that DNA methylation changes are the most prevalent among the various epigenetic processes, vitamin C likely has great value in the regulation of gene expression.

5. Vitamin C in Adjuvant Cancer Therapy

Vitamin C has been frequently prescribed as a complementary or alternative treatment for cancer patients in previous decades. Following the report that intravenous ascorbic acid administration is safe [105], there has been an increasing amount of literature on implementing ascorbic acid therapy in various cancers. However, one question that needs to be asked is whether vitamin C influences conventional chemotherapy or radiotherapy. Vitamin C seems to be effective in preventing the side effects of chemotherapy and radiotherapy [106,107]. However, the ROS generated during radiation may be eliminated by vitamin C, which can diminish the therapeutic effect of radiotherapy. Similarly, chemotherapeutic agents whose pharmacological actions are based on ROS generation may also be inefficient under vitamin C supplementation [108]. Therefore, there is still a need for further research in this field.

5.1. Hematological Malignancies

In vitro studies on leukemia cells proved that ascorbic acid plays an important role in modifying the growth of cancer cells [109]. Moreover, even a pharmacological concentration of ascorbic acid is sufficient to particularly kill the primary cancer cells in blood samples from multiple myeloma patients [110]. A recent in vitro study suggested that vitamin C can contribute to increased chemosensitivity in the lymphoma cell line via the induction of SMAD1 expression, which is frequently silenced by methylation in diffuse large B-cell lymphoma [111]. Moreover, the stage of lymphoma is inversely associated with the vitamin C level [111]. Ascorbic acid was also successfully used as an adjunct therapy for hypomethylating agents in AML patients [97]. Additionally, a recent clinical report supports the beneficial role of the intravenous administration of ascorbate in cases of AML with TET2 mutation [112]. Moreover, the parenteral use of vitamin C in AML with a relapse significantly improves blood cell counts and quality of life [113].

5.2. Breast Cancer

Similar to hematological malignancies, vitamin C is decreased in more severe cases of breast cancer [114]. Furthermore, a decreased level of vitamin C in breast tumors is linked with higher HIF-1 pathway activity and a more advanced stage of necrosis [114]. Moreover, recent studies indicated that ascorbic acid can induce apoptosis in breast cancer cell lines. According to the authors, vitamin C is associated with the upregulation of TRAIL, which is proven to be an apoptosis inducer [115]. Ascorbic acid also contributes to suppressing the invasion and migration of breast cancer cell lines by inhibiting the epithelial–mesenchymal transition [116]. Interestingly, in vitro studies on a triple-negative breast cancer cell line demonstrated that the concentration of vitamin C obtainable by oral intake is sufficient to inhibit metastatic activity [100]. Furthermore, in vivo studies indicated that the dietary supplementation of ascorbic acid may reduce the mortality of breast cancer patients [117]. Surprisingly, the dietary intake of ascorbic acid in postmenopausal women may actually enhance the risk of breast carcinogenesis [118].

5.3. Melanoma

In vitro studies and murine models indicated that vitamin C inhibits invasion and growth in melanoma cells [70,71,92]. According to Chen et al., ascorbic acid promotes the apoptosis of melanoma cells by stimulating the Bax/Bcl-2 pathway, which leads to the activation of caspases followed by protein degradation and cell death [119]. Moreover, a recent study by Yang et al. suggested that ascorbic acid induces cytotoxicity in melanoma cells in a dose-dependent manner [120]. Only high concentrations of vitamin C are sufficient to induce cell death, whereas at lower concentrations, vitamin C can, in fact, promote invasiveness and tumor growth [120]. Vitamin C also plays an important role in the regulation of the HIF1-α protein under normoxic conditions. However, the expression of HIF1-α in cancer cells is extensive, so it may be conducive to the expression of particular proteins associated with melanoma cell motility and invasion [121]. Moreover, in vitro studies indicated that the melanogenesis process induced in melanoma cells may, in fact, be a trigger for an increase in HIF1-α expression [122]. The supplementation of ascorbic acid in melanoma cell lines contributes to the regulation of HIF1-α activity and accumulation [123,124]. Interestingly, a similar effect was not visible for DHA supplementation. Therefore, it seems possible that the ascorbic acid control of HIF1-α stability is reliant on SVCT activity. Moreover, it has been suggested that HIF1-α may interact with the TET2 protein in the melanoma and glioblastoma cell lines [123]. Supplementation of ascorbic acid in melanoma cell lines with TET2 knockdown resulted in an increase in 5-hmC. In addition, HIF1-α knockdown contributed to enhancing TET2 expression in melanoma and glioblastoma cells [123], which shed new light on the plausible regulation of expression between these two proteins in malignant cells.

5.4. Glioma and Glioblastoma

Millimolar doses of sodium ascorbate are also believed to have a relevant impact on the inhibition of glioblastoma cell invasion and viability in both in vitro and in vivo models [125]. However, according to the authors, a specific form of cell death provoked by sodium ascorbate called autoschizis needs further examination before using vitamin C as an adjunctive cancer therapy [125]. Nonetheless, a meta-analysis by Zhou et al. indicated that vitamin C intake may help to diminish the chance of glioma incidence [126]. Moreover, several studies indicated that, in glioma patients, intravenous supplementation may successfully serve as an adjuvant tumor therapy and significantly increase survival, as well as reduce and stabilize the tumor [127,128].

5.5. Prostate Cancer

Similar to the aforementioned in vitro studies, the effect of vitamin C on prostate cancer cell lines restrains the proliferation and movement of those cell lines [125]. However, the experimental data from in vivo studies are rather controversial, and there is no general agreement about the effects of ascorbic acid on prostate tumors. The parenteral administration of vitamin C to rats with prostate cancer yielded promising results. The ascorbic acid contributed to tumor suppression and the inhibition of metastasis [98]. Favorable results were also achieved in a meta-analysis comprising over 18 prostate cancer studies, indicating the association between vitamin C and a reduction in prostate cancer incidence [129]. Interestingly, according to The Prostate Cancer and Environment Study, ascorbic acid through dietary administration does not decrease the risk of prostate cancer or lower its aggressiveness at diagnosis [130]. Similar results were obtained in a posttrial study by Wang et al., who indicated that vitamin C supplementation did not contribute to prostate cancer occurrence [131].

6. Impaired SVCT Function in Cancer

6.1. Polymorphisms of SVCT

The vitamin C concentration in plasma and tissues has been identified as a one of the major contributing factors for cancer incidence. As mentioned above, cancer patients often exhibit a lower level of vitamin C in their plasma [8,68,69]. Apart from ROS generation and a changed redox status in cancer cells, it was suggested that this phenomenon may be linked to the single nucleotide polymorphisms (SNPs) of the vitamin C transporters SVCT1 and SVCT2. SNPs in the coding regions of *SLC23A1* and *SLC23A2* are implicated in the vitamin C level in plasma and its transport inhibition [132,133]. A cohort study involving 15000 participants by Timpson et al. conclusively demonstrated that *SLC23A1* rs33972313 is involved in decreasing of vitamin C circulating concentrations, which decreased by over 4 μmol [132]. According to a murine study by Corpe et al., *SLC23A1* rs33972313 is associated with a 40–50% reduction in ascorbate accumulation in cells [52]. Furthermore, a European Prospective Investigation into Cancer and Nutrition (EPIC) cohort study revealed that both SVCT1 and SVCT2 SNPs are implicated in the vitamin C plasma concentration [133]. This study determined that two *SLC23A1* SNPs, rs11950646 and rs33972313, are involved in vitamin C decreases of 10–13% and 24%, respectively. Interestingly, two *SLC23A2* SNPs, rs6053005 and rs6133175, were both found to be associated with an ascorbic acid increase of 24% [133]. This discrepancy may be due to the different roles and types of localization among vitamin C transporters. Although this subject needs further research, SVCT1 and SVCT2 SNPs may serve as ascorbic acid level predictors.

While this process is still being explored, previous studies reported the involvement of SVCT SNPs in several cancers. Since SVCT1 is responsible for vitamin C absorption and reabsorption, it is possible to find the *SLC23A1* SNP in gastric cancers. Surprisingly, none of the SVCT1 genetic polymorphisms are associated with gastric cancer risk [133,134]. However, polymorphisms of the second vitamin C transporter SVCT2: *SLC23A2* (*SLC23A2* rs6116568 and *SLC23A2* rs12479919) were correlated with gastric cancer incidence [133,134]. The concentration of vitamin C in the gastric juice and mucosa is significantly higher than that observed in plasma [135], which highlights vitamin C's important role in stomach function. However, previous studies indicated that rat gastric glands are rich in SVCT2 instead of SVCT1 [44]. Thus, SVCT2 alone may play a crucial role in vitamin C absorption.

The involvement of a genetic polymorphism of SVCT1 in cancer was detected in follicular lymphoma. A large population-based case–control study revealed that *SLC23A1* rs6596472 and *SLC23A1* rs11950646 may increase the risk of follicular lymphoma by up to 80% [136]. An elevated risk of follicular lymphoma was also associated with a genetic variant of SVCT2 (*SLC23A2* rs1776948). The same variant and two others (*SLC23A2* rs6133175 and *SLC23A2* rs1715364) were also identified in chronic lymphocytic leukemia (CLL) [136]. A study involving over 400 CLL cases detected a significant correlation between the same two SVCT2 polymorphisms (*SLC23A2* rs6133175 and *SLC23A2* rs1776948) with CLL development [137]. Moreover, these genetic variants of *SLC23A2* could not be modulated by fruit and vegetable intake as a dietary principal source of vitamin C. However, the CLL patients had greater fruit administration than healthy subjects [137]. Dietary vitamin C consumption was also not found to be associated with a risk of advanced colorectal adenoma [138]. However, incidence of this cancer was correlated with two genetic variations of SVCT2, *SLC23A2* rs4987219 and *SLC23A2* rs1110277 [138]. The genetic variant *SLC23A2* rs4987219 was also found to be a possible modifier of human papillomavirus 16 (HPV16)-associated head and neck cancer [139]. According to this study, predispositions for HPV16 infection followed by this type of head and neck cancer are strongly associated with vitamin C metabolism. It was suggested that genetic variations of SVCT transporters have distinct exposures to HPV16 [139]. It cannot be excluded that SNPs found in the *SLC23A1* and *SLC23A2* genes may have an impact on transcription regulation. All known effects of SVCT polymorphisms are collected in Table 1.

Table 1. SVCT polymorphisms and their implications.

SVCT Type	SNP ID	Effect	References
SVCT1	*SLC23A1* rs33972313	decrease in circulating vitamin C	Timpson et al., 2010 [132]
		40–50% reduction in ascorbate accumulation in murine cells	Corpe et al., 2010 [52]
		24% decrease in vitamin C's plasma concentration	Duell et al., 2013 [133]
	SLC23A1 rs11950646	10–13% decrease in vitamin C's plasma concentration	Duell et al., 2013 [133]
	SLC23A1 rs6596472	higher risk of follicular lymphoma	Skibola et al., 2008 [136]
	SLC23A1 rs11950646	higher risk of follicular lymphoma	Skibola et al., 2008 [136]
SVCT2	*SLC23A2* rs6053005	24% increase in vitamin C's plasma concentration	Duell et al., 2013 [133]
	SLC23A2 rs6133175	24% increase in vitamin C's plasma concentration	Duell et al., 2013 [133]
	SLC23A2 rs6116568	higher risk of gastric cancer	Duell et al., 2013 [133]
	SLC23A2 rs12479919	higher risk of gastric cancer	Wright et al., 2009 [134]
	SLC23A2 rs1776948	higher risk of follicular lymphoma	Skibola et al., 2008 [136]
		higher risk of chronic lymphocytic leukemia (CLL)	Skibola et al., 2008 [136] Casabonne et al., 2017 [137]
	SLC23A2 rs6133175	higher risk of chronic lymphocytic leukemia (CLL)	Skibola et al., 2008 [136] Casabonne et al., 2017 [137]
	SLC23A2 rs1715364	higher risk of chronic lymphocytic leukemia (CLL)	Skibola et al., 2008 [136]
	SLC23A2 rs4987219	higher risk of colorectal adenoma	Erichsen et al., 2008 [138]
		plausible modifying factor of HPV16-associated head and neck cancer	Chen et al., 2009 [139]
	SLC23A2 rs1110277	higher risk of colorectal adenoma	Erichsen et al., 2008 [138]

6.2. Altered Expression of SVCT

The location of SVCT1 is mostly limited to epithelial tissues; hence, SVCT1 is primarily responsible for vitamin C homeostasis and circulation in the whole body [44,51]. Given that a loss of *SLC23A1* contributes to serious vitamin C deficiency in mice [52], it seems possible that alterations in SVCT1 may be far more severe in humans. To date, there is no study on SVCT1 loss in humans. On the other hand, SVCT2 is located in the vast majority of metabolically active tissues and conceivably controls vitamin C accumulation [44,51]. Hence, it seems possible that alterations in SVCT2 may be involved in carcinogenesis. Therefore, several studies analyzed SVCT2 expression. SVCT2 expression has been detected in multiple tumor samples, with a significantly higher percentage of intracellular, rather than membrane, immunoreactivity [67]. Moreover, studies on breast cancer have indicated the differential expression of SVCT2 in breast tumors, with the highest level in hormone-independent breast cancer. Normal breast epithelium samples, however, have not shown SVCT2 expression. Interestingly, the expression of SVCT1 in breast tumor samples has not been detected [66]. Further examination of the breast cancer cell lines revealed that these cell lines are incapable of vitamin C intake in an ascorbic acid form via SVCT transporters and can only intake in ascorbic acid form as DHA using GLUT transporters. This observation indicates SVCT2 deficiency in the cell membrane. However, the expression of this transporter has been identified in the mitochondria, where it is presumably responsible for low affinity vitamin C transport [66]. According to a study by Hong et al., SVCT2 is crucial for ascorbate-induced cancer cell death [140]. Ascorbate transport via SVCT2 to cancer cells is associated with enhanced intracellular ROS generation, which eventually leads to breast cancer cell termination. Furthermore, SVCT2 knockdown in breast cancer cells with previously high SVCT2 expression resulted in resistance to ascorbic acid treatment [140]. The association between SVCT2 expression and ascorbic acid treatment has also been evaluated in colorectal cancer cell lines [141]. Similar to a previous study, the cytotoxicity of ascorbic acid was proportional to the expression of SVCT2. Moreover, the cellular response to ascorbic acid treatment was dependent on SVCT2 expression. Cancer cells with low SVCT2 expression levels exhibited anti-cancer effects at high doses of ascorbic acid and a proliferative effect at low doses of this compound. In contrast, cancer cells with high SVCT2 expression exerted anti-cancer outcomes at all ascorbic acid concentrations. A possible explanation for this discrepancy is the insufficient ROS generation at low ascorbic acid concentrations in colorectal cancer cells with low SVCT2 expression [141]. The intensified cytotoxicity induced by ascorbic acid, which depends on SVCT2 expression, has also been investigated in hepatocellular cancer [142] and cholangiocarcinoma [143]. Moreover, colorectal cancers with KRAS mutations are often resistant to cetuximab, which is a major drug used in the therapy of these cancers [144]. An in vitro study on colon cancer cells with KRAS mutations showed that vitamin C can partner with cetuximab to induce cell death depending on SVCT2 expression [145]. According to the authors, ascorbic acid combined with cetuximab may impact the MAPK/ERK signaling pathway, which is disturbed in colon cancers with a KRAS mutation. However, specific changes in MAPK/ERK signaling after ascorbic acid and cetuximab exposure were observed only in colorectal cancer cells with SVCT2 expression [145]. Furthermore, the impact of ascorbic acid on MAPK/ERK signaling, which depends on SVCT2 expression, was also discovered in mouse neuroblastoma cells [146]. It was suggested that the overexpression of SVCT2 is associated with the differentiated phenotype of N2a mouse neuroblastoma cells. The supplementation of ascorbic acid to neuroblastoma cells with SVCT2 overexpression resulted in the promotion of MAPK/ERK phosphorylation, which may eventually lead to central nervous system development [146].

7. Conclusions

Since its conception, the possibility of treating cancer with vitamin C has been a controversial and much-disputed subject. Some published data have indicated promising findings for vitamin C's role in cancer therapy, as well as its bioavailability in cancers. Its clinical anticancer potential is reflected in the number of clinical trials involving vitamin C. The level of vitamin C in cells may be related to vitamin C transporter expression and its polymorphism in cells. Therefore, mutations of the two main vitamin C transporters may contribute to their impaired function and thus may plausibly contribute to cancer development, as suggested in this review. Further investigations are needed to estimate the actual association between polymorphisms of SVCT, cancer risk and incidence. Additionally, the positions of genetic polymorphisms in the SLC23A1 and SLC23A2 genes include introns and exons [147]. Hence, the reason why polymorphisms located in introns play a role in vitamin C regulation remains ambiguous. It seems possible that genetic variations may have an impact on the regulation of SVCT transcription. According to Skibola et al., in silico models indicate that the polymorphisms of SLC23A2 (SLC23A2 rs1715364) may increase SLC23A2 expression, which may consequently intensify vitamin C bioavailability [136]. Vitamin C appears to be a promising candidate for cancer prevention and treatment. However, there is still a need for further research, especially on the role of vitamin C transporter polymorphisms in different types of cancers and cancer treatments.

Author Contributions: All authors equally contributed to this work. All authors have read and agreed to the published version of the manuscript.

Acknowledgments: The authors would like to thank Lukasz Czarnecki for preparing figures for this review.

References

1. Nishikimi, M.; Yagi, K. Biochemistry and molecular biology of ascorbic acid biosynthesis. *Subcell. Biochem.* **1996**, *25*, 17–39. [CrossRef] [PubMed]
2. Cui, J.; Pan, Y.-H.; Zhang, Y.; Jones, G.; Zhang, S. Progressive pseudogenization: Vitamin C synthesis and its loss in bats. *Mol. Biol. Evol.* **2010**, *28*, 1025–1031. [CrossRef] [PubMed]
3. Du, J.; Cullen, J.J.; Buettner, G.R. Ascorbic acid: Chemistry, biology and the treatment of cancer. *Biochim. Biophys. Acta* **2012**, *1826*, 443–457. [CrossRef] [PubMed]
4. Bielski, B.H.J. Chemistry of ascorbic acid radicals. In *Ascorbic Acid: Chemistry, Metabolism, and Uses*; Advances in Chemistry; American Chemical Society: Washington, WA, USA, 1982; Volume 200, pp. 81–100. ISBN 978-0-8412-0632-8.
5. Jackson, T.S.; Xu, A.; Vita, J.A.; Keaneyjr, J.F. Ascorbate prevents the interaction of superoxide and nitric oxide only at very high physiological concentrations. *Circ. Res.* **1998**, *83*, 916–922. [CrossRef]
6. Buettner, G.R. In the absence of catalytic metals ascorbate does not autoxidize at pH 7: Ascorbate as a test for catalytic metals. *J. Biochem. Biophys. Methods* **1988**, *16*, 27–40. [CrossRef]
7. Chen, Q.; Espey, M.G.; Sun, A.Y.; Lee, J.-H.; Krishna, M.C.; Shacter, E.; Choyke, P.L.; Pooput, C.; Kirk, K.L.; Buettner, G.R.; et al. Ascorbate in pharmacologic concentrations selectively generates ascorbate radical and hydrogen peroxide in extracellular fluid in vivo. *Proc. Natl. Acad. Sci. USA* **2007**, *104*, 8749–8754. [CrossRef]
8. Liu, M.; Ohtani, H.; Zhou, W.; Ørskov, A.D.; Charlet, J.; Zhang, Y.W.; Shen, H.; Baylin, S.B.; Liang, G.; Grønbæk, K.; et al. Vitamin C increases viral mimicry induced by 5-aza-2'-deoxycytidine. *Proc. Natl. Acad. Sci. USA* **2016**, *113*, 10238–10244. [CrossRef]
9. Clifton, I.J.; McDonough, M.A.; Ehrismann, D.; Kershaw, N.J.; Granatino, N.; Schofield, C.J. Structural studies on 2-oxoglutarate oxygenases and related double-stranded β-helix fold proteins. *J. Inorg. Biochem.* **2006**, *100*, 644–669. [CrossRef]
10. A McDonough, M.; Loenarz, C.; Chowdhury, R.; Clifton, I.J.; Schofield, C.J. Structural studies on human 2-oxoglutarate dependent oxygenases. *Curr. Opin. Struct. Biol.* **2010**, *20*, 659–672. [CrossRef]
11. Gorres, K.L.; Raines, R.T. Prolyl 4-hydroxylase. *Crit. Rev. Biochem. Mol. Biol.* **2010**, *45*, 106–124. [CrossRef]
12. Ono, R.; Taki, T.; Taketani, T.; Taniwaki, M.; Kobayashi, H.; Hayashi, Y. LCX, leukemia-associated protein with a CXXC domain, is fused to MLL in acute myeloid leukemia with trilineage dysplasia having t(10;11)(q22;q23). *Cancer Res.* **2002**, *62*, 4075–4080.
13. Lorsbach, R.B.; Moore, J.; Mathew, S.; Raimondi, S.C.; Mukatira, S.T.; Downing, J.R. TET1, a member of a novel protein family, is fused to MLL in acute myeloid leukemia containing the t(10;11)(q22;q23). *Leukemia* **2003**, *17*, 637–641. [CrossRef]
14. Tahiliani, M.; Koh, K.P.; Shen, Y.; Pastor, W.A.; Bandukwala, H.; Brudno, Y.; Agarwal, S.; Iyer, L.M.; Liu, D.R.; Aravind, L.; et al. Conversion of 5-Methylcytosine to 5-Hydroxymethylcytosine in mammalian DNA by MLL partner TET1. *Science* **2009**, *324*, 930–935. [CrossRef] [PubMed]
15. Ito, S.; Shen, L.; Dai, Q.; Wu, S.C.; Collins, L.B.; Swenberg, J.A.; He, C.; Zhang, Y. Tet proteins can convert 5-Methylcytosine to 5-Formylcytosine and 5-Carboxylcytosine. *Science* **2011**, *333*, 1300–1303. [CrossRef] [PubMed]
16. Minor, E.A.; Court, B.L.; Young, J.I.; Wang, G. Ascorbate Induces Ten-Eleven Translocation (Tet) methylcytosine dioxygenase-mediated generation of 5-Hydroxymethylcytosine. *J. Biol. Chem.* **2013**, *288*, 13669–13674. [CrossRef] [PubMed]
17. Yin, R.; Mao, S.-Q.; Zhao, B.; Chong, Z.; Yang, Y.; Zhao, C.; Zhang, D.; Huang, H.; Gao, J.; Li, Z.; et al. Ascorbic acid enhances tet-mediated 5-Methylcytosine oxidation and promotes DNA demethylation in mammals. *J. Am. Chem. Soc.* **2013**, *135*, 10396–10403. [CrossRef]
18. Tsukada, Y.-I.; Fang, J.; Erdjument-Bromage, H.; Warren, M.E.; Borchers, C.H.; Tempst, P.; Zhang, Y. Histone demethylation by a family of JmjC domain-containing proteins. *Nat. Cell Biol.* **2006**, *439*, 811–816. [CrossRef]
19. Klose, R.J.; Kallin, E.M.; Zhang, Y. JmjC-domain-containing proteins and histone demethylation. *Nat. Rev. Genet.* **2006**, *7*, 715–727. [CrossRef]
20. Miller, J.L.; Grant, P.A. The role of DNA methylation and histone modifications in transcriptional regulation in humans. *Subcell. Biochem.* **2013**, *61*, 289–317. [CrossRef]
21. Martin, C.; Zhang, Y. The diverse functions of histone lysine methylation. *Nat. Rev. Mol. Cell Biol.* **2005**, *6*, 838–849. [CrossRef]

22.   Clark, S.; Melki, J. DNA methylation and gene silencing in cancer: Which is the guilty party? *Oncogene* **2002**, *21*, 5380–5387. [CrossRef] [PubMed]

23.   Haffner, M.C.; Chaux, A.; Meeker, A.K.; Esopi, D.M.; Gerber, J.; Pellakuru, L.G.; Toubaji, A.; Argani, P.; Iacobuzio-Donahue, C.; Nelson, W.G.; et al. Global 5-hydroxymethylcytosine content is significantly reduced in tissue stem/progenitor cell compartments and in human cancers. *Oncotarget* **2011**, *2*, 627–637. [CrossRef] [PubMed]

24.   Kudo, Y.; Tateishi, K.; Yamamoto, K.; Yamamoto, S.; Asaoka, Y.; Ijichi, H.; Nagae, G.; Yoshida, H.; Aburatani, H.; Koike, K. Loss of 5-hydroxymethylcytosine is accompanied with malignant cellular transformation. *Cancer Sci.* **2012**, *103*, 670–676. [CrossRef] [PubMed]

25.   Yildirim, O.; Li, R.; Hung, J.-H.; Chen, P.B.; Dong, X.; Ee, L.-S.; Weng, Z.; Rando, O.J.; Fazzio, T.G. Mbd3/NURD complex regulates expression of 5-Hydroxymethylcytosine marked genes in embryonic stem cells. *Cell* **2011**, *147*, 1498–1510. [CrossRef]

26.   Andricovich, J.; Kai, Y.; Tzatsos, A. Lysine-specific histone demethylases in normal and malignant hematopoiesis. *Exp. Hematol.* **2016**, *44*, 778–782. [CrossRef]

27.   Delhommeau, F.; Dupont, S.; Della Valle, V.; James, C.; Trannoy, S.; Massé, A.; Kosmider, O.; Le Couedic, J.-P.; Robert, F.; Alberdi, A.; et al. Mutation inTET2in myeloid cancers. *N. Engl. J. Med.* **2009**, *360*, 2289–2301. [CrossRef]

28.   Kosmider, O.; Gelsi-Boyer, V.; Ciudad, M.; Racoeur, C.; Jooste, V.; Vey, N.; Quesnel, B.; Fenaux, P.; Bastie, J.-N.; Beyne-Rauzy, O.; et al. TET2 gene mutation is a frequent and adverse event in chronic myelomonocytic leukemia. *Haematologica* **2009**, *94*, 1676–1681. [CrossRef]

29.   Brahimi-Horn, M.C.; Pouysségur, J. HIF at a glance. *J. Cell Sci.* **2009**, *122*, 1055–1057. [CrossRef]

30.   Postovit, L.-M.; Abbott, D.E.; Payne, S.L.; Wheaton, W.W.; Margaryan, N.V.; Sullivan, R.; Jansen, M.K.; Csiszar, K.; Hendrix, M.J.; Kirschmann, D.A. Hypoxia/reoxygenation: A dynamic regulator of lysyl oxidase-facilitated breast cancer migration. *J. Cell. Biochem.* **2008**, *103*, 1369–1378. [CrossRef]

31.   Vaupel, P.; Höckel, M.; Mayer, A. Detection and characterization of tumor hypoxia using pO2 histography. *Antioxid. Redox Signal.* **2007**, *9*, 1221–1236. [CrossRef]

32.   Carreau, A.; El Hafny-Rahbi, B.; Matejuk, A.; Grillon, C.; Kieda, C. Why is the partial oxygen pressure of human tissues a crucial parameter? Small molecules and hypoxia. *J. Cell. Mol. Med.* **2011**, *15*, 1239–1253. [CrossRef] [PubMed]

33.   Harris, A.L. Hypoxia—A key regulatory factor in tumour growth. *Nat. Rev. Cancer* **2002**, *2*, 38–47. [CrossRef] [PubMed]

34.   Semenza, G.L. Signal transduction to hypoxia-inducible factor 1. *Biochem. Pharmacol.* **2002**, *64*, 993–998. [CrossRef]

35.   Pugh, C.W.; Ratcliffe, P.J. Regulation of angiogenesis by hypoxia: Role of the HIF system. *Nat. Med.* **2003**, *9*, 677–684. [CrossRef] [PubMed]

36.   Downes, N.L.; Laham-Karam, N.; Kaikkonen-Määttä, M.; Ylä-Herttuala, S. Differential but complementary HIF1α and HIF2α transcriptional regulation. *Mol. Ther.* **2018**, *26*, 1735–1745. [CrossRef] [PubMed]

37.   Holmquist-Mengelbier, L.; Fredlund, E.; Löfstedt, T.; Noguera, R.; Navarro, S.; Nilsson, H.; Pietras, A.; Vallon-Christersson, J.; Borg, Å.; Gradin, K.; et al. Recruitment of HIF-1α and HIF-2α to common target genes is differentially regulated in neuroblastoma: HIF-2α promotes an aggressive phenotype. *Cancer Cell* **2006**, *10*, 413–423. [CrossRef]

38.   Cameron, E.; Pauling, L. Supplemental ascorbate in the supportive treatment of cancer: Reevaluation of prolongation of survival times in terminal human cancer. *Proc. Natl. Acad. Sci. USA* **1978**, *75*, 4538–4542. [CrossRef]

39.   Creagan, E.T.; Moertel, C.G.; O'Fallon, J.R.; Schutt, A.J.; O'Connell, M.J.; Rubin, J.; Frytak, S. Failure of High-Dose Vitamin C (Ascorbic Acid) Therapy to Benefit Patients with Advanced Cancer. A controlled trial. *N. Engl. J. Med.* **1979**, *301*, 687–690. [CrossRef]

40.   Moertel, C.G.; Fleming, T.R.; Creagan, E.T.; Rubin, J.; O'Connell, M.J.; Ames, M.M. High-Dose Vitamin C versus Placebo in the Treatment of Patients with Advanced Cancer Who Have Had No Prior Chemotherapy. A randomized double-blind comparison. *N. Engl. J. Med.* **1985**, *312*, 137–141. [CrossRef]

41.   Levine, M.; Conry-Cantilena, C.; Wang, Y.; Welch, R.W.; Washko, P.W.; Dhariwal, K.R.; Park, J.B.; Lazarev, A.; Graumlich, J.F.; King, J.; et al. Vitamin C pharmacokinetics in healthy volunteers: Evidence for a recommended dietary allowance. *Proc. Natl. Acad. Sci. USA* **1996**, *93*, 3704–3709. [CrossRef]

42. Graumlich, J.F.; Ludden, T.M.; Conry-Cantilena, C.; Cantilena, J.L.R.; Wang, Y.; Levine, M. Pharmacokinetic model of ascorbic acid in healthy male volunteers during depletion and repletion. *Pharm. Res.* **1997**, *14*, 1133–1139. [CrossRef] [PubMed]

43. Levine, M.; Wang, Y.; Padayatty, S.J.; Morrow, J. A new recommended dietary allowance of vitamin C for healthy young women. *Proc. Natl. Acad. Sci. USA* **2001**, *98*, 9842–9846. [CrossRef] [PubMed]

44. Tsukaguchi, H.; Tokui, T.; MacKenzie, B.; Berger, U.V.; Chen, X.-Z.; Wang, Y.; Brubaker, R.F.; Hediger, M.A. A family of mammalian Na+-dependent L-ascorbic acid transporters. *Nat. Cell Biol.* **1999**, *399*, 70–75. [CrossRef] [PubMed]

45. Wilson, J.X. Regulation of Vitamin C transport. *Annu. Rev. Nutr.* **2005**, *25*, 105–125. [CrossRef]

46. Godoy, A.; Ormazabal, V.; Moraga-Cid, G.; Zúñiga, F.A.; Sotomayor, P.; Barra, V.; Vasquez, O.; Montecinos, V.; Mardones, L.; Guzmán, C.; et al. Mechanistic Insights and Functional Determinants of the Transport Cycle of the Ascorbic Acid Transporter SVCT2. Activation by sodium and absolute dependence on bivalent cations. *J. Biol. Chem.* **2006**, *282*, 615–624. [CrossRef]

47. Daruwala, R.; Song, J.; Koh, W.S.; Rumsey, S.C.; Levine, M. Cloning and functional characterization of the human sodium-dependent vitamin C transporters hSVCT1 and hSVCT2. *FEBS Lett.* **1999**, *460*, 480–484. [CrossRef]

48. Rivas, C.I.; Zúñiga, F.A.; Salas-Burgos, A.; Mardones, L.; Ormazabal, V.; Vera, J.C. Vitamin C transporters. *J. Physiol. Biochem.* **2008**, *64*, 357–375. [CrossRef]

49. A Stratakis, C.; E Taymans, S.; Daruwala, R.; Song, J.; Levine, M. Mapping of the human genes (SLC23A2 and SLC23A1) coding for vitamin C transporters 1 and 2 (SVCT1 and SVCT2) to 5q23 and 20p12, respectively. *J. Med. Genet.* **2000**, *37*, E20. [CrossRef]

50. Bürzle, M.; Suzuki, Y.; Ackermann, D.; Miyazaki, H.; Maeda, N.; Clémençon, B.; Burrier, R.; Hediger, M.A. The sodium-dependent ascorbic acid transporter family SLC23. *Mol. Asp. Med.* **2013**, *34*, 436–454. [CrossRef]

51. Savini, I.; Rossi, A.; Pierro, C.; Avigliano, L.; Catani, M.V. SVCT1 and SVCT2: Key proteins for vitamin C uptake. *Amino Acids* **2007**, *34*, 347–355. [CrossRef]

52. Corpe, C.P.; Tu, H.; Eck, P.K.; Wang, J.; Faulhaber-Walter, R.; Schnermann, J.; Margolis, S.; Padayatty, S.; Sun, H.; Wang, Y.; et al. Vitamin C transporter Slc23a1 links renal reabsorption, vitamin C tissue accumulation, and perinatal survival in mice. *J. Clin. Investig.* **2010**, *120*, 1069–1083. [CrossRef]

53. Wang, H.; Dutta, B.; Huang, W.; DeVoe, L.D.; Leibach, F.H.; Ganapathy, V.; Prasad, P.D. Human Na$^+$-dependent vitamin C transporter 1 (hSVCT1): Primary structure, functional characteristics and evidence for a non-functional splice variant. *Biochim. Biophys. Acta* **1999**, *1461*, 1–9. [CrossRef]

54. Sotiriou, S.; Gispert, S.; Cheng, J.; Wang, Y.; Chen, A.; Hoogstraten-Miller, S.; Miller, G.F.; Kwon, O.; Levine, M.; Guttentag, S.H.; et al. Ascorbic-acid transporter Slc23a1 is essential for vitamin C transport into the brain and for perinatal survival. *Nat. Med.* **2002**, *8*, 514–517. [CrossRef]

55. Parker, W.H.; Qu, Z.-C.; May, J.M. Ascorbic acid transport in brain microvascular pericytes. *Biochem. Biophys. Res. Commun.* **2015**, *458*, 262–267. [CrossRef] [PubMed]

56. Rumsey, S.C.; Kwon, O.; Xu, G.W.; Burant, C.F.; Simpson, I.; Levine, M. Glucose transporter isoforms GLUT1 and GLUT3 transport dehydroascorbic acid. *J. Biol. Chem.* **1997**, *272*, 18982–18989. [CrossRef]

57. Rumsey, S.C.; Daruwala, R.; Al-Hasani, H.; Zarnowski, M.J.; Simpson, I.A.; Levine, M. Dehydroascorbic acid transport by GLUT4 in xenopus oocytes and isolated rat adipocytes. *J. Biol. Chem.* **2000**, *275*, 28246–28253. [CrossRef] [PubMed]

58. Corpe, C.P.; Eck, P.K.; Wang, J.; Al-Hasani, H.; Levine, M. Intestinal Dehydroascorbic Acid (DHA) transport mediated by the facilitative sugar transporters, GLUT2 and GLUT8*. *J. Biol. Chem.* **2013**, *288*, 9092–9101. [CrossRef]

59. Linster, C.L.; Schaftingen, E.V. Vitamin C. *FEBS J.* **2007**, *274*, 1–22. [CrossRef] [PubMed]

60. Washko, P.W.; Wang, Y.; Levine, M. Ascorbic acid recycling in human neutrophils. *J. Biol. Chem.* **1993**, *268*, 15531–15535.

61. Litwack, G. Chapter 6—Insulin and sugars. In *Human Biochemistry*; Litwack, G., Ed.; Academic Press: Boston, MA, USA, 2018; pp. 131–160. ISBN 978-0-12-383864-3.

62. Agus, D.B.; Gambhir, S.S.; Pardridge, W.M.; Spielholz, C.; Baselga, J.; Vera, J.C.; Golde, D.W. Vitamin C Crosses the Blood-Brain Barrier in the Oxidized Form through the Glucose Transporters. Available online: https://www.jci.org/articles/view/119832/pdf (accessed on 26 August 2020).

63. Nualart, F.J.; Rivas, C.I.; Montecinos, V.P.; Godoy, A.S.; Guaiquil, V.H.; Golde, D.W.; Vera, J.C. Recycling of Vitamin C by a Bystander Effect. *J. Biol. Chem.* **2002**, *278*, 10128–10133. [CrossRef]

64. Tu, H.; Li, H.; Wang, Y.; Niyyati, M.; Wang, Y.; Leshin, J.; Levine, M. Low Red Blood Cell Vitamin C Concentrations Induce Red Blood Cell Fragility: A Link to Diabetes Via Glucose, Glucose Transporters, and Dehydroascorbic Acid. *EBioMedicine* **2015**, *2*, 1735–1750. [CrossRef]

65. Kim, H.-R.; Park, S.-W.; Cho, H.-J.; Chae, K.-A.; Sung, J.-M.; Kim, J.-S.; Landowski, C.P.; Sun, D.; El-Aty, A.M.A.; Amidon, G.L.; et al. Comparative gene expression profiles of intestinal transporters in mice, rats and humans. *Pharmacol. Res.* **2007**, *56*, 224–236. [CrossRef]

66. Peña, E.; Roa, F.J.; Inostroza, E.; Sotomayor, K.; González, M.; Gutierrez-Castro, F.A.; Maurin, M.; Sweet, K.; Labrousse, C.; Gatica, M.; et al. Increased expression of mitochondrial sodium-coupled ascorbic acid transporter-2 (mitSVCT2) as a central feature in breast cancer. *Free. Radic. Biol. Med.* **2019**, *135*, 283–292. [CrossRef]

67. Roa, F.J.; Peña, E.; Inostroza, E.; Sotomayor, K.; González, M.; Gutierrez-Castro, F.A.; Maurin, M.; Sweet, K.; Labrousse, C.; Gatica, M.; et al. Data on SVCT2 transporter expression and localization in cancer cell lines and tissues. *Data Brief* **2019**, *25*, 103972. [CrossRef] [PubMed]

68. Mayland, C.R.; Bennett, M.I.; Allan, K. Vitamin C deficiency in cancer patients. *Palliat. Med.* **2005**, *19*, 17–20. [CrossRef] [PubMed]

69. Choi, M.-A.; Kim, B.-S.; Yu, R. Serum antioxidative vitamin levels and lipid peroxidation in gastric carcinoma patients. *Cancer Lett.* **1999**, *136*, 89–93. [CrossRef]

70. Cha, J.; Roomi, M.W.; Ivanov, V.; Kalinovsky, T.; Niedzwiecki, A.; Rath, M. Ascorbate depletion increases growth and metastasis of melanoma cells in vitamin C deficient mice. *Exp. Oncol.* **2011**, *33*, 226–230. [PubMed]

71. Cha, J.; Roomi, M.W.; Ivanov, V.; Kalinovsky, T.; Niedzwiecki, A.; Rath, M. Ascorbate supplementation inhibits growth and metastasis of B16FO melanoma and 4T1 breast cancer cells in vitamin C-deficient mice. *Int. J. Oncol.* **2013**, *42*, 55–64. [CrossRef]

72. Gupta, S.C.; Hevia, D.; Patchva, S.; Park, B.; Koh, W.; Aggarwal, B.B. Upsides and downsides of reactive oxygen species for cancer: The roles of reactive oxygen species in tumorigenesis, prevention, and therapy. *Antioxid. Redox Signal.* **2012**, *16*, 1295–1322. [CrossRef]

73. Schieber, M.; Chandel, N.S. ROS function in redox signaling and oxidative stress. *Curr. Biol.* **2014**, *24*, R453–R462. [CrossRef]

74. Galloway, S.P.; McMillan, D.C.; Sattar, N. Effect of the inflammatory response on trace element and vitamin status. *Ann. Clin. Biochem.* **2000**, *37*, 289–297. [CrossRef]

75. Chen, Q.; Espey, M.G.; Krishna, M.C.; Mitchell, J.B.; Corpe, C.P.; Buettner, G.R.; Shacter, E.; Levine, M. Pharmacologic ascorbic acid concentrations selectively kill cancer cells: Action as a pro-drug to deliver hydrogen peroxide to tissues. *Proc. Natl. Acad. Sci. USA* **2005**, *102*, 13604–13609. [CrossRef]

76. Takemura, Y.; Satoh, M.; Satoh, K.; Hamada, H.; Sekido, Y.; Kubota, S. High dose of ascorbic acid induces cell death in mesothelioma cells. *Biochem. Biophys. Res. Commun.* **2010**, *394*, 249–253. [CrossRef] [PubMed]

77. Chen, Q.; Espey, M.G.; Sun, A.Y.; Pooput, C.; Kirk, K.L.; Krishna, M.C.; Khosh, D.B.; Drisko, J.; Levine, M. Pharmacologic doses of ascorbate act as a prooxidant and decrease growth of aggressive tumor xenografts in mice. *Proc. Natl. Acad. Sci. USA* **2008**, *105*, 11105–11109. [CrossRef] [PubMed]

78. Uetaki, M.; Tabata, S.; Nakasuka, F.; Soga, T.; Tomita, M. Metabolomic alterations in human cancer cells by vitamin C-induced oxidative stress. *Sci. Rep.* **2015**, *5*, 13896. [CrossRef]

79. Otto, A.M. Warburg effect(s)—A biographical sketch of Otto Warburg and his impacts on tumor metabolism. *Cancer Metab.* **2016**, *4*, 1–8. [CrossRef]

80. Yun, J.; Rago, C.; Cheong, I.; Pagliarini, R.; Angenendt, P.; Rajagopalan, H.; Schmidt, K.; Willson, J.K.V.; Markowitz, S.; Zhou, S.; et al. Glucose deprivation contributes to the development of KRAS pathway mutations in tumor cells. *Science* **2009**, *325*, 1555–1559. [CrossRef]

81. Yun, J.; Mullarky, E.; Lu, C.; Bosch, K.N.; Kavalier, A.; Rivera, K.D.; Roper, J.; Chio, I.I.C.; Giannopoulou, E.G.; Rago, C.; et al. Vitamin C selectively kills KRAS and BRAF mutant colorectal cancer cells by targeting GAPDH. *Science* **2015**, *350*, 1391–1396. [CrossRef] [PubMed]

82. Kawada, K.; Nakamoto, Y.; Kawada, M.; Hida, K.; Matsumoto, T.; Murakami, T.; Hasegawa, S.; Togashi, K.; Sakai, Y. Relationship between 18F-Fluorodeoxyglucose accumulation and KRAS/BRAF mutations in colorectal cancer. *Clin. Cancer Res.* **2012**, *18*, 1696–1703. [CrossRef] [PubMed]

83. Pouysségur, J.; Dayan, F.; Mazure, N.M. Hypoxia signalling in cancer and approaches to enforce tumour regression. *Nat. Cell Biol.* **2006**, *441*, 437–443. [CrossRef]

84. Sinnberg, T.; Noor, S.; Venturelli, S.; Berger, A.; Schuler, P.; Garbe, C.; Busch, C. The ROS-induced cytotoxicity of ascorbate is attenuated by hypoxia and HIF-1alpha in the NCI60 cancer cell lines. *J. Cell. Mol. Med.* **2014**, *18*, 530–541. [CrossRef] [PubMed]

85. Ngo, B.; Van Riper, J.M.; Cantley, L.C.; Yun, J. Targeting cancer vulnerabilities with high-dose vitamin C. *Nat. Rev. Cancer* **2019**, *19*, 271–282. [CrossRef] [PubMed]

86. Feinberg, A.P.; Vogelstein, B. Hypomethylation distinguishes genes of some human cancers from their normal counterparts. *Nat. Cell Biol.* **1983**, *301*, 89–92. [CrossRef] [PubMed]

87. Gama-Sosa, M.A.; Slagel, V.A.; Trewyn, R.W.; Oxenhandler, R.; Kuo, K.C.; Gehrke, C.W.; Ehrlich, M. The 5-methylcytosine content of DNA from human tumors. *Nucleic Acids Res.* **1983**, *11*, 6883–6894. [CrossRef] [PubMed]

88. Li, J.; Huang, Q.; Zeng, F.; Li, W.; He, Z.; Chen, W.; Zhu, W.; Zhang, B. The prognostic value of global DNA hypomethylation in cancer: A meta-analysis. *PLoS ONE* **2014**, *9*, e106290. [CrossRef] [PubMed]

89. Han, L.; Hou, L.; Zhou, M.-J.; Ma, Z.; Lin, D.-L.; Wu, L.; Ge, Y. Aberrant NDRG1 methylation associated with its decreased expression and clinicopathological significance in breast cancer. *J. Biomed. Sci.* **2013**, *20*, 52. [CrossRef] [PubMed]

90. Starczak, M.; Zarakowska, E.; Modrzejewska, M.; Dziaman, T.; Szpila, A.; Linowiecka, K.; Guz, J.; Szpotan, J.; Gawronski, M.; Labejszo, A.; et al. In vivo evidence of ascorbate involvement in the generation of epigenetic DNA modifications in leukocytes from patients with colorectal carcinoma, benign adenoma and inflammatory bowel disease. *J. Transl. Med.* **2018**, *16*, 204. [CrossRef]

91. Blaschke, K.; Ebata, K.T.; Karimi, M.M.; Zepeda-Martínez, J.A.; Goyal, P.; Mahapatra, S.; Tam, A.; Laird, D.J.; Hirst, M.; Rao, A.; et al. Vitamin C induces Tet-dependent DNA demethylation and a blastocyst-like state in ES cells. *Nat. Cell Biol.* **2013**, *500*, 222–226. [CrossRef]

92. Gustafson, C.B.; Yang, C.; Dickson, K.M.; Shao, H.; Van Booven, D.; Harbour, J.W.; Liu, Z.-J.; Wang, G. Epigenetic reprogramming of melanoma cells by vitamin C treatment. *Clin. Epigenet.* **2015**, *7*, 51. [CrossRef]

93. Modrzejewska, M.; Gawronski, M.; Skonieczna, M.; Zarakowska, E.; Starczak, M.; Foksinski, M.; Rzeszowska-Wolny, J.; Gackowski, D.; Olinski, R. Vitamin C enhances substantially formation of 5-hydroxymethyluracil in cellular DNA. *Free. Radic. Biol. Med.* **2016**, *101*, 378–383. [CrossRef]

94. Peng, D.; Ge, G.; Gong, Y.; Zhan, Y.; He, S.; Guan, B.; Li, Y.; Xu, Z.; Hao, H.; He, Z.-S.; et al. Vitamin C increases 5-hydroxymethylcytosine level and inhibits the growth of bladder cancer. *Clin. Epigenet.* **2018**, *10*, 94. [CrossRef] [PubMed]

95. Liu, J.; Hong, J.; Han, H.; Park, J.; Kim, D.; Park, H.; Ko, M.; Koh, Y.; Shin, D.-Y.; Yoon, S.-S. Decreased vitamin C uptake mediated by SLC2A3 promotes leukaemia progression and impedes TET2 restoration. *Br. J. Cancer* **2020**, *122*, 1445–1452. [CrossRef] [PubMed]

96. Cimmino, L.; Dolgalev, I.; Wang, Y.; Yoshimi, A.; Martin, G.H.; Wang, J.; Ng, V.; Xia, B.; Witkowski, M.T.; Mitchell-Flack, M.; et al. Restoration of TET2 function blocks aberrant self-renewal and leukemia progression. *Cell* **2017**, *170*, 1079–1095.e20. [CrossRef] [PubMed]

97. Zhao, H.; Zhu, H.; Huang, J.; Zhu, Y.; Hong, M.; Zhu, H.; Zhang, J.; Li, S.; Yang, L.; Lian, Y.; et al. The synergy of Vitamin C with decitabine activates TET2 in leukemic cells and significantly improves overall survival in elderly patients with acute myeloid leukemia. *Leuk. Res.* **2018**, *66*, 1–7. [CrossRef]

98. Pollard, H.B.; A Levine, M.; Eidelman, O.; Pollard, M. Pharmacological ascorbic acid suppresses syngeneic tumor growth and metastases in hormone-refractory prostate cancer. *In Vivo* **2010**, *24*, 249–255.

99. Polireddy, K.; Dong, R.; Reed, G.; Yu, J.; Chen, P.; Williamson, S.; Violet, P.-C.; Pessetto, Z.; Godwin, A.K.; Fan, F.; et al. High dose parenteral ascorbate inhibited pancreatic cancer growth and metastasis: Mechanisms and a phase I/IIa study. *Sci. Rep.* **2017**, *7*, 17188. [CrossRef]

100. Gan, L.; Camarena, V.; Mustafi, S.; Wang, G. Vitamin C inhibits triple-negative breast cancer metastasis by affecting the expression of YAP1 and synaptopodin 2. *Nutrients* **2019**, *11*, 2997. [CrossRef]

101. Zhang, T.; Huang, K.; Zhu, Y.; Wang, T.; Shan, Y.; Long, B.; Li, Y.; Chen, Q.; Wang, P.; Zhao, S.; et al. Vitamin C–dependent lysine demethylase 6 (KDM6)-mediated demethylation promotes a chromatin state that supports the endothelial-to-hematopoietic transition. *J. Biol. Chem.* **2019**, *294*, 13657–13670. [CrossRef]

102. Wang, T.; Chen, K.; Zeng, X.; Yang, J.; Wu, Y.; Shi, X.; Qin, B.; Zeng, L.; Esteban, M.A.; Pan, G.; et al. The histone demethylases Jhdm1a/1b enhance somatic cell reprogramming in a Vitamin-C-Dependent manner. *Cell Stem Cell* **2011**, *9*, 575–587. [CrossRef]

103. Ebata, K.; Mesh, K.; Liu, S.; Bilenky, M.; Fekete, A.; Acker, M.G.; Hirst, M.; Garcia, B.A.; Ramalho-Santos, M. Vitamin C induces specific demethylation of H3K9me2 in mouse embryonic stem cells via Kdm3a/b. *Epigenet. Chromatin* **2017**, *10*, 36. [CrossRef]

104. Yong-Hee, R.; Kim, M.; Kim, S.-Y.; Yi, S.-H.; Rhee, Y.-H.; Kim, T.; Lee, E.-H.; Park, C.-H.; Dixit, S.; Harrison, F.E.; et al. Vitamin C Facilitates Dopamine Neuron Differentiation in Fetal Midbrain Through TET1- and JMJD3-Dependent Epigenetic Control Manner. *STEM CELLS* **2015**, *33*, 1320–1332. [CrossRef]

105. Hoffer, L.J.; Levine, M.; Assouline, S.; Melnychuk, D.; Padayatty, S.J.; Rosadiuk, K.; Rousseau, C.; Robitaille, L.; Miller, W.H. Phase I clinical trial of i.v. ascorbic acid in advanced malignancy. *Ann. Oncol.* **2008**, *19*, 1969–1974. [CrossRef] [PubMed]

106. Carr, A.; Vissers, M.C.M.; Cook, J.S. The effect of intravenous vitamin c on cancer- and chemotherapy-related fatigue and quality of life. *Front. Oncol.* **2014**, *4*, 283. [CrossRef]

107. Park, H.; Kang, J.; Choi, J.; Heo, S.; Lee, D.-H. The effect of high dose intravenous Vitamin C during radiotherapy on breast cancer patients' neutrophil–lymphocyte ratio. *J. Altern. Complement. Med.* **2020**, *26*, 1039–1046. [CrossRef]

108. Carr, A.; Cook, J. Intravenous Vitamin C for cancer therapy—Identifying the current gaps in our knowledge. *Front. Physiol.* **2018**, *9*, 1182. [CrossRef] [PubMed]

109. Park, C.H.; Kimler, B.F.; Yi, S.Y.; Park, S.H.; Kim, K.; Jung, C.W.; Kim, S.H.; Lee, E.R.; Rha, M.; Kim, S.; et al. Depletion of l-ascorbic acid alternating with its supplementation in the treatment of patients with acute myeloid leukemia or myelodysplastic syndromes. *Eur. J. Haematol.* **2009**, *83*, 108–118. [CrossRef]

110. Xia, J.; Xu, H.; Zhang, X.; Allamargot, C.; Coleman, K.L.; Nessler, R.; Frech, I.; Tricot, G.; Zhan, F. Multiple myeloma tumor cells are selectively killed by pharmacologically-dosed ascorbic acid. *EBioMedicine* **2017**, *18*, 41–49. [CrossRef] [PubMed]

111. Shenoy, N.; Bhagat, T.; Nieves, E.; Stenson, M.; Lawson, J.; Choudhary, G.S.; Habermann, T.; Nowakowski, G.; Singh, R.; Wu, X.; et al. Upregulation of TET activity with ascorbic acid induces epigenetic modulation of lymphoma cells. *Blood Cancer J.* **2017**, *7*, e587. [CrossRef] [PubMed]

112. Das, A.B.; Kakadia, P.M.; Wojcik, D.; Pemberton, L.; Browett, P.J.; Bohlander, S.; Vissers, M.C.M. Clinical remission following ascorbate treatment in a case of acute myeloid leukemia with mutations in TET2 and WT1. *Blood Cancer J.* **2019**, *9*, 82. [CrossRef]

113. Foster, M.N.; Carr, A.; Antony, A.; Peng, S.; Fitzpatrick, M. Intravenous Vitamin C Administration improved blood cell counts and health-related quality of life of patient with history of relapsed acute myeloid leukaemia. *Antioxidants* **2018**, *7*, 92. [CrossRef]

114. Campbell, E.J.; Dachs, G.U.; Morrin, H.R.; Davey, V.C.; Robinson, B.A.; Vissers, M.C.M. Activation of the hypoxia pathway in breast cancer tissue and patient survival are inversely associated with tumor ascorbate levels. *BMC Cancer* **2019**, *19*, 307. [CrossRef] [PubMed]

115. Sant, D.W.; Mustafi, S.; Gustafson, C.B.; Chen, J.; Slingerland, J.M.; Wang, G. Vitamin C promotes apoptosis in breast cancer cells by increasing TRAIL expression. *Sci. Rep.* **2018**, *8*, 5306. [CrossRef] [PubMed]

116. Zeng, L.-H.; Wang, Q.-M.; Feng, L.-Y.; Ke, Y.-D.; Xu, Q.-Z.; Wei, A.-Y.; Zhang, C.; Ying, R.-B. High-dose vitamin C suppresses the invasion and metastasis of breast cancer cells via inhibiting epithelial-mesenchymal transition. *OncoTargets Ther.* **2019**, *12*, 7405–7413. [CrossRef]

117. Harris, H.R.; Orsini, N.; Wolk, A. Vitamin C and survival among women with breast cancer: A Meta-analysis. *Eur. J. Cancer* **2014**, *50*, 1223–1231. [CrossRef] [PubMed]

118. Cadeau, C.; Fournier, A.; Mesrine, S.; Clavel-Chapelon, F.; Fagherazzi, G.; Boutron-Ruault, M.-C. Vitamin C supplement intake and postmenopausal breast cancer risk: Interaction with dietary vitamin C. *Am. J. Clin. Nutr.* **2016**, *104*, 228–234. [CrossRef] [PubMed]

119. Chen, X.; Chen, Y.; Qu, C.; Pan, Z.; Qin, Y.; Zhang, X.; Liu, W.; Li, D.; Zheng, Q. Vitamin C induces human melanoma A375 cell apoptosis via Bax- and Bcl-2-mediated mitochondrial pathways. *Oncol. Lett.* **2019**, *18*, 3880–3886. [CrossRef] [PubMed]

120. Yang, G.; Yan, Y.; Ma, Y.; Yang, Y. Vitamin C at high concentrations induces cytotoxicity in malignant melanoma but promotes tumor growth at low concentrations. *Mol. Carcinog.* **2017**, *56*, 1965–1976. [CrossRef] [PubMed]

121. Zbytek, B.; Peacock, D.L.; Seagroves, T.N.; Slominski, A.T. Putative role of HIF transcriptional activity in melanocytes and melanoma biology. *Derm. Endocrinol.* **2013**, *5*, 239–251. [CrossRef]

122. Slominski, A.T.; Kim, T.-K.; Brożyna, A.; Janjetovic, Z.; Brooks, D.; Schwab, L.; Skobowiat, C.; Jóźwicki, W.; Seagroves, T. The role of melanogenesis in regulation of melanoma behavior: Melanogenesis leads to stimulation of HIF-1α expression and HIF-dependent attendant pathways. *Arch. Biochem. Biophys.* **2014**, *563*, 79–93. [CrossRef]

123. Fischer, A.P.; Miles, S.L. Ascorbic acid, but not dehydroascorbic acid increases intracellular vitamin C content to decrease Hypoxia Inducible Factor -1 alpha activity and reduce malignant potential in human melanoma. *Biomed. Pharmacother.* **2017**, *86*, 502–513. [CrossRef]

124. Miles, S.L.; Fischer, A.P.; Joshi, S.S.; Niles, R.M. Ascorbic acid and ascorbate-2-phosphate decrease HIF activity and malignant properties of human melanoma cells. *BMC Cancer* **2015**, *15*, 867. [CrossRef] [PubMed]

125. Ryszawy, D.; Pudełek, M.; Catapano, J.; Ciarach, M.; Setkowicz, Z.; Konduracka, E.; Madeja, Z.; Czyż, J. High doses of sodium ascorbate interfere with the expansion of glioblastoma multiforme cells in vitro and in vivo. *Life Sci.* **2019**, *232*, 116657. [CrossRef]

126. Zhou, S.; Wang, X.; Tan, Y.; Qiu, L.; Fang, H.; Li, W. Association between Vitamin C intake and glioma risk: Evidence from a meta-analysis. *Neuroepidemiology* **2015**, *44*, 39–44. [CrossRef] [PubMed]

127. Baillie, N.; Carr, A.; Peng, S. The Use of Intravenous Vitamin C as a supportive therapy for a patient with glioblastoma multiforme. *Antioxidants* **2018**, *7*, 115. [CrossRef] [PubMed]

128. A Mikirova, N.; Hunnunghake, R.; Scimeca, R.C.; Chinshaw, C.; Ali, F.; Brannon, C.; Riordan, N. High-dose intravenous vitamin c treatment of a child with neurofibromatosis Type 1 and optic pathway glioma: A case report. *Am. J. Case Rep.* **2016**, *17*, 774–781. [CrossRef]

129. Bai, X.-Y.; Qu, X.; Jiang, X.; Xu, Z.; Yang, Y.; Su, Q.; Wang, M.; Wu, H. Association between dietary Vitamin C intake and risk of prostate cancer: A meta-analysis involving 103,658 subjects. *J. Cancer* **2015**, *6*, 913–921. [CrossRef]

130. Parent, M.-E.; Richard, H.; Rousseau, M.-C.; Trudeau, K. Vitamin C intake and risk of prostate cancer: The montreal PROtEuS study. *Front. Physiol.* **2018**, *9*, 1218. [CrossRef] [PubMed]

131. Wang, L.; Sesso, H.D.; Glynn, R.J.; Christen, W.G.; Bubes, V.; Manson, J.E.; Buring, J.E.; Gaziano, J.M. Vitamin E and C supplementation and risk of cancer in men: Posttrial follow-up in the Physicians' Health Study II randomized trial. *Am. J. Clin. Nutr.* **2014**, *100*, 915–923. [CrossRef] [PubMed]

132. Timpson, N.J.; Forouhi, N.G.; A Brion, M.-J.; Harbord, R.M.; Cook, D.G.; Johnson, P.; McConnachie, A.; Morris, R.; Rodriguez, S.; Luan, J.; et al. Genetic variation at the SLC23A1 locus is associated with circulating concentrations of l-ascorbic acid (vitamin C): Evidence from 5 independent studies with >15,000 participants. *Am. J. Clin. Nutr.* **2010**, *92*, 375–382. [CrossRef] [PubMed]

133. Duell, E.J.; Lujan-Barroso, L.; Llivina, C.; Muñoz, X.; Jenab, M.; Boutron-Ruault, M.-C.; Clavel-Chapelon, F.; Racine, A.; Boeing, H.; Buijsse, B.; et al. Vitamin C transporter gene (SLC23A1 and SLC23A2) polymorphisms, plasma vitamin C levels, and gastric cancer risk in the EPIC cohort. *Genes Nutr.* **2013**, *8*, 549–560. [CrossRef]

134. Wright, M.E.; Andreotti, G.; Lissowska, J.; Yeager, M.; Zatonski, W.; Chanock, S.J.; Chow, W.-H.; Hou, L. Genetic variation in sodium-dependent ascorbic acid transporters and risk of gastric cancer in Poland. *Eur. J. Cancer* **2009**, *45*, 1824–1830. [CrossRef] [PubMed]

135. Waring, A.J.; Drake, I.M.; Schorah, C.J.; White, K.L.; A Lynch, D.; Axon, A.T.; Dixon, M.F. Ascorbic acid and total vitamin C concentrations in plasma, gastric juice, and gastrointestinal mucosa: Effects of gastritis and oral supplementation. *Gut* **1996**, *38*, 171–176. [CrossRef] [PubMed]

136. Skibola, C.F.; Bracci, P.M.; Halperin, E.; Nieters, A.; Hubbard, A.; Paynter, R.A.; Skibola, D.R.; Agana, L.; Becker, N.; Tressler, P.; et al. Polymorphisms in the estrogen receptor 1 and Vitamin C and matrix metalloproteinase gene families are associated with susceptibility to lymphoma. *PLoS ONE* **2008**, *3*, e2816. [CrossRef]

137. Casabonne, D.; Gracia, E.; Espinosa, A.; Bustamante, M.; Benavente, Y.; Robles, C.; Costas, L.; Alonso, E.; Gonzalez-Barca, E.; Tardón, A.; et al. Fruit and vegetable intake and vitamin C transporter gene (SLC23A2) polymorphisms in chronic lymphocytic leukaemia. *Eur. J. Nutr.* **2017**, *56*, 1123–1133. [CrossRef] [PubMed]

138. Erichsen, H.C.; Peters, U.; Eck, P.K.; Welch, R.; Schoen, R.E.; Yeager, M.; Levine, M.; Hayes, R.B.; Chanock, S. Genetic variation in sodium-dependent Vitamin C Transporters SLC23A1 and SLC23A2 and risk of advanced colorectal adenoma. *Nutr. Cancer* **2008**, *60*, 652–659. [CrossRef]

139. Chen, A.A.; Marsit, C.J.; Christensen, B.C.; Houseman, E.A.; McClean, M.; Smith, J.F.; Bryan, J.T.; Posner, M.R.; Nelson, H.H.; Kelsey, K. Genetic variation in the vitamin C transporter, SLC23A2, modifies the risk of HPV16-associated head and neck cancer. *Carcinogenesis* **2009**, *30*, 977–981. [CrossRef]

140. Hong, S.-W.; Lee, S.-H.; Moon, J.-H.; Hwang, J.J.; Kim, D.E.; Ko, E.; Kim, H.-S.; Cho, I.J.; Kang, J.-S.; Kim, J.-E.; et al. SVCT-2 in breast cancer acts as an indicator for L-ascorbate treatment. *Oncogene* **2012**, *32*, 1508–1517. [CrossRef]

141. Cho, S.; Chae, J.S.; Shin, H.; Shin, Y.; Song, H.; Kim, Y.; Yoo, B.C.; Roh, K.; Cho, S.; Kil, E.-J.; et al. Hormetic dose response to L-ascorbic acid as an anti-cancer drug in colorectal cancer cell lines according to SVCT-2 expression. *Sci. Rep.* **2018**, *8*, 11372. [CrossRef]

142. Lv, H.; Wang, C.; Fang, T.; Li, T.; Lv, G.; Han, Q.; Yang, W.; Wang, H.-Y. Vitamin C preferentially kills cancer stem cells in hepatocellular carcinoma via SVCT-2. *NPJ Precis. Oncol.* **2018**, *2*, 1–13. [CrossRef]

143. Wang, C.; Lv, H.; Yang, W.; Li, T.; Fang, T.; Lv, G.; Han, Q.; Dong, L.; Jiang, T.; Jiang, B.; et al. SVCT-2 determines the sensitivity to ascorbate-induced cell death in cholangiocarcinoma cell lines and patient derived xenografts. *Cancer Lett.* **2017**, *398*, 1–11. [CrossRef]

144. Lièvre, A.; Bachet, J.-B.; Le Corre, D.; Boige, V.; Landi, B.; Emile, J.-F.; Côté, J.-F.; Tomasic, G.; Penna, C.; Ducreux, M.; et al. KRAS mutation status is predictive of response to cetuximab therapy in colorectal cancer. *Cancer Res.* **2006**, *66*, 3992–3995. [CrossRef] [PubMed]

145. Jung, S.-A.; Lee, D.-H.; Moon, J.-H.; Hong, S.-W.; Shin, J.-S.; Hwang, I.Y.; Shin, Y.J.; Kim, J.H.; Gong, E.-Y.; Kim, S.-M.; et al. L-Ascorbic acid can abrogate SVCT-2-dependent cetuximab resistance mediated by mutant KRAS in human colon cancer cells. *Free. Radic. Biol. Med.* **2016**, *95*, 200–208. [CrossRef] [PubMed]

146. Salazar, K.; Martinez, M.; Ulloa, V.; Bertinat, R.; Martínez, F.; Jara, N.; Espinoza, F.; Bongarzone, E.R.; Nualart, F. SVCT2 overexpression in neuroblastoma cells induces cellular branching that is associated with ERK signaling. *Mol. Neurobiol.* **2016**, *53*, 6668–6679. [CrossRef] [PubMed]

147. Eck, P.K.; Erichsen, H.C.; Taylor, V.J.G.; Yeager, M.; Hughes, A.L.; Levine, M.; Chanock, S.J. Comparison of the genomic structure and variation in the two human sodium-dependent vitamin C transporters, SLC23A1 and SLC23A2. *Qual. Life Res.* **2004**, *115*, 285–294. [CrossRef]

2

Vitamin C Deficiency Reduces Muscarinic Receptor Coronary Artery Vasoconstriction and Plasma Tetrahydrobiopterin Concentration in Guinea Pigs

Gry Freja Skovsted *, Pernille Tveden-Nyborg, Maiken Marie Lindblad, Stine Normann Hansen and Jens Lykkesfeldt 🆔

Department of Veterinary and Animal Sciences, Faculty of Health and Medical Sciences, University of Copenhagen, Ridebanevej 9, 1870 Frederiksberg C, Denmark; ptn@sund.ku.dk (P.T.-N.); mali@sund.ku.dk (M.M.L.); snoha@sund.ku.dk (S.N.H.); jopl@sund.ku.dk (J.L.)
* Correspondence: gryfreja@sund.ku.dk

Abstract: Vitamin C (vitC) deficiency is associated with increased cardiovascular disease risk, but its specific interplay with arteriolar function is unclear. This study investigates the effect of vitC deficiency in guinea pigs on plasma biopterin status and the vasomotor responses in coronary arteries exposed to vasoconstrictor/-dilator agents. Dunkin Hartley female guinea pigs ($n = 32$) were randomized to high (1500 mg/kg diet) or low (0 to 50 mg/kg diet) vitC for 10–12 weeks. At euthanasia, coronary artery segments were dissected and mounted in a wire-myograph. Vasomotor responses to potassium, carbachol, sodium nitroprusside (SNP), U46619, sarafotoxin 6c (S6c) and endothelin-1 (ET-1) were recorded. Plasma vitC and tetrahydrobiopterin were measured by HPLC. Plasma vitC status reflected the diets with deficient animals displaying reduced tetrahydrobiopterin. Vasoconstrictor responses to carbachol were significantly decreased in vitC deficient coronary arteries independent of their general vasoconstrictor/vasodilator capacity ($p < 0.001$). Moreover, in vitC deficient animals, carbachol-induced vasodilator responses correlated with coronary artery diameter ($p < 0.001$). Inhibition of cyclooxygenases with indomethacin increased carbachol-induced vasoconstriction, suggesting an augmented carbachol-induced release of vasodilator prostanoids. Atropine abolished carbachol-induced vasomotion, supporting a specific muscarinic receptor effect. Arterial responses to SNP, potassium, S6c, U46619 and ET-1 were unaffected by vitC status. The study shows that vitC deficiency decreases tetrahydrobiopterin concentrations and muscarinic receptor mediated contraction in coronary arteries. This attenuated vasoconstrictor response may be linked to altered production of vasoactive arachidonic acid metabolites and reduced muscarinic receptor expression/signaling.

Keywords: Vitamin C; ascorbic acid; vascular responses; biopterins

---

1. Introduction

The association between vitamin C (vitC) deficiency and an increased risk of cardiovascular disease (CVD) in humans is well-established [1–6], though a mechanistic link is yet to be elucidated. VitC is an essential nutrient for humans and an estimated 10–15% of adults in the Western populations suffer from hypovitaminosis C (plasma concentration <23 μM) [7]. Pathologies of vascular diseases are characterized by changed vasomotion as a consequence of an imbalance in vasodilation and vasoconstriction, leading to abnormal blood flow regulation and organ dysfunction. In the vasculature, vitC is a key component in maintaining collagen integrity of blood vessels; prolonged severe deficiency ultimately leads to the development of bleedings and haematoma hallmarking scurvy. However, little is known about how non-scorbutic vitC deficiency affects the function of the vascular cells and the vasomotion of arterioles proximal to the capillaries.

In human endothelial cells in vitro, vitC has been shown to act as specific redox modulator in the nitric oxide (NO) synthesis essential for vasodilation [8]. Furthermore, vitC provides reducing equivalents in the conversion of dihydrobiopterin (BH_2) to tetrahydrobiopterin (BH_4) [9,10], which in turn acts as co-factor for endothelial nitric oxide syntase (eNOS) to ensure the generation of NO [11]. Reduced BH_4 levels lead to eNOS uncoupling, and generation of superoxide rather than NO [12], likely to form the strong oxidant peroxynitrite and decreasing NO bioavailability [9]. We have previously shown that vitC deficiency in guinea pigs leads to decreased BH_4 plasma concentration in vivo [13], potentially weakening the vasodilator capacity.

Another important aspect of vitC is its antioxidant function, serving as a scavenger of reactive oxygen species (ROS) [14]. ROS play key roles in signal transduction related to both vasodilation and vasoconstiction [15] and can inhibit the two major endothelium-derived relaxing factors, NO and prostacyclin [15]. While eNOS uncoupling reduces NO bioavailability, peroxynitrite can inactivate prostacyclin synthase by tyrosin nitration of its active site [16,17]. Thus, as the primary vascular antioxidant, vitC protects the endothelium from oxidative stress [18].

A third mechanism of vitC-associated action could be on the cholinergic response of vascular smooth muscle cells (VSMCs). Increased oxidative stress has been found to reduce muscarinic receptor function in smooth muscle cells of the urinary bladder [19], and studies have shown an attenuated parasympathetic response [20] and muscarinic-cholinergic receptor density [21] in submandibular gland acinar cells in vitC deficient guinea pigs. As coronary arteries express muscarinic receptors in the endothelium and VSMCs, and an extensive network of cholinergic perivascular nerve fibres in the coronary artery tree is present in guinea pigs [22], the acetylcholine analogue carbachol was applied to study both vasodilator and vasoconstrictor responses.

In contrast to rats and mice, guinea pigs and humans share a requirement for dietary vitC. This makes the guinea pig an excellent in vivo model for studying effects of diet-imposed vitC deficiency. In this study, we examined a causal relationship between chronic vitC deficiency and plasma biopterin redox status, and putative consequences on the vasodilator and vasoconstrictor responses in isolated coronary arteries.

2. Materials and Methods

2.1. Animal Study

All experimental animal procedures were performed following protocols approved by the Danish Animal Experimental Inspectorate under the Ministry of Environment and Food of Denmark (No. 2012-15-2934-00205). Group sizes were determined by power analysis of sample size, applying a power of 80% and a 5% significance level. A difference of 30% was considered biologically relevant and variations of the chosen end-points were based on our previous experience with the model [23,24]. Animals were selected by randomization from a larger, extensive, study of diet imposed vitC deficiency in guinea pigs intended to investigate vitC transport to the brain (unpublished results). Thus, the current data-set depicts findings from a randomly defined subset of animals, representing high vitC intake (control) and low (deficient), thereby, reflecting the extremes of the imposed interventions of the main study.

Seven-day old, Dunkin Hartley female guinea pigs (Envigo, Horst, The Netherlands) were equipped with subcutaneous microchip implant for identification (Uno Pico Transponder, Zevenaar, The Netherlands) upon arrival to the facility. Animals were randomized into weight stratified groups and subjected to either high ($n = 16$; 1500 mg vitC/kg feed; Controls) or low vitC ($n = 16$, 0 mg vitC/kg feed for 3 weeks, followed by 50 mg vitC/kg feed until study termination; Deficient). All diets were chow based standard guinea pig diets for growing animals (Ssniff Spezialdiäten, Soesst, Germany), differing only in vitC levels as confirmed by post production analysis. Animals were group-housed in identical floor pens and allowed free access to feed, dried hay (devoid of vitC by analysis) and drinking water. Body-weight was monitored throughout the study period, and though vitC deficient animals experienced a brief period (1–3 days) of weight stagnation immediately prior to changing from 0 mg to 50 mg vitC/kg feed, clinical signs of vitC deficiency were absent and body weight was comparable between groups at the time of euthanasia, 10–12 weeks after study start.

2.2. Euthanasia

Guinea pigs were sedated with Torbugesic Vet (2 mL/kg) (Butorphanol 10 mg/mL; ScanVet Animal Health, Fredernsborg, Denmark) and anesthetized with 5% isofluorane (Isoba Vet 100%, Intervet International, Boxmeer, The Netherlands) in oxygen (Conoxia® 100%, AGA A/S, Copenhagen, Denmark) until cessation of voluntary reflexes. Blood was collected by cardiac puncture through the apex using a 18 G needle fitted onto a 1 mL syringe previously flushed with 15% tripotassium EDTA. Immediately hereafter, the guinea pig was euthanized by decapitation.

2.3. Wire Myography and Tissue Preparation

Immediately following euthanasia, the heart was isolated and placed into cold physiological buffer (in mM: 117.8 NaCl, 4.0 KCl, 2.0 $CaCl_2$, 0.9 $MgCl_2$, 1.25 NaH_2PO_4, 20 $NaHCO_3$, and 5.0 glucose). The left anterior descending (LAD) coronary artery was dissected from surrounding myocardial tissue, cut into 2 mm segments and directly mounted in a wire myograph (Danish Myo Technology, Aarhus, Denmark). The anatomical localization of the LAD coronary artery is illustrated in Supplemental Figure S1. Wire myography experiments were initiated by normalisation to an internal circumference corresponding to 0.9 of the circumference at 13.3 kPa. Following a 15 min equilibration period in physiological buffer the artery segments were contracted 2–3 times using 60 mM potassium (similar composition as the above physiological buffer, except that NaCl was exchanged with KCl on equimolar basis) to measure the vasoconstrictor reactivity of the arteries. Only segments with potassium induced contraction >0.5 mN/mm were included in the study. After washing to obtain baseline relaxation, the ETB receptor agonist, Sarafotoxin 6c (S6c) was added in a cumulative fashion (10^{-12} to 10^{-7} M). Carbachol induced vasodilation and vasoconstriction (10^{-12} to 3×10^{-4} M) was tested following pre-constriction with potassium (40 mM). In order to elucidate the carbachol vasomotor responses, carbachol concentration-response curves were acquired either in absence (controls) or in presence of the muscarinic receptor antagonist, atropine (10^{-5} M), the COX-inhibitor indomethacin (10^{-4} M) or the eNOS inhibitor L-NAME (10^{-5} M). Endothelium-independent vasodilation was tested by sodium nitroprusside (10^{-9} to 10^{-5} M) following pre-constriction with 40 mM potassium. U46619 (10^{-12} to 10^{-5} M) and endothelin-1 (ET-1)-induced (10^{-12} to 10^{-7} M) vasoconstriction were tested using cumulative additions.

2.4. Biochemical Analysis

EDTA-stabilized blood samples were centrifuged ($16,000 \times g$, 1 min, 4 °C). Plasma for ascorbate and dehydroascorbic acid (DHA) analysis was stabilized with meta-phosphoric acid prior to storage at −80 °C. Previous studies have shown that both ascorbate and DHA are stable under these conditions for at least five years [23]. Concentrations were measured by HPLC with colorimetric detection as previously described [25,26]. The remaining plasma aliquots were stored neat at −80 °C until further analysis, except for samples for BH_2 and BH_4 determination, where the blood was stabilized in 0.1% dithioerythritol prior to centrifugation ($2000 \times g$, 4 min, 4 °C), yielding a plasma fraction, which was analyzed by HPLC, as previously described [13].

2.5. Data and Statistical Analysis

Force data (mN) were transformed to tension (Nm^{-1}) by dividing by twice the artery segment length and subtracting the baseline tension values [24]. Active tension was calculated by subtracting the passive tension from the potassium-induced active tension. Agonist-induced tension was normalized to the potassium induced active tension. Carachol-induced relaxation was calculated by subtracting the active tensions from the potassium-induced (40 mM) active tension. All statistical analysis and graphs were performed in GraphPad Prism 7.00 (GraphPad Software, La Jolla, CA, USA). Differences between two groups were evaluated by a two-sided Student's t-test. For multiple comparisons (in functional myography data), two-way ANOVA repeated-measures with Sidak's multiple comparisons was applied. Correlations between specific outcomes were evaluated by Pearson correlation (r) coefficient with two-tailed p-values.

2.6. Materials

Endothelin-1, human, porcine (Catalogue No. SC324, PolyPeptide Group, Strassbourg, France), Sarafotoxin S6c (SC457, PolyPeptide Group, Strassbourg, France), 9,11-dideoxy-11α,9α-epoxy-methanoprostaglandin F2α (BML-PG023-0001, Enzo Life Sciences, Exeter, UK). Carbamoylcholine chloride (C4382-1G SIGMA, Sigma-Aldrich, St. Louis, MO, USA), indomethacin (I7378-5G SIGMA, Sigma-Aldrich, St. Louis, MO, USA), Nω-nitro-L-arginine methylester hydrochloride (N5751 Sigma, Sigma-Aldrich, St. Louis, MO, USA), atropine (A0132 SIGMA, Sigma-Aldrich, St. Louis, MO, USA), meta-phosphoric acid (239275, Sigma, Sigma-Aldrich, St. Louis, MO, USA), 1,4-dithioerythritol (D9680, Sigma, Sigma-Aldrich, St. Louis, MO, USA).

3. Results

3.1. Effects of Vitamin C Deficiency on Weight Gain of Animals, Plasma Ascorbate Concentration and Plasma BH_4 Concentration

Plasma vitC concentrations were measured at euthanasia, following 11 weeks on the experimental diets. The dietary regimen was reflected in plasma ascorbate and DHA concentrations, with marked ($p < 0.001$) reduction in plasma ascorbate concentration in the deficient group compared to the control group (Table 1). VitC deficiency also led to a significant reduction in plasma BH_4 concentration ($p < 0.0001$) (Figure 1).

Table 1. Animal weight and plasma analyses. Data are expressed as means ± SEM, N is number of animals, **** Different from controls, $p < 0.0001$, unpaired t-test.

	N	Controls	N	VitC Deficient
Weight (g)	16	625 ± 14	16	602 ± 16
Ascorbate concentration, (μM)	16	60.2 ± 5.1	16	2.3 ± 0.1 ****
Ascorbate total, (μM)	16	61.5 ± 5.3	16	2.3 ± 0.1 ****
% DHA	16	1.9 ± 0.5	16	2.2 ± 1.0

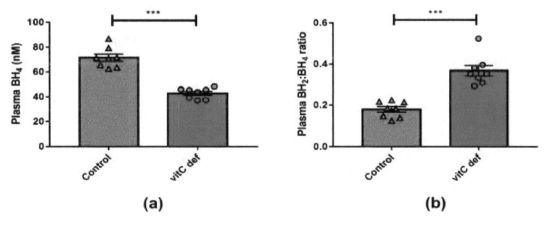

(a)   (b)

Figure 1. (a) Plasma concentrations of BH_4; (b) plasma BH_2:BH_4-ratio. Means ± SEM, *** $p < 0.0001$ ($n = 8$).

3.2. Contractile Reactivity

The potency and efficacy of ET-1 was significantly higher than that of U46619 ($p < 0.05$), and the selective ETB receptor agonist, S6c, induced only a negligible contraction in the coronary artery segments (Table 2). VitC status did not have a significant effect on the potassium, ET-1, U46619 or S6c vasoconstrictor responses (Figure 2a,b). In contrast to the other vasoconstrictors, potassium induced a long-lasting vasocontractile response persisting for at least 10 min and potassium was therefore used as a pre-constrictor in the studies of the relaxation-inducing agonists. Coronary arteries from vitC deficient guinea pigs were significantly smaller than the controls ($p < 0.05$, Table 2). Additionally, we found that for the vitC deficient group, the animal weight was positively correlated with the coronary artery diameter ($p < 0.002$, Table 3 and Figure 3a).

Table 2. Artery segment properties, diameter (μm), potassium tension (Nm^{-1}), agonist induced contraction (% of potassium contraction). Data are expressed as means ± SEM, N is number of animals, n is number of artery segments, NC = not calculated. * Different from controls, $p < 0.05$, unpaired *t*-test.

	N, n	Controls	N, n	VitC Deficient
Diameter	16, 35	366 ± 16	16, 35	312 ± 12 *
Potassium, tension	16, 35	3.2 ± 0.2	16, 35	3.1 ± 0.3
Endothelin-1	12, 17	Emax 116 ± 16 pEC50 8.2 ± 0.1	12, 17	Emax 108 ± 8 pEC50 8.3 ± 0.1
Sarafotoxin 6c	8, 20	Emax NC pEC50 NC	8, 20	Emax 3 ± 1.6 pEC50 8.5 ± 0.7
U46619	16, 35	Emax 58 ± 9 pEC50 6.6 ± 0.1	16, 35	Emax 64 ± 13 pEC50 6.7 ± 0.2

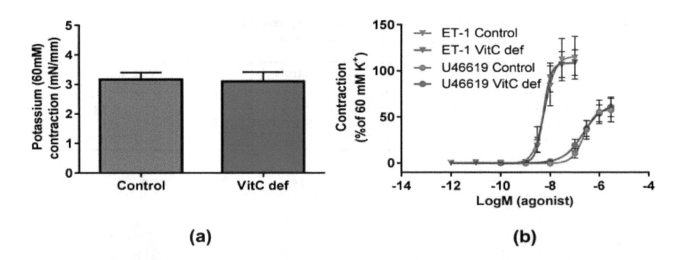

(a)   **(b)**

Figure 2. Contractile responses in coronary arteries. (**a**) Contractile responses to 60 mM extracellular potassium; (**b**) contractile responses to cumulative concentrations of ET-1 and U46610 in coronary arteries from control guinea pigs (green) and vitC deficient (red). Means ± SEM (K⁺, *n* = 16; ET-1, *n* = 12; U46619, *n* = 16).

Table 3. Correlation analyses of specific outcomes in the control and vitC deficient groups. Pearson correlation analyses, N is number of animals, n is number of artery segments, r is Pearson correlation coefficient, ** $p <0.002$, *** $p < 0.001$.

	Controls			VitC Deficient		
	N, n	Pearson r	p Values	N, n	Pearson r	p Values
Diameter vs. weight	16, 35	0.182	0.500	16, 35	0.729	0.001 **
Diameter vs. carb induced dilatation	16, 35	0.010	0.954	16, 35	0.555	0.0005 ***
Diameter vs. carb induced contraction	16, 35	−0.174	0.518	16, 35	−0.286	0.284
BH$_4$ vs. carb induced dilatation	8, 15	0.403	0.105	8, 15	0.057	0.840
BH$_4$ vs. carb induced contraction	8, 15	−0.372	0.172	8, 15	0.232	0.406

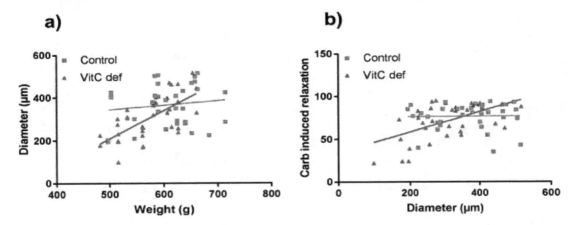

Figure 3. Scatter plots of coronary artery diameter vs. guinea pig body weight (**a**) and carbachol-induced vasorelaxation compared with coronary artery diameter (**b**). Control guinea pigs (green squares) and VitC deficient (red triangles).

3.3. Vascular Responses to Carbachol

Cumulative concentrations of carbachol in the range of 1 nM to 1 μM markedly relaxed coronary artery segments pre-contracted with 40 mM potassium (Figure 4a) and higher concentrations (1 μM to 0.3 mM) caused a rise in the isometric tension in a concentration-dependent fashion. Carbachol-induced relaxation and sensitivity was not significantly different in coronary arteries from vitC deficient guinea pigs compared to controls (Figure 3a); however, a significantly positive correlation between coronary artery diameter and carbachol-induced relaxation was found in coronary arteries from vitC deficient guinea pigs, but not in controls ($p < 0.001$), Table 3 and Figure 3b). The maximal carbachol-induced contraction response was significantly lower in segments from vitC deficient compared to controls ($p < 0.001$; Figure 4a) and in both vitC deficient and control animals the contractions were independent on coronary artery diameter ($p > 0.05$, Table 3). The muscarinic receptor antagonist, atropine (10 μM), blocked both the carbachol-induced vasodilation and vasoconstriction from both diet groups (Figure 2b). To evaluate the contribution of NO and prostanoids to carbachol-induced vasodilation and vasoconstriction, carbachol concentration- response curves were recorded during pre-contraction induced by potassium and in the presence of the COX inhibitor, indomethacin (10 μM), NOS inhibitor, L-NAME (100 μM) or in the presence of both indomethacin (10 μM) and L-NAME (100 μM). The presences of inhibitors alone or in combination revealed no differences in the vasodilator responses in control compared with vitC deficient animals, and the augmented vasoconstrictor responses in arteries from control animals compared to segments from vitC deficient animals were maintained in the presence of the inhibitors (Figure 4b–d).

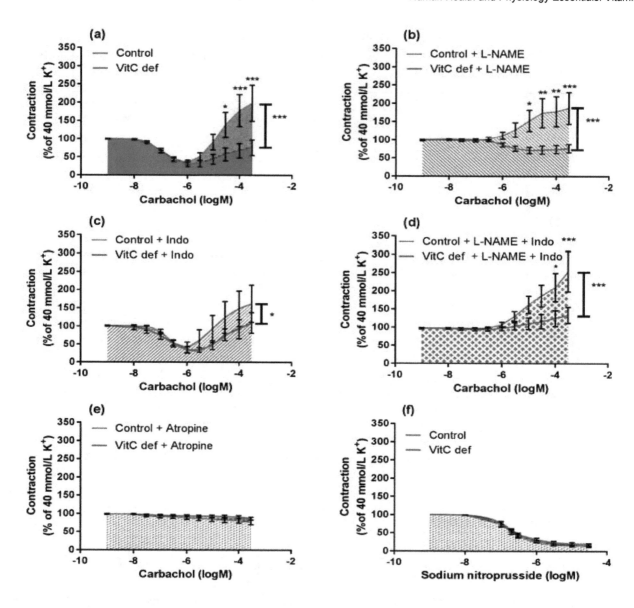

Figure 4. Log-concentration-response curves of coronary artery segments from vitC versus control guinea pigs. (**a**) Vasomotor responses to carbachol in coronary artery segments pre-constricted with 40 mM extracellular potassium; (**b**) in presence of L-NAME; (**c**) indomethacin; (**d**) both L-NAME and indomethacin; (**e**) atropine. (**f**) Vasodilator responses to sodium nitroprusside (SNP) in coronary arteries pre-constricted with 40 mM extracellular potassium. Control guinea pigs (green) and VitC deficient (red). Means ± SEM (n = 8–16), * $p < 0.05$, ** $p < 0.01$, *** $p < 0.001$.

L-NAME significantly inhibited the vasodilatory response to carbachol in segments from both control and vitC deficient guinea pigs ($p < 0.001$; Figure 5a,b); however L-NAME alone had no effect on the subsequent vasoconstrictor response compared to non-treated segments. In the presence of indomethacin alone, both carbachol-induced vasodilatation and vasoconstriction were restored (Figure 5c,d) in arteries from both groups compared to non-treated segments.

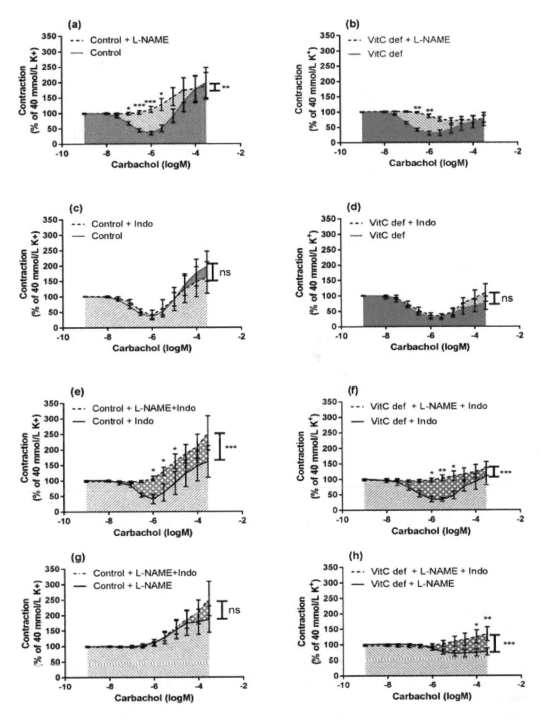

Figure 5. Log-concentration-response curves of coronary artery segments after treatment with L-NAME and/or indomethacin. The figures illustrate how the combination of inhibitors in artery segments from the same animal modulates the carbachol-induced vasodilator and constrictor responses. Vasomotor responses to carbachol in artery segments pre-constricted with 40 mM extracellular potassium: in absence versus presence of L-NAME in (**a**) control guinea pigs; (**b**) vitC deficient. In absence versus presence of indomethacin in (**c**) control; and (**d**) vitC deficient, in absence of L-NAME versus presence both L-NAME and indomethacin in (**e**) control guinea pigs; (**f**) VitC deficient, and in absence of indomethacin versus presence both L-NAME and indomethacin in (**g**) control guinea pigs; (**h**) VitC deficient. Means ± SEM ($n = 8$–16), * $p < 0.05$, ** $p < 0.01$, *** $p < 0.001$.

In the presence of L-NAME, indomethacin amplified the carbachol-induced vasoconstriction only in segments from vitC deficient guinea pigs, suggesting a potential effect arachidonic acid metabolites e.g., vasodilator prostanoids counteracting the vasoconstrictor effect of carbachol in coronary arteries from vitC deficient guinea pigs or increased production of vasoconstrictor leukotrienes, which is unmasked in the presence of indomethacine. This effect was not recorded for control animals.

In summary, we found that carbachol-induced vasodilator and constrictor responses were mediated by muscarinic receptors. In vitC deficient guinea pigs, the diameter of the coronary arteries were significantly and positively correlated with the weight of the animals and the endothelium-dependent vasorelaxation. These correlations were not present in the control group. In vitC deficient guinea pigs the muscarinic receptor-induced vasoconstrictor responses were significantly attenuated compared to controls and partly restored by COX-inhibition.

3.4. Relaxing Responses to SNP

To evaluate the endothelium-independent response to NO, relaxing response to the NO donor SNP (1 nM to 30 μM) was measured in potassium pre-contracted arteries. SNP induced a concentration dependent relaxation and the maximal relaxation and the sensitivity to SNP were not affected by the vitC status in the animals (Figure 4f).

4. Discussion

The present study shows that vasoconstrictor responses to carbachol are significantly decreased in arteries from vitC deficient guinea pigs as compared to arteries from control animals, proposing a link between vitC deficiency and compromised vascular function in vivo. Interestingly, contractions induced by other constrictors: potassium, S6c, U46619 and ET-1 were not affected by vitC status, suggesting that the contractile apparatus *per se* is not affected. Although vitC deficiency decreased plasma BH_4 levels, there was no significantly decreased vasodilator capacity compared to controls. However, vitC deficient guinea pigs had significantly smaller coronary artery diameters than controls, and in vitC deficient guinea pigs, the decreased diameter correlated with decreased carbachol-induced vasodilatation. Consequently, it appears that impaired vitC status affects the diameter of the coronary arteries and the endothelial function; furthermore vitC status induces a specific effect on the parasympathetic muscarinic receptor system, as measured by attenuated vasoconstrictor responses.

The parasympathetic neurotransmitter, acetylcholine and its analogue carbachol are widely used to study endothelial dependent/independent vasodilation and vasoconstriction, and the agonist is relevant since guinea pigs have an extensive network of cholinergic perivascular nerve fibres in the coronary artery tree [22]. In isolated coronary artery segments, carbachol induced a biphasic concentration-response pattern with an initial vasodilator response at low concentrations (from 10 nM to 1 μM) followed by a vasoconstrictor response at higher concentrations (from 1 μM to 0.3 mM). Carbachol-responses in the presence of atropine, indomethacin and/or L-NAME in the organ bath were assessed, revealing that atropine blocked both the carbachol-induced vasodilatation and vasoconstriction over the entire carbachol concentration interval. This suggests that carbachol elicits its effect via muscarinic receptors on guinea pig coronary arteries. This is consistent with previous studies showing that acetylcholine-induced vasodilator responses in bovine [25], simian [26] and mice [27] coronary arteries are mediated predominantly by endothelial muscarinic M_3 receptors, and that acetylcholine induced vasoconstrictor responses are mediated by vascular M_3 receptors in bovine [28,29] and porcine [30,31] coronary arteries.

In this study, we found that in vitC deficient guinea pigs, the endothelial-dependent vasodilation was significantly correlated with coronary artery diameter; a correlation that was not present in controls. Furthermore, we found coronary artery diameters were significantly smaller in vitC deficient guinea pigs as compared to control guinea pigs, despite sampling at uniform, anatomically defined, orientation. These results suggest that vitC deficiency potentially impair coronary artery growth and endothelial function of young guinea pigs. Hence, those guinea pigs that responded most sensitively to vitC restriction further developed more overall growth retardation with consequently impaired coronary artery growth and endothelial function. In the control group, in contrast, the variation in artery diameter did not reflect a pathophysiological response, but rather, a random variation in growth. Previously, degenerative changes in the capillary endothelium have been found in scorbutic guinea pigs whereas the larger arteries showed no abnormalities [32]. However, although we found this correlation between artery diameter and endothelial function in vitC deficient animals and not in controls; we found no overall effect of vitC deficiency when comparing the two groups. Treatment of the coronary artery segments with L-NAME abolished the initial carbachol-induced vasodilator response in both diet groups. In contrast, indomethacin did not significantly affect the vasodilator response between groups, suggesting that carbachol-induced vasodilator response was predominantly driven by endothelial-dependent NO release. Importantly, the vasodilator responses were investigated in arteries preconstricted with high extracellular concentration of potassium. High potassium concentrations depolarize VSMC and endothelial cells [33] which consequently hide a putative endothelium-derived hyperpolarizing factor (EDHF) mediated vasodilator effect [34]. Therefore, blocking the contribution of EDHF to vasodilation allowed the isolation of the effects of NO and prostaglandins on carbachol induced vasodilation.

Muscarinic receptors are widely expressed in smooth muscle cells in several organs, and diet-induced ascorbate deficiency in guinea pigs has previously been shown to reduce muscarinic-cholinergic receptor density [21]. Increased oxidative stress has been found to acutely reduce muscarinic receptor-mediated smooth muscle cell constriction in guinea pigs [19], and increased ROS production in ischemia/reperfusion reduce efficacy and sensitivity to cholinergic stimulation [35,36], linking redox imbalance to functional consequences mediated via muscarinic receptors.

Stimulating the arteries with the NO donor sodium nitroprussid revealed vasodilation with similar sensitivity and maximal effect in arteries from vitC deficient and control guinea pigs (Figure 4f). NO mediates a vasodilator effect by binding to soluble guanylyl cyclase (sGC) in VSMC. Guanylyl then catalyses the production of cGMP, which activates protein kinase G that via dephosphorylation of myosin light chain leads to vasorelaxation [37]. Oxidative stress has been showed to down-regulate soluble guanylyl cyclase expression and activity [38]. In present study, we found no effect of vitC deficiency on the NO-mediated vasodilation, indicating that the sGC activity was unaltered by the vitC status.

When coronary artery segments were treated with L-NAME and/or indomethacin, the carbachol-induced vasoconstrictor response remained reduced in arteries from vitC deficient compared to control animals. However, indomethacin increased the carbachol-induced vasoconstrictor response in eNOS blocked segments from vitC deficient animals, which was not present in arteries from control animals. This suggests that vitC deficiency promotes the release of vasodilator prostanoids in coronary arteries when stimulated with carbachol. Vasodilator prostanoids have previously been found to negate the effect of coronary vasoconstrictors after myocardial infarction [39], a condition known to induce oxidative stress [40] and be detrimental to cellular function and survival. In contrast, inhibition of prostanoid production has been found to have little effect in healthy humans [41] and dogs [42]. In this study, prostanoid-induced suppression of carbachol vasoconstrictor responses in coronary arteries were increased in vitC deficient guinea pigs, suggesting a compensatory role in the regulation of coronary vascular tone under vitC and BH_4 deficiency. The contractile responses induced by either extracellular potassium, U46619, S6c or ET-1 were not affected by vitC status, supporting the idea that the general vasoconstrictor capacity is not affected by vitC deficiency.

VitC deficiency (defined as plasma concentrations <23 µM) is surprisingly common, affecting ~15% of adults in the Western World with even higher prevalence among individuals who smoke, have high BMI, low socioeconomic status [7] as well as children with underlying medical conditions [43,44]. Epidemiological studies have shown an association between vitC deficiency and an increased risk of cardiovascular disease; however, the mechanistic link has not been elucidated [45,46]. Altered vasomotion and reactivity of coronary arteries plays an important role in pathophysiologic mechanisms involved in heart disease. The parasympathetic nervous system is known to provide a modulating influence on the response of coronary arteries to local metabolic requirements in the heart [47]. Moreover, muscarinic receptors are known to be expressed in human coronary arteries [48]. Patients with variant angina or coronary stenosis have been found to have altered coronary vasoconstriction after injection of acetylcholine, pointing toward a causal relationship with altered muscarinic receptor response and disease [49,50]. The observation that muscarinic receptor mediated contraction is impaired as a result of vitC deficiency is of potential importance, not only in regulation of coronary artery vasomotion, but also in other tissues that are highly dependent on parasympathetic-muscarinic receptor-mediated contraction (bladder, esophagus, intestines, pancreas, and salivary glands). For obvious ethical reasons, it is impossible to perform long-term controlled trials on humans to establish the consequence of vitC deficiency on vasculature and present knowledge is therefore restricted to indirect evidence. Applying the guinea pig as a unique and validated model of diet-induced vitC deficiency, this study shows that chronic vitC deficiency in vivo alters the response of the coronary arteries to parasympathetic stimuli. This provides a link between vitC deficiency and cardiovascular disease, proposing a yet undisclosed, specific, effect of vitC in the modulation of muscarinic receptor-modulated response within the vascular wall. Though requiring further investigation, the apparent association between vitC status and coronary artery contraction may prove relevant in the prevention and treatment of cardiovascular diseases in humans with poor vitC status.

The present study has several limitations. Based on existing literature, we expected that vitC deficiency reduced NO-mediated vasodilation as a consequence of the decreased BH_4 plasma concentration. The potential reason for the lack of correlation between the BH_4 plasma concentrations and endothelial function could be that we determined biopterines and vitC in the plasma, rather than in the arteries, which could potentially more adequately have reflected the vessel status. Interestingly, a correlation between animal weight, artery diameter and endothelial function in vitC deficient guinea pigs was found. Future studies are needed to elaborate on a causal relationship and putative functional consequences e.g., clarifying if vitC deficiency induces morphological changes of the heart muscle and vessels. Furthermore, measurements of intracellular calcium concentrations would be highly relevant to determine if vitC deficiency alters cytosolic calcium levels and handling, which can lead to increased tone and decreased vessel diameter. Here, the effect of vitC deficiency was evaluated in young guinea pigs—reproductive maturity is reached at around 10 weeks of age—with no other underlying pathophysiological condition. We found that the coronary arteries were highly resistant to mechanically endothelial denudation, suggesting that the animals, despite vitC deficiency, retained a high NO capacity and/or sensitivity in the coronary arteries. However, it could be speculated that in the presence of an additional vascular disease, such as atherosclerosis, left ventricular hypertension [51] or even age-related reductions in compensatory abilities, a decreased vitC concentration and consequently, a reduced capacity to recycle BH_4, may be crucial in preserving an adequate vasodilator capacity [52].

Our finding, that the muscarinic receptor system is highly sensitive to vitC deficiency, is a novel and so far unrecognized effect of in vivo vitC deficiency. Future studies are needed to elucidate the mechanisms underlying the impaired muscarinic receptor mediated contraction observed here and to study other tissues with highly dependent parasympathetic-muscarinic receptor-mediated contraction (e.g., bladder, esophagus, intestines, pancreas, and salivary glands).

5. Conclusions

The present study shows that chronic vitC deficiency impairs vasomotor function of coronary arteries. During vitC deficiency, the endothelial function is reduced, with decreasing vessel diameter and carbachol-induced vasoconstrictor responses being significantly impaired. The carbachol-induced effects are apparently mediated by altered muscarinic receptor activity. Although further studies are required to evaluate the underlying mechanisms and the potential clinical implications, these findings may provide a link between chronic vitC deficiency and increased risk of cardiovascular disease reported in numerous epidemiological studies.

Acknowledgments: We thank Joan Elisabeth Frandsen for her excellent technical expertise and assistance in the ascorbate measurements. This study was supported by the LIFEPHARM Centre for In Vivo Pharmacology.

Author Contributions: G.F.S., P.T.N. and J.L. conceived and designed the experiments; G.F.S. carried out the myography experiments and data analysis. P.T.N., M.M.L. and S.N.H. performed the animal study. G.F.S., P.T.N. and J.L. interpreted the data and wrote the manuscript. All authors read and commented on the final draft of the manuscript.

References

1. Myint, P.K.; Luben, R.N.; Wareham, N.J.; Khaw, K.-T. Association Between Plasma Vitamin C Concentrations and Blood Pressure in the European Prospective Investigation Into Cancer-Norfolk Population-Based Study. *Hypertension* **2011**, *58*, 372–379. [CrossRef] [PubMed]
2. Myint, P.K.; Luben, R.N.; Welch, A.A.; Bingham, S.A.; Wareham, N.J.; Khaw, K.T. Plasma vitamin C concentrations predict risk of incident stroke over 10 years in 20,649 participants of the European Prospective Investigation into Cancer Norfolk prospective population study. *Am. J. Clin. Nutr.* **2008**, *87*, 64–69. [PubMed]
3. NyyssÖnen, K.; Parviainen, M.T.; Salonen, R.; Tuomilehto, J.; Salonen, J.T. Vitamin C deficiency and risk of myocardial infarction: Prospective population study of men from eastern Finland. *BMJ* **1997**, *314*, 634–638. [CrossRef] [PubMed]
4. Pfister, R.; Michels, G.; Bragelmann, J.; Sharp, S.J.; Luben, R.; Wareham, N.J.; Khaw, K.T. Plasma vitamin C and risk of hospitalisation with diagnosis of atrial fibrillation in men and women in EPIC-Norfolk prospective study. *Int. J. Cardiol.* **2014**, *177*, 830–835. [CrossRef] [PubMed]
5. Pfister, R.; Sharp, S.J.; Luben, R.; Wareham, N.J.; Khaw, K.T. Plasma vitamin C predicts incident heart failure in men and women in European Prospective Investigation into Cancer and Nutrition-Norfolk prospective study. *Am. Heart J.* **2011**, *162*, 246–253. [CrossRef] [PubMed]
6. Wannamethee, S.G.; Bruckdorfer, K.R.; Shaper, A.G.; Papacosta, O.; Lennon, L.; Whincup, P.H. Plasma Vitamin C, but Not Vitamin E, Is Associated With Reduced Risk of Heart Failure in Older Men. *Circ. Heart Fail.* **2013**, *6*, 647–654. [CrossRef] [PubMed]
7. Schleicher, R.L.; Carroll, M.D.; Ford, E.S.; Lacher, D.A. Serum vitamin C and the prevalence of vitamin C deficiency in the United States: 2003–2004 National Health and Nutrition Examination Survey (NHANES). *Am. J. Clin. Nutr.* **2009**, *90*, 1252–1263. [CrossRef] [PubMed]
8. Heller, R.; Unbehaun, A.; Schellenberg, B.; Mayer, B.; Werner-Felmayer, G.; Werner, E.R. L-ascorbic acid potentiates endothelial nitric oxide synthesis via a chemical stabilization of tetrahydrobiopterin. *J. Biol. Chem.* **2001**, *276*, 40–47. [CrossRef] [PubMed]
9. Mortensen, A.; Lykkesfeldt, J. Does vitamin C enhance nitric oxide bioavailability in a tetrahydrobiopterin-dependent manner? In vitro, in vivo and clinical studies. *Nitric Oxide Biol. Chem. Off. J. Nitric Oxide Soc.* **2014**, *36*, 51–57. [CrossRef] [PubMed]
10. Baker, T.A.; Milstien, S.; Katusic, Z.S. Effect of vitamin C on the availability of tetrahydrobiopterin in human endothelial cells. *J. Cardiovasc. Pharmacol.* **2001**, *37*, 333–338. [CrossRef] [PubMed]
11. Tejero, J.; Stuehr, D. Tetrahydrobiopterin in nitric oxide synthase. *IUBMB Life* **2013**, *65*, 358–365. [CrossRef] [PubMed]
12. Vasquez-Vivar, J.; Martasek, P.; Whitsett, J.; Joseph, J.; Kalyanaraman, B. The ratio between tetrahydrobiopterin and oxidized tetrahydrobiopterin analogues controls superoxide release from endothelial nitric oxide synthase: An EPR spin trapping study. *Biochem. J.* **2002**, *362*, 733–739. [CrossRef] [PubMed]
13. Mortensen, A.; Hasselholt, S.; Tveden-Nyborg, P.; Lykkesfeldt, J. Guinea pig ascorbate status predicts tetrahydrobiopterin plasma concentration and oxidation ratio in vivo. *Nutr. Res.* **2013**, *33*, 859–867. [CrossRef] [PubMed]
14. Chen, X.; Touyz, R.M.; Park, J.B.; Schiffrin, E.L. Antioxidant effects of vitamins C and E are associated with altered activation of vascular NADPH oxidase and superoxide dismutase in stroke-prone SHR. *Hypertension* **2001**, *38*, 606–611. [CrossRef] [PubMed]

15. Lee, M.Y.; Griendling, K.K. Redox signaling, vascular function, and hypertension. *Antioxid. Redox Signal.* **2008**, *10*, 1045–1059. [CrossRef] [PubMed]

16. Zou, M.H. Peroxynitrite and protein tyrosine nitration of prostacyclin synthase. *Prostaglandins Lipid Mediat.* **2007**, *82*, 119–127. [CrossRef] [PubMed]

17. Zou, M.H.; Li, H.; He, C.; Lin, M.; Lyons, T.J.; Xie, Z. Tyrosine nitration of prostacyclin synthase is associated with enhanced retinal cell apoptosis in diabetes. *Am. J. Pathol.* **2011**, *179*, 2835–2844. [CrossRef] [PubMed]

18. Frei, B.; Stocker, R.; England, L.; Ames, B.N. Ascorbate: The most effective antioxidant in human blood plasma. *Adv. Exp. Med. Biol.* **1990**, *264*, 155–163. [PubMed]

19. De Jongh, R.; Haenen, G.R.; van Koeveringe, G.A.; Dambros, M.; De Mey, J.G.; van Kerrebroeck, P.E. Oxidative stress reduces the muscarinic receptor function in the urinary bladder. *Neurourol. Urodyn.* **2007**, *26*, 302–308. [CrossRef] [PubMed]

20. Sawiris, P.; Chanaud, N.; Enwonwu, C.O. Impaired inositol trisphosphate generation in carbachol-stimulated submandibular gland acinar cells from ascorbate deficient guinea pigs. *J. Nutr. Biochem.* **1995**, *6*, 557–563. [CrossRef]

21. Sawiris, P.G.; Enwonwu, C.O. Ascorbate deficiency impairs the muscarinic-cholinergic and ss-adrenergic receptor signaling systems in the guinea pig submandibular salivary gland. *J. Nutr.* **2000**, *130*, 2876–2882. [PubMed]

22. Gulbenkian, S.; Edvinsson, L.; Saetrum Opgaard, O.; Valenca, A.; Wharton, J.; Polak, J.M. Neuropeptide Y modulates the action of vasodilator agents in guinea-pig epicardial coronary arteries. *Regul. Pept.* **1992**, *40*, 351–362. [CrossRef]

23. Lykkesfeldt, J. Ascorbate and dehydroascorbic acid as reliable biomarkers of oxidative stress: Analytical reproducibility and long-term stability of plasma samples subjected to acidic deproteinization. *Cancer Epidemiol. Biomark. Prev.* **2007**, *16*, 2513–2516. [CrossRef] [PubMed]

24. DMT Normalization Guide. Available online: https://www.dmt.dk/uploads/6/5/6/8/65689239/dmt_normalization_guide.pdf (accessed on 22 June 2017).

25. Brunner, F.; Kuhberger, E.; Groschner, K.; Poch, G.; Kukovetz, W.R. Characterization of muscarinic receptors mediating endothelium-dependent relaxation of bovine coronary artery. *Eur. J. Pharmacol.* **1991**, *200*, 25–33. [CrossRef]

26. Ren, L.M.; Nakane, T.; Chiba, S. Muscarinic receptor subtypes mediating vasodilation and vasoconstriction in isolated, perfused simian coronary arteries. *J. Cardiovasc. Pharmacol.* **1993**, *22*, 841–846. [CrossRef] [PubMed]

27. Lamping, K.G.; Wess, J.; Cui, Y.; Nuno, D.W.; Faraci, F.M. Muscarinic (M) receptors in coronary circulation: Gene-targeted mice define the role of M_2 and M_3 receptors in response to acetylcholine. *Arterioscler. Thromb. Vasc. Biol.* **2004**, *24*, 1253–1258. [CrossRef] [PubMed]

28. Brunner, F.; Kuhberger, E.; Schloos, J.; Kukovetz, W.R. Characterization of muscarinic receptors of bovine coronary artery by functional and radioligand binding studies. *Eur. J. Pharmacol.* **1991**, *196*, 247–255. [CrossRef]

29. Duckles, S.P.; Garcia-Villalon, A.L. Characterization of vascular muscarinic receptors: Rabbit ear artery and bovine coronary artery. *J. Pharmacol. Exp. Ther.* **1990**, *253*, 608–613. [PubMed]

30. Entzeroth, M.; Doods, H.N.; Mayer, N. Characterization of porcine coronary muscarinic receptors. *Naunyn-Schmiedeberg's Arch. Pharmacol.* **1990**, *341*, 432–438. [CrossRef]

31. Van Charldorp, K.J.; van Zwieten, P.A. Comparison of the muscarinic receptors in the coronary artery, cerebral artery and atrium of the pig. *Naunyn-Schmiedeberg's Arch. Pharmacol.* **1989**, *339*, 403–408. [CrossRef]

32. Findlay, G.M. The Effects of an Unbalanced Diet in the Production of Guinea-pig Scurvy. *Biochem. J.* **1921**, *15*, 355–357. [CrossRef] [PubMed]

33. Karaki, H.; Urakawa, N.; Kutsky, P. Potassium-induced contraction in smooth muscle. *Nihon Heikatsukin Gakkai Zasshi* **1984**, *20*, 427–444. [CrossRef] [PubMed]

34. Mombouli, J.V.; Illiano, S.; Nagao, T.; Scott-Burden, T.; Vanhoutte, P.M. Potentiation of endothelium-dependent relaxations to bradykinin by angiotensin I converting enzyme inhibitors in canine coronary artery involves both endothelium-derived relaxing and hyperpolarizing factors. *Circ. Res.* **1992**, *71*, 137–144. [CrossRef] [PubMed]

35. Saito, M.; Wada, K.; Kamisaki, Y.; Miyagawa, I. Effect of ischemia-reperfusion on contractile function of rat urinary bladder: Possible role of nitric oxide. *Life Sci.* **1998**, *62*, PL149–PL156. [CrossRef]

36. Hisadome, Y.; Saito, M.; Kono, T.; Satoh, I.; Kinoshita, Y.; Satoh, K. Beneficial effect of preconditioning on ischemia-reperfusion injury in the rat bladder in vivo. *Life Sci.* **2007**, *81*, 347–352. [CrossRef] [PubMed]

37. Kots, A.Y.; Martin, E.; Sharina, I.G.; Murad, F. A short history of cGMP, guanylyl cyclases, and cGMP-dependent protein kinases. *Handb. Exp. Pharmacol.* **2009**, *191*, 1–14.

38. Priviero, F.B.; Zemse, S.M.; Teixeira, C.E.; Webb, R.C. Oxidative stress impairs vasorelaxation induced by the soluble guanylyl cyclase activator BAY 41-2272 in spontaneously hypertensive rats. *Am. J. Hypertens.* **2009**, *22*, 493–499. [CrossRef] [PubMed]

39. De Beer, V.J.; Taverne, Y.J.; Kuster, D.W.; Najafi, A.; Duncker, D.J.; Merkus, D. Prostanoids suppress the coronary vasoconstrictor influence of endothelin after myocardial infarction. *Am. J. Physiol. Heart Circ. Physiol.* **2011**, *301*, H1080–H1089. [CrossRef] [PubMed]

40. Hori, M.; Nishida, K. Oxidative stress and left ventricular remodelling after myocardial infarction. *Cardiovasc. Res.* **2009**, *81*, 457–464. [CrossRef] [PubMed]

41. Edlund, A.; Sollevi, A.; Wennmalm, A. The role of adenosine and prostacyclin in coronary flow regulation in healthy man. *Acta Physiol. Scand.* **1989**, *135*, 39–46. [CrossRef] [PubMed]

42. Dai, X.Z.; Bache, R.J. Effect of indomethacin on coronary blood flow during graded treadmill exercise in the dog. *Am. J. Physiol.* **1984**, *247*, H452–H458. [PubMed]

43. Lykkesfeldt, J.; Poulsen, H.E. Is vitamin C supplementation beneficial? Lessons learned from randomised controlled trials. *Br. J. Nutr.* **2010**, *103*, 1251–1259. [CrossRef] [PubMed]

44. Frei, B.; Birlouez-Aragon, I.; Lykkesfeldt, J. Authors' perspective: What is the optimum intake of vitamin C in humans? *Crit. Rev. Food Sci. Nutr.* **2012**, *52*, 815–829. [CrossRef] [PubMed]

45. Frikke-Schmidt, H.; Lykkesfeldt, J. Role of marginal vitamin C deficiency in atherogenesis: In vivo models and clinical studies. *Basic Clin. Pharmacol. Toxicol.* **2009**, *104*, 419–433. [CrossRef] [PubMed]

46. Tveden-Nyborg, P.; Lykkesfeldt, J. Does vitamin C deficiency increase lifestyle-associated vascular disease progression? Evidence based on experimental and clinical studies. *Antioxid. Redox Signal.* **2013**, *19*, 2084–2104. [CrossRef] [PubMed]

47. Dart, A.M.; Du, X.J.; Kingwell, B.A. Gender, sex hormones and autonomic nervous control of the cardiovascular system. *Cardiovasc. Res.* **2002**, *53*, 678–687. [CrossRef]

48. Niihashi, M.; Esumi, M.; Kusumi, Y.; Sato, Y.; Sakurai, I. Expression of muscarinic receptor genes in the human coronary artery. *Angiology* **2000**, *51*, 295–300. [PubMed]

49. Ludmer, P.L.; Selwyn, A.P.; Shook, T.L.; Wayne, R.R.; Mudge, G.H.; Alexander, R.W.; Ganz, P. Paradoxical vasoconstriction induced by acetylcholine in atherosclerotic coronary arteries. *N. Engl. J. Med.* **1986**, *315*, 1046–1051. [CrossRef] [PubMed]

50. Yasue, H.; Horio, Y.; Nakamura, N.; Fujii, H.; Imoto, N.; Sonoda, R.; Kugiyama, K.; Obata, K.; Morikami, Y.; Kimura, T. Induction of coronary artery spasm by acetylcholine in patients with variant angina: Possible role of the parasympathetic nervous system in the pathogenesis of coronary artery spasm. *Circulation* **1986**, *74*, 955–963. [CrossRef] [PubMed]

51. Bell, J.P.; Mosfer, S.I.; Lang, D.; Donaldson, F.; Lewis, M.J. Vitamin C and quinapril abrogate LVH and endothelial dysfunction in aortic-banded guinea pigs. *Am. J. Physiol. Heart Circ. Physiol.* **2001**, *281*, H1704–H1710. [PubMed]

52. LeBlanc, A.J.; Hoying, J.B. Adaptation of the Coronary Microcirculation in Aging. *Microcirculation* **2016**, *23*, 157–167. [CrossRef] [PubMed]

3

High Dose Ascorbate Causes Both Genotoxic and Metabolic Stress in Glioma Cells

Maria Leticia Castro [1], Georgia M. Carson [1], Melanie J. McConnell [1,2] and Patries M. Herst [2,3,*

[1] School of Biological Sciences, Victoria University, P.O.Box 600, Wellington 6140, New Zealand;
   leticia.castro@vuw.ac.nz (M.L.C.); georgia.carson@hotmail.co.nz (G.M.C.);
   Melanie.McConnell@vuw.ac.nz (M.J.M.)
[2] Malaghan Institute of Medical Research, P.O.Box 7060, Wellington 6242, New Zealand
[3] Department of Radiation Therapy, University of Otago, P.O.Box 7343, Wellington 6242, New Zealand
* Correspondence: patries.herst@otago.ac.nz

Abstract: We have previously shown that exposure to high dose ascorbate causes double stranded breaks (DSBs) and a build-up in S-phase in glioblastoma (GBM) cell lines. Here we investigated whether or not this was due to genotoxic stress as well as metabolic stress generated by exposure to high dose ascorbate, radiation, ascorbate plus radiation and H_2O_2 in established and primary GBM cell lines. Genotoxic stress was measured as phosphorylation of the variant histone protein, H2AX, 8-oxo-7,8-dihydroguanine (8OH-dG) positive cells and cells with comet tails. Metabolic stress was measured as a decrease in NADH flux, mitochondrial membrane potential (by CMXRos), ATP levels (by ATP luminescence) and mitochondrial superoxide production (by mitoSOX). High dose ascorbate, ascorbate plus radiation, and H_2O_2 treatments induced both genotoxic and metabolic stress. Exposure to high dose ascorbate blocked DNA synthesis in both DNA damaged and undamaged cell of ascorbate sensitive GBM cell lines. H_2O_2 treatment blocked DNA synthesis in all cell lines with and without DNA damage. DNA synthesis arrest in cells with damaged DNA is likely due to both genotoxic and metabolic stress. However, arrest in DNA synthesis in cells with undamaged DNA is likely due to oxidative damage to components of the mitochondrial energy metabolism pathway.

Keywords: high dose ascorbate; H_2O_2; radiation; oxidative stress; genotoxic stress; metabolic stress; DNA synthesis arrest

---

1. Introduction

The last decade has seen a renewed interest in intravenous high dose (pharmacological) ascorbate (AA) as an anticancer treatment. Most authors in the field attribute the anticancer effect of high dose AA to its pro-oxidant effect. In the extracellular acidic and metal-rich tumour environment, high dose AA generates extracellular hydrogen peroxide (H_2O_2), which diffuses into adjacent cancer cells and overwhelms the anti-oxidant defence system (reviewed by [1]). The resulting oxidative stress damages macromolecules [1] as well as depleting NAD^+ and ATP levels [2–5]. Yun and colleagues reported recently that the oxidised form of AA, dehydroascorbate (DHA) rather than AA was responsible for selectively killing glycolysis-driven colorectal cancer cells with BRAF and KRAS mutations [6]. DHA is transported into cells through glucose transporters (GLUT-1), where it is reduced back to AA at the expense of glutathione (GSH), causing oxidative stress and inhibition of glyceraldehyde-3-phosphate dehydrogenase (GAPDH) and thus glycolysis, leading to ATP depletion [6,7]. In addition to causing oxidative stress, AA has been shown to increase hypoxia inducible factor, HIF-1, hydroxylase activity, leading to a decrease in HIF-1 pathway activation and a less aggressive phenotype in colorectal [8] and endometrial cancer [9], and inhibit the proliferation of breast cancer MCF-7 mammospheres [10].

Most authors have reported that high dose AA has little or no effect on non-cancerous cell lines (reviewed by [11]) and few side effects in animal models [12,13] or clinical trials [4,14,15]. Cancer specificity has been attributed to the acidic and metal-rich tumour micro-environment combined with the inferior anti-oxidant capacity and compromised DNA repair pathways of tumour cells [16–19]. Combining high dose AA with ionizing radiation should therefore radio-sensitize highly radiation resistant glioblastoma (GBM) cells [20,21] and improve the dismal prognosis for GBM patients [22].

Our group has studied the effect of high dose AA on radio-sensitization of GBMs in several studies. We initially showed that a GBM cell line isolated from a GBM patient was much more sensitive to high dose AA, radiation and combined treatments than a mouse-derived normal glial cell line [23]. However, a subsequent more detailed study showed that six human GBM cell lines, a human glial cell line and human umbilical vein endothelial cells were similarly sensitive to high dose AA and/or radiation. Sensitivity depended on their antioxidant and DNA repair capacity regardless of their cancerous status [24]. We further showed that exposure to high dose AA caused accumulation in S-phase as well as genotoxic stress. Genotoxic stress was demonstrated by a higher percentage of cells with foci caused by phosphorylation of the variant histone protein (H2AX) associated with the DNA damage response (γH2AX) as well as more γH2AX foci per cell [23,24]. The number of γH2AX foci correlates well with the number of double strand breaks (DSBs) generated by ionising radiation [25–28]. However, fewer than half of γH2AX foci induced by H_2O_2 [25–27] and UV [28] are associated with DSBs; with foci produced during replication likely representing stalled replication forks, which can either be repaired or progress to DSBs [25–28]. Another type of DNA lesion that causes genotoxic stress are 8-oxo-7,8-dihydroguanine (8OH-dG) lesions caused by aggressive hydroxyl free radicals generated by H_2O_2 in the close vicinity of DNA [18]. Although these lesions are also present in some untreated GBM cell lines and many GBM tumours [21], they are generated specifically in response to H_2O_2 [25–27]. The lesions are rapidly repaired by base excision repair (BER) and if unrepaired may generate single stranded breaks [18] or double stranded breaks [25–28]. Metabolic stress, in the form of low NAD^+ and low ATP levels as a result of high dose AA exposure, has been shown by several authors [2–5]. In this paper, we analysed the extent of genotoxic and metabolic stress and the effect on DNA synthesis by high dose AA in established and patient-derived GBM cell lines and compared these effects to those of radiation, H_2O_2 and combined treatments.

2. Materials and Methods

2.1. Materials

Unless otherwise noted, tissue plasticware was purchased from Corning (In Vitro Technologies, Auckland, New Zealand); all cell culture reagents were from Gibco BRL (Thermo Fisher Scientific, Auckland, New Zealand). Alexa Fluor 488 anti-H2AX-Phosphorylated (Ser139) Antibody was from BioLegend (Norrie Biotech, Auckland, New Zealand). Rabbit anti-8-OHdG polyclonal antibody (J-1: sc-139586) was from, Santa Cruz Biotech (Dallas, Texas, USA) and isotype control (IgG/10500C) was from Thermofisher Scientific (Wellington, New Zealand). Goat Polyclonal Anti-Rabbit IgG H&L (Alexa Fluor® 488) secondary antibody was from Abcam (Cambridge, MA, USA). Foxp3/Transcription Factor Fixation/Permeabilization Concentrate and Diluent was purchased from eBioscience (Huntingtree Bioscience Supplies, Auckland, New Zealand). Click-iT EdU Alexa Fluor Flow Cytometry Assay Kits, Vybrant DyeCycle Stains, MitoSOX™ Red Mitochondrial Superoxide Indicator and MitoTracker® Red CMXRos were purchased from Life Technologies (Thermo Fisher Scientific, Auckland, New Zealand). CellTiter 96® AQueous One Solution Cell Proliferation Assay (MTS) was sourced from Promega Corporation (Madison, WI, USA). Luminescent ATP Detection Assay Kit was obtained from Abcam (Cambridge, MA, USA). Sodium ascorbate, and all other chemicals and reagents were from Sigma Chemical Company (St. Louis, MO, USA).

2.2. Cell Lines

GBM cell lines, LN18, U87MG and T98G were obtained from the American Type Culture Collection. Primary GBM cells (NZG0809, NZG1003) were isolated and cultured from GBM material as previously described [29]. GBMs were grown in RPMI-1640 supplemented with 5% (*v/v*) FBS. All cells were maintained in a humidified incubator at 37 °C/5% CO_2.

2.3. Ascorbate Treatment

Exponentially growing cells (30–40% confluent) were seeded 24 h prior to treatment in 6 well plates (3–5 × 10^4 cells/well). Cells were exposed to 5 mM AA in media for 1 h, washed in Dulbecco's Phosphate Buffer Saline (PBS, 1.4 M NaCl, 27 mM KCl, 170 mM NaH_2PO_4, 17.6 mM KH_2PO_4) and re-incubated in fresh medium. Cells that received radiation were irradiated in the presence of AA.

2.4. Radiation Treatment

Exponentially growing cells (30–40% confluent) were irradiated fully immersed in medium with 6 Gy using Cesium-137 γ-rays (Gammacell 3000 Elan, Best Theratronics, Kanata, ON, Canada). After irradiation, cells were re-incubated in fresh medium.

2.5. DNA Synthesis: EdU Incorporation

Fluorescent detection of incorporated thymidine analogue EdU (5-ethynyl-2'-deoxyuridine) was used as a measure of DNA synthesis. Cells were pulse-labelled with 4 μM EdU for 1 h prior to analysis. Incorporated EdU was detected using a copper catalyzed covalent reaction between Click-iT® EdU Alexa Fluor® 488 or Alexa Fluor® 647 dye azide and an alkyne on the ethynyl moiety of EdU. Briefly, cells were pulse labelled with EdU for 1hr prior to harvesting, washed twice in FACS buffer (PBS + 1% Bovine Serum Albumin (BSA), and incubated in Click-iT fixative at room temperature for 15 min in the dark. Cells were washed and resuspended in saponin-based permeabilisation buffer for 15 min prior to incubation in the Click-iT AF647 reaction cocktail for 30 min in the dark at room temperature. For DNA content staining, these cells were incubated in a 5 μM Vybrant Dye Cycle Green/HBSS staining solution for 30 min at 37 °C prior to analysis by flow cytometry using a BD FACSCanto II (Becton Dickinson, San Jose, CA, USA). Data were analysed using FlowJo (TreeStar, Ashland, OR, USA).

2.6. γH2AX Labelling

Genotoxic stress was determined by measuring the extent of phosphorylation of the histone protein, H2AX, using Alexa Fluor 488 labelled anti-γH2AX antibody in permeabilised cells. EdU labelled cells were harvested and washed in PBS buffer, distributed into 96 well plates (5 × 10^5 cells/well), washed in 200 μL FACS buffer (PBS + 1% BSA), pelleted at 400× *g* (in a Megafuge 2.0R, Heraeus centrifuge, Labcare, Buckinghamshire, UK) for 4 min and fixed in 200 μL Forkhead box P3 (FoxP3)/Transcription Factor Fixation/ Permeabilization solution for 45 min at room temperature. Cells were washed twice in 200 μL 1x Permeabilization/Wash buffer (PBS, 1% BSA, 0.5% Saponin), pelleted and incubated in Click-iT® AF647 reaction cocktail for 30 min in the dark. Cells were then washed twice in Perm/Wash buffer and incubated in antibody solution (50 μL anti-γH2AX antibody or isotype control diluted 1:200 in 1x Perm/Wash buffer) at 4 °C overnight. Following this, cells were washed twice in Perm/Wash buffer and resuspended in 400 μL FACS buffer. Cells were analysed by flow cytometry using a BD FACSCanto II (Becton Dickinson, San Jose, CA, USA) and FlowJo software (TreeStar, Ashland, OR, USA).

2.7. 8OH-dG Lesions

Harvested cells were washed in PBS buffer and distributed into 96 well plates (5 × 10^5 cells/well), washed in 200 μL FACS buffer (PBS + 1% BSA), pelleted at 400× *g* (in a Megafuge 2.0R, Heraeus centrifuge, Labcare, Buckinghamshire, UK) for 4 min and fixed in 200 µL Foxp3/Transcription Factor Fix/Perm solution for 45 min at room temperature. Cells were washed twice in 200 µL 1x Permeabilization/Wash buffer (PBS, 1% BSA, 0.5% Saponin), pelleted and resuspended in primary antibody solution (50 µL rabbit anti-8OH-dG polyclonal antibody or isotype control (diluted at 400 ng/mL in 1x Perm/Wash buffer) at 4 °C overnight, washed twice in Perm/Wash buffer and resuspended in secondary antibody solution (Goat Polyclonal Anti-Rabbit IgG H&L (Alexa Fluor® 488), Abcam) at 1000 ng/mL) for an hour at room temperature. Cells were then washed twice in Perm/wash buffer and resuspended in 400 µL FACS buffer for analysis by flow cytometry using a BD FACSCanto II (Becton Dickinson, San Jose, CA, USA) and FlowJo software (TreeStar, Ashland, OR, USA).

2.8. Comet Tail Assay

Glass slides (LabServ Superfrost Plus) were pre-coated with 1% normal melting point agarose (Invitrogen UltraPure Agarose) and air-dried for 24 h. Cells were added to 1% low melting point agarose at a ratio of 1:10 (v/v) to final cell concentration 1×10^4 cells/mL, and dropped onto agarose coated slides. Agarose and cells were air dried for 30 min at room temperature, then lysed in pre-chilled lysis solution (2.5 M NaCl, 100 mM EDTA pH 10, 10 mM Trizma, 1% sodium lauryl sarcosinate, and 1% Triton X-100, pH 10) for 1 h at 4 °C. Slides were rinsed in 1x Tris-Borate-EDTA buffer TBE, and equilibrated for 30 min in 1x TBE before electrophoresis at 30 volts/cm for 60 min. Slides were stained with 10 µg/mL propidium iodide for 20 min at 4 °C, rinsed in TBE, and imaged on a fluorescent microscope (Olympus BX51 microscope with TXRED filter). Cell nuclei were analysed using ImageJ Comet Assay plugin, based on an NIH Image Comet Assay by H.M. Miller (https://www.med.unc.edu/microscopy/resources/imagej-plugins-and-macros/comet-assay) from Robert Bagnell. Briefly, tight ovals are drawn around the head and the tail. The tail length is the distance from the centre of the head (defined as the average of XY coordinates of all pixels in the head oval) to the centre of mass of the tail (defined as the brightness-weighted average of XY coordinates of the selected tail oval). Tail length is calculated as the Pythagorean distance between the two points. ImageJ outputs were imported into Microsoft Excel and averages were imported into Prism (Graphpad) V6.0 for analysis.

2.9. MTS Assay

The colorimetric CellTiter 96® AQueous One Solution Cell Proliferation Assay containing the soluble tetrazolium compound MTS (3-(4,5-dimethylthiazol-2-yl)-5-(3-carboxymethoxyphenyl) -2-(4-sulfophenyl)-2H-tetrazolium, inner salt) and electron coupling reagent PES (phenazine ethosulfate) were utilised for assessment of NADH flux in cells. Cells (5×10^3 cells/well) were plated into 96 well plates and incubated overnight. Cells were treated and washed three times in 300 µL of PBS. 100 µL of culture media was replaced and 20 µL of CellTiter 96® AQueous One Solution Reagent was added. Plates were incubated for 1−4 h at 37 °C and absorbance was measured at 490 nm on an Enspire 2300 plate reader (Perkin-Elmer, Shelton, CT, USA).

2.10. MitoTracker® Red CMXRos

Mitochondrial membrane potential was assessed using the cell-permeant X-rosamine derived MitoTracker® Red CMXRos dye. Treated cells and untreated cells were harvested and incubated in 50 nM CMXRos in PBS for 30 min at 37 °C. Cells were analysed by flow cytometry using a BD FACSCanto II (Becton Dickinson, San Jose, CA, USA) and FlowJo software (TreeStar, OR, USA).

2.11. MitoSOX™ Red Mitochondrial Superoxide Indicator

Live-cell permeant MitoSOX Red superoxide indicator targets mitochondria, where it is selectively oxidized by mitochondrial superoxide to exhibit red fluorescence. Treated and untreated cells were harvested and incubated in 5 µM MitoSOX in PBS for 10 min at 37 °C, fluorescent signal detected by flow cytometry using a FACSCanto II (Becton Dickinson, San Jose, CA, USA) with FlowJo software (TreeStar, OR, USA).

2.12. ATP Measurements

Cellular ATP was assessed using the firefly luciferase based Luminescent ATP Detection Assay Kit (Abcam, Cambridge, UK) according to manufacturer's instruction. Cells (2×10^3 cells/well) were plated into 96 well cell culture treated white plates and incubated overnight. Cells were treated, washed, and lysed in 50 µL of detergent for 5 min on an orbital shaker at 700 rpm. Substrate solution (50 µL) was added and cells were incubated in the dark for a further 5 min on an orbital shaker at 700 rpm. The plate was dark adapted for 10 min prior to luminescent reading using an Enspire plate reader (Perkin-Elmer, Shelton, CT, USA).

2.13. Cell Viability

GL261 cells were collected 48 h after treatment by trypsinization, washed in PBS and resuspended in 1 µg/mL propidium iodide, for cell count and dye exclusion using flow cytometry using a BD FACSCanto II (Becton Dickinson, San Jose, CA, USA) and FlowJo software (TreeStar, Ashland, OR, USA). All viability assays were completed at least three times in triplicate.

2.14. Statistical Analysis

Data were analysed using Excel (Microsoft v. 2010; Redmond Campus, Redmond, WA, USA) or Prism (Graphpad) V6.0. All experiments were done at least three times in triplicate; values are averages ± standard error of the means (SEM). Flow cytometry plots are representative of at least 3 separate experiments.

3. Results

3.1. GBM Cells Have Different Sensitivities to High Dose Ascorbate

Our previous research showed that TG98G cells were less sensitive to 5 mM AA as evidenced by higher clonogenicity than other GBM cells, most likely because of its very high antioxidant content [26]. A more in-depth analysis of AA sensitivity (Figure 1) showed that the IC_{50} of T98G cells was much higher (16.5 mM AA) than that of LN18, NZG0809 and NZG1003 cells (5.8, 6.8 and 7.6 mM AA respectively).

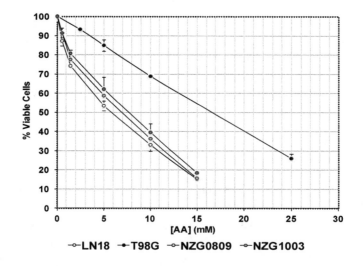

Figure 1. Sensitivities of different glioblastoma (GBM) cells to high dose ascorbic acid (AA). Cells were exposed to different concentrations of AA. Viability was measured by Trypan blue exclusion after 48 h. Values are averages ± standard error of the means (SEM) of at least 3 independent experiments in triplicate.

3.2. High Dose Ascorbate Generates Oxidative Damage and Double-Stranded DNA Breaks

We have previously used γH2AX foci as a measure of DSBs [23,24]. However, less than half of γH2AX foci after H_2O_2 exposure correlate closely with DSBs [25–27]. As most of the high dose AA effects are thought to be mediated though H_2O_2 formation and H_2O_2 has been shown to generate 8OH-dG lesions, we determined the level of 8OH-dG lesions in our cell lines before and after exposure to 5 mM AA, 6 Gy radiation, a combination of AA and radiation and 500 μM H_2O_2. We saw very few lesions 1–2 h after treatments (results not shown) but increasing numbers after 48 h (Figure 2A,B). We performed single cell gel electrophoresis to confirm that high dose AA does generate some DSBs, as evidenced by the presence of "tails" in the comet tail assay (Figure 2C,D). Notably, there were cells without comet tails (and thus DSBs) after exposure to AA, consistent with previous data demonstrating the presence of γH2AX-negative cells [24].

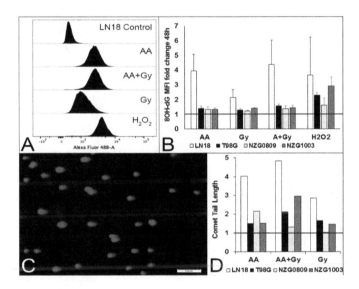

Figure 2. Different types of DNA damage after a 1h exposure to 5 mM AA, 6 Gy, 5 mM AA + 6 Gy and 500 μM H_2O_2. (**A**) Histograms of 8OH-dG lesions 48 h after treatments of LN18 cells. (**B**) Median fluorescence intensity (MFI) fold change compared with untreated cells of LN18, T98G, NZG0809 and NZG1003 cells. Values are averages ± SEM of at least 3 independent experiments in triplicate. Increased 8OH-dG lesions for H_2O_2 treatment over AA, Gy and AA + Gy was statistically significant ($p < 0.05$: unpaired two-tailed student t-test) for T98G and NZG1003. C. Representative photograph of comet tails (DSBs) of LN18 cells after a 1 h exposure to 5 mM AA. D. Fold change compared with controls of comet tail length of the different cell lines after a 1 h exposure to 5 mM AA, 6 Gy, 5 mM AA + 6 Gy compared to untreated controls (set at 1). Average number of comet tails measured per cell line: 278 (controls), 162 (AA), 220 (Gy) and 272 (AA + Gy).

3.3. High Dose Ascorbate Abrogates DNA Replication Which Does Not Resolve over Time

We previously showed that GBM cells accumulate in S-phase 24 h after transient exposure to high dose AA [23,24], suggestive of replication fork collapse [25–28]. Here, we measured the extent of DNA synthesis by incorporation of the modified nucleotide ethynyl deoxyuridine (EdU) at early (Figure 3A) and late (Figure 3B) time points after treatments. Plotting EdU incorporation against DNA content resulted in a typical distribution for dividing cells, where the strongly EdU positive cells were predominantly in S-phase with an intermediate DNA content. Strikingly, a 1 h AA exposure completely arrested DNA replication within 2 h in three of the four cell types tested, which was not resolved by 96 h. DNA synthesis in T98G was much less affected by AA, consistent with previous data suggesting this cell line is less sensitive to AA (Figure 1, [24]. In most cells, radiation resulted in a G2 arrest by 24 h with a resumption of normal cell cycle by later time points, in stark contrast to the sustained AA-induced block in DNA synthesis. NZG0809 showed low level of EdU incorporation after AA exposure which was not specifically associated with S-phase.

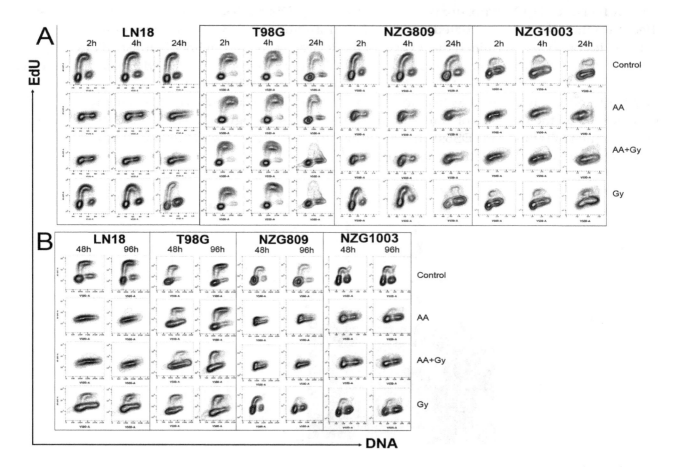

Figure 3. DNA synthesis indicated by EdU incorporation (*y*-axis) and DNA content by nucleic acid content (*x*-axis). G1 cells, with half the content of G2 cells are EdU negative, whereas cells undergoing synthesis have incorporated EdU into the newly synthesised DNA with subsequent increased signal. Cells were harvested at early time points (**A**) and late time points (**B**) after treatments. Flow cytometry plots are representative of at least three independent experiments.

3.4. High Dose Ascorbate Blocks Replication in Both Damaged and Undamaged Cells

The loss of DNA synthesis in AA-treated cells was profound and long-lasting with no recovery of affected cell lines over a four day period. However, the DNA damage data indicated that a small proportion of cells did not sustain any DNA damage, neither γH2AX, DSBs nor 8OH-dG. We therefore directly compared DNA damage with DNA synthesis. DNA damage in untreated controls was visible in both replicating and non-replicating cells, as expected from genetically unstable GBMs [21]. Both damaged and undamaged cells continued to synthesize DNA after radiation. However, almost no DNA synthesis was seen after AA or combined treatment, not even in undamaged cells in LN18 and NZG0809. A small amount of DNA synthesis was seen in NZG1003, particularly at later time points in DNA damaged cells. Despite sustaining moderate amounts of DNA damage, DNA synthesis in T98G was relatively unaffected by AA treatment (Figure 4A). Interestingly, a 1 h exposure to 50–100 μM H_2O_2 stopped DNA synthesis, even in T98G (Figure 4B).

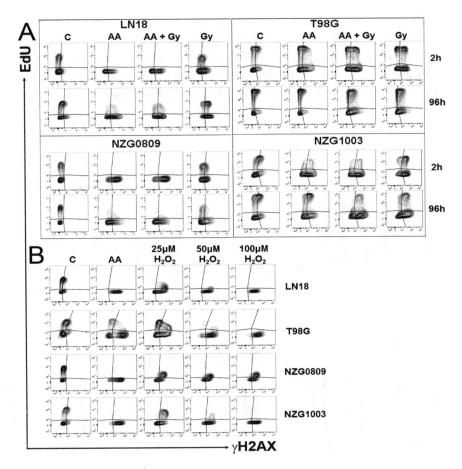

Figure 4. DNA synthesis indicated by EdU incorporation (*y*-axis) versus DNA damage by γH2AX foci (*x*-axis). Cells were treated as indicated and harvested after 2 h (A and B) or 96 h (**A**). (**B**) Effect of a 1 h exposure to 5 mM AA compared with that of different concentrations of H_2O_2. Flow cytometry plots are representative of at least three independent experiments.

3.5. High Dose Ascorbate Causes Metabolic Stress

Cells with damaged DNA can no longer replicate because of genotoxic stress. However, the observation that replication had also stopped in cells without apparent genotoxic stress was unexpected. It suggests that DNA damage, at least for some cells, is not the primary driver to replication loss, and subsequent cell death. High dose AA has also been shown to decrease ATP levels [3–6,16]. We also found that ATP levels declined significantly after a 1 h exposure to 5 mM AA in LN18, NZG0809 and NZG1003 but not in T98G. In comparison, 500 μM H_2O_2 decreased ATP levels more than 5 mM AA in all cell lines, including T98G (Figure 5A). We next determined the effect of treatments on cellular NADH flux by measuring reduction of the water soluble tetrazolium salt, MTS [30]. We found a substantial decrease in MTS reduction 1 h after AA treatment, combined treatment and after 500 μM H_2O_2 in LN18, NZG0809 and NZG1003. MTS reduction in T98G was only minimally affected by 5 mM AA but strongly inhibited by 500 μM H_2O_2 (Figure 5B). Robust mitochondrial electron transport (MET) activity results in a strong potential across the inner mitochondrial membrane. We found a decrease in mitochondrial membrane potential in LN18, NZG0809 and NZG1003 1 h after exposure to AA treatments, whereas H_2O_2 treatment decreased the mitochondrial membrane potential in all four cell lines (Figure 5C). Interestingly, we found an increase in mitochondrial superoxide levels after exposure to AA and H_2O_2 treatments (Figure 5D). Exposure to radiation did not affect ATP levels, MTS reduction, mitochondrial membrane potential or mitochondrial superoxide production in any of the cell lines at such early time points. This was not unexpected as the effects of radiation only become evident at later time points [20]. We previously measured viability 48 h after treatments and found that viability of LN18, NZG0809 and NZG1003 cells decreased substantially after AA treatments. T98G was relatively insensitive to AA whereas NZG1003 was relatively insensitive to radiation (Figure 5E). Correlational analysis (Figure 5F) showed that 1 h after exposure to AA, cellular ATP levels strongly correlated with MTS reduction and mitochondrial membrane potential; MTS reduction strongly correlated with mitochondrial membrane potential; 1 h ATP levels and MTS reduction correlated strongly with 48 h survival.

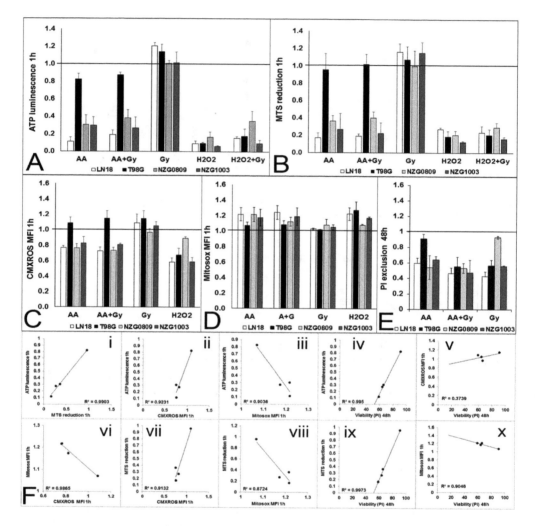

Figure 5. Metabolic stress after 1 h exposure to 5 mM AA, 6 Gy, 5 mM AA + 6 Gy and 500 μM H_2O_2 compared to untreated controls (set at 1). (**A**) Cellular ATP levels measured by luminescence; (**B**) Cellular NADH flux measured by MTS reduction; (**C**) Mitochondrial membrane potential measured by CMXROS; (**D**) Mitochondrial superoxide production measured by Mitosox. (**E**) Viability measured as PI exclusion 48 h after treatments. Fold change compared with untreated control cells. ATP luminescence, MTS reduction and CMXRos MFI were all significantly higher after 6 Gy treatment compared with all other treatments for LN18, NZG0809 and NZG1003. Viability after 5 mM AA treatment was significantly higher for T98G and after 6 Gy treatment for NZG0809. ($p < 0.05$: un-paired two-tailed student t-test). Values are averages ± SEM of at least 3 independent experiments in triplicate. (**F**) Correlations between cellular ATP levels, MTS reduction, mitochondrial membrane potential, mitochondrial superoxide production (all at 1 h) and cell viability at 48 h. Each dot represents one of the four cell lines.

4. Discussion

We previously showed that high dose AA generates γH2AX lesions and causes accumulation of cells in S phase [23,24]. In this paper, we analysed the extent of genotoxic and metabolic stress and the effect on DNA synthesis by high dose AA, radiation and combined treatments. With respect to genotoxic stress, we verified that high dose AA can indeed generate DSBs (as measured by comet tail assay) as well as 8OH-dG lesions. The increase in 8OH-dG lesions over time suggests effective base excision repair at early time points, but sustained free radical production combined with a lack of effective base excision repair at later time points. This may be caused by low cellular ATP levels. The small amount of EdU incorporation in NZG0809 throughout the cell cycle after AA exposure most likely reflects DNA synthesis as part of base excision repair, or other repair mechanisms, rather than DNA replication [31].

DNA synthesis blockade was expected in cells with DNA damage. However, the fact that undamaged cells were also unable to synthesise DNA in a sustained manner was unexpected and suggests that high dose AA directly affects cell metabolism. AA has been previously reported to decrease ATP levels in neuroblastoma cells [2], prostate cancer [3], ovarian cancer [4] pancreatic cancer [5]. This decrease in ATP was shown to be a result of genotoxic stress in the form of 8OH-dG lesions, which were repaired by PARP-1, leading to consumption of cytoplasmic NAD^+ (a cofactor of PARP-1). Decreased levels of NAD^+ inhibited glycolysis and glycolytic ATP production [2–5]. However, the cells that remained undamaged also stopped synthesising DNA and yet they have no need to activate PARP-1 with subsequent depletion of NAD^+ levels. We hypothesise that undamaged cells do not synthesise DNA because of depleted cellular ATP, due to direct oxidative damage to components of the energy metabolism pathways. In support of this hypothesis, Yun and colleagues recently showed that intracellular reduction of DHA to AA killed glycolysis-driven KRAS and BRAF mutated colorectal cancer cells through inhibition of glycolysis resulting in ATP depletion [6,7].

Intracellular NADH flux is a good measure of overall cellular energy metabolism. The tetrazolium dye MTS is reduced intracellularly (predominantly by NADH generated during glycolysis) as well as extracellularly (predominantly by NADH originating from the mitochondria) in the presence of an intermediate electron acceptor [30]. The strong decrease in MTS reduction at 1 h closely mimicked the strong drop in cellular ATP levels as well as a decrease in mitochondrial membrane potential. This may reflect both a lack of NAD^+ (required to fix 8OH-dG lesions) and/or a direct inhibition of glycolysis, Krebs cycle and MET activity, possibly due to oxidative damage to their components. In this respect it is of interest to note that H_2O_2 was previously shown to specifically damage the adenine nucleotide translocase (ANT) [32]. ANT is an inner mitochondrial membrane translocase which delivers ATP from the mitochondrial matrix to hexokinase II to facilitate the first step in glycolysis [33]. Oxidative damage to ANT inhibits glycolysis and thus glycolytic ATP production [32]. Declining glycolytic rates limit the amount of pyruvate entering the mitochondria which limits Krebs cycle activity, decreasing NADH and FADH2 levels that fuel MET, oxidative phosphorylation (OXPHOS), mitochondrial membrane potential and generate mitochondrial ATP. Superoxide is produced in the mitochondria during MET as a result of premature leakage of electrons at respiratory complexes I and III [34]. The small increase in superoxide levels we observed, combined with a decrease in membrane potential after AA and H_2O_2 treatments, suggests increased leakage due to oxidative damage to respiratory complexes. Both ATP level and MTS reduction 1 h after AA exposure were excellent predictors for cell survival 48 h later. Results presented in this paper show that both damaged and undamaged cells halt DNA synthesis within 2 h of exposure to AA which is not resolved 4 days later. This suggests that high dose AA and H_2O_2 generate both genotoxic and metabolic stress which contribute to blocking DNA synthesis in AA sensitive GBM cell lines. The specific contribution of each type of stress is likely to differ between cell lines and between cells of the same cell line.

The effect of H_2O_2 and high dose AA as mediators of genotoxic and metabolic stress were very similar in three of the four cell lines—T98G cells were less affected by AA than by H_2O_2 in all respects. This was expected, as this cell line is less sensitive to AA due to its high antioxidant capacity with an IC_{50} that is at least two times higher than that of the other cell lines [24]. It is possible that the antioxidant capacity of T98G was overwhelmed by a H_2O_2 bolus but able to cope with the H_2O_2 generated over a period of time from external AA.

5. Conclusions

This paper confirms that the mechanism of action of high dose AA is likely mediated by H_2O_2 generation as exposure to high dose AA and H_2O_2 abrogated DNA synthesis in cells with damaged and undamaged DNA. Both genotoxic stress and metabolic stress contributed to DNA synthesis arrest in DNA damaged cells. However, DNA synthesis arrest in undamaged cells can only be explained by direct oxidative damage to components of mitochondrial energy production.

Acknowledgments: This research was supported by Genesis Oncology Trust and the Neurological Foundation of New Zealand.

Author Contributions: Patries M. Herst, Melanie J. McConnell and Maria Leticia Castro conceived and designed the experiments; Maria Leticia Castro and Georgia M. Carson performed the experiments; Maria Leticia Castro and Patries M. Herst analyzed the data; Patries M. Herst wrote the manuscript with constructive feedback from Melanie J. McConnell, Maria Leticia Castro and Georgia M. Carson and all authors approved the final manuscript.

References

1. Parrow, N.L.; Leshin, J.A.; Levine, M. Parenteral ascorbate as a cancer therapeutic: A reassessment based on pharmacokinetics. *Antioxid. Redox Signal.* **2013**, *19*, 2141–2156. [CrossRef] [PubMed]
2. Bruchelt, G.; Schraufstätter, I.U.; Niethammer, D.; Cochrane, C. Ascorbic Acid Enhances the Effects of 6-Hydroxydopamine and H_2O_2 on Iron-dependent DNA Strand Breaks and Related Processes in the Neuroblastoma Cell Line SK-N-SH. *Cancer Res.* **1991**, *51*, 6066–6072.
3. Chen, P.; Yu, J.; Chalmers, B.; Drisko, J.; Yang, J.; Li, B.; Chen, Q. Pharmacological ascorbate induces cytotoxicity in prostate cancer cells through ATP depletion and induction of autophagy. *Anticancer Drugs* **2012**, *23*, 437–444. [CrossRef] [PubMed]
4. Ma, Y.; Chapman, J.; Levine, M.; Polireddy, K.; Drisko, J. High dose parenteral ascorbate enhanced chemosensitivity of ovarian cancer and reduced toxicity of chemotherapy. *Sci. Transl. Med.* **2014**, *6*, 222ra18. [CrossRef] [PubMed]
5. Du, J.; Martin, S.M.; Levine, M.; Wagner, B.A.; Buettner, G.R.; Wang, S.H.; Taghiyev, A.F.; Du, C.; Knudson, C.M.; Cullen, J.J. Mechanisms of Ascorbate-Induced Cytotoxicity in Pancreatic Cancer. *Clin. Cancer Res.* **2010**, *16*, 509–520. [CrossRef] [PubMed]
6. Yun, J.; Mullarky, E.; Lu, C.; Bosch, K.; Kavalier, A.; Rivera, K.; Roper, J.; Chio, I.I.C.; Giannopoulou, E.G.; Rago, C.; et al. Vitamin C selectively kills *KRAS* and *BRAF* mutant colorectal cancer cells by targeting GAPDH. *Science* **2015**, *350*, 1391–1396. [CrossRef] [PubMed]
7. Van der Reest, J.; Gottlieb, E. Anti-cancer effects of vitamin C revisited. *Cell Res.* **2016**, *26*, 269–270. [CrossRef] [PubMed]
8. Kuiper, C.; Dachs, G.U.; Munn, D.; Currie, M.J.; Robinson, B.A.; Pearson, J.F.; Vissers, M.C.M. Increased Tumor Ascorbate is Associated with Extended Disease-Free Survival and Decreased Hypoxia-Inducible Factor-1 Activation in Human Colorectal Cancer. *Front Oncol.* **2014**, *4*, 1–10. [CrossRef] [PubMed]
9. Kuiper, C.; Molenaar, I.G.M.; Dachs, G.U.; Currie, M.J.; Sykes, P.H.; Vissers, M.C.M. Low ascorbate levels are associated with increased hypoxia-inducible factor-1 activity and an aggressive tumor phenotype in endometrial cancer. *Cancer Res.* **2010**, *70*, 5749–5758. [CrossRef] [PubMed]
10. Bonuccelli, G.; De Francesco, E.M.; DeBoer, R.; Tanowitz, H.B.; Lisanti, M.P. NADH autofluorescence, a new metabolic biomarker for cancer stem cells: Identification of Vitamin C and CAPE as natural products targeting "stemness". *Oncotarget* **2017**, *8*, 20667–20678. [CrossRef] [PubMed]
11. Du, J.; Cullen, J.J.; Buettner, G.R. Ascorbic acid: Chemistry, biology and the treatment of cancer. *Buochim. Biophys. Acta* **2012**, *1826*, 443–457. [CrossRef] [PubMed]
12. Du, J.; Cieslak, J.A.; Welsh, J.L.; Sibenaller, Z.A.; Allen, B.G.; Wagner, B.A.; Kalen, A.L.; Doskey, C.M.; Strother, R.K.; Button, A.M.; et al. Pharmacological Ascorbate Radiosensitizes Pancreatic Cancer. *Cancer Res.* **2015**, *75*, 3314–3326. [CrossRef] [PubMed]

13. Chen, Q.; Espey, M.G.; Sun, A.Y.; Pooput, C.; Kirk, K.L.; Krishna, M.C.; Khosh, D.B.; Drisko, J.; Levine, M. Pharmacologic doses of ascorbate act as a prooxidant and decrease growth of aggressive tumor xenografts in mice. *Proc. Natl. Acad. Sci. USA* **2008**, *105*, 11105–11109. [CrossRef] [PubMed]

14. Monti, D.A.; Mitchell, E.; Bazzan, A.J.; Littman, S.; Zabrecky, G.; Yeo, C.J.; Pillai, M.V.; Newberg, A.B.; Deshmukh, S.; Levine, M. Phase I evaluation of intravenous ascorbic acid in combination with gemcitabine and erlotinib in patients with metastatic pancreatic cancer. *PLoS ONE* **2012**, *7*, e29794. [CrossRef] [PubMed]

15. Welsh, J.L.; Wagner, B.A.; van't Erve, T.J.; Zehr, P.S.; Berg, D.J.; Halfdanarson, T.R.; Yee, N.S.; Bodeker, K.L.; Du, J.; Roberts, L.J., II; et al. Pharmacological ascorbate with gemcitabine for the control of metastatic and node-positive pancreatic cancer (PACMAN): results from a phase I clinical trial. *Cancer Chemother. Pharmacol.* **2013**, *71*, 765–775. [CrossRef] [PubMed]

16. Deubzer, B.; Mayet, F.; Kuçi, Z.; Niewisch, M.; Merkel, G.; Handgretinger, R.; et al. H_2O_2-mediated cytotoxicity of pharmacologic ascorbate concentrations to neuroblastoma cells: potential role of lactate and ferritin. *Cell. Physiol. Biochem.* **2010**, *25*, 767–774. [CrossRef] [PubMed]

17. Duarte, T.L.; Almeida, G.M.; Jones, G.D.D. Investigation of the role of extracellular H_2O_2 and transition metal ions in the genotoxic action of ascorbic acid in cell culture models. *Toxicol. Lett.* **2007**, *170*, 57–65. [CrossRef] [PubMed]

18. Valko, M.; Rhodes, C.J.; Moncol, J.; Izakovic, M.; Mazur, M. Free radicals, metals and antioxidants in oxidative stress-induced cancer. *Chem. Biol. Interact.* **2006**, *160*, 1–40. [CrossRef] [PubMed]

19. Baader, S.L.; Bruchelt, G.; Carmine, T.C.; Lode, H.N.; Rieth, A.G.; Niethammer, D. Ascorbic acid mediated iron release from cellular ferritin and its relation to DNA strand break formation in neuroblastoma cells. *J. Cancer Res. Clin. Oncol.* **1994**, *120*, 415–421. [CrossRef] [PubMed]

20. Wouters, B.; Begg, A. Irradiation-induced damage and the DNA damage response. In *Basic Clinical Radiobiology*, 4th, ed.; Joiner, M.C., van der Kogel, A.J., Eds.; Hodder & Arnold: London, UK, 2009; pp. 11–41.

21. Bartkova, J.; Hamerlik, P.; Stockhausen, M.-T.; Ehrmann, J.; Hlobilkova, A.; Laursen, H.; Kalita, O.; Kolar, Z.; Poulsen, H.S.; Broholm, H.; et al. Replication stress and oxidative damage contribute to aberrant constitutive activation of DNA damage signalling in human gliomas. *Oncogene* **2010**, *29*, 5095–5102. [CrossRef] [PubMed]

22. Stupp, R.; Hegi, M.; Mason, W.; van den Bent, M.; Taphoorn, M.; Janzer, R.; Ludwin, S.K.; Allgeier, A.; Fisher, B.; Belanger, K.; et al. Effects of radiotherapy with concomitant and adjuvant temozolomide versus radiotherapy alone on survival in glioblastoma in a randomised phase III study: 5-year analysis of the EORTC-NCIC trial. *Lancet Oncol.* **2009**, *10*, 459–466. [CrossRef]

23. Herst, P.M.; Broadley, K.W.R.; Harper, J.L.; McConnell, M.J. Pharmacological concentrations of ascorbate radiosensitize glioblastoma multiforme primary cells by increasing oxidative DNA damage and inhibiting G2/M arrest. *Free Radic. Biol. Med.* **2012**, *52*, 1486–1493. [CrossRef] [PubMed]

24. Castro, M.; McConnell, M.; Herst, P. Radio-sensitisation by pharmacological ascorbate in glioblastoma multiforme cells, human glial cells and HUVECs depends on their antioxidant and DNA repair capabilities and is not cancer specific. *Free Radic. Biol. Med.* **2014**, *75*, 200–209. [CrossRef] [PubMed]

25. Katsube, T.; Mori, M.; Tsuji, H.; Shiomi, T.; Wang, B.; Liu, Q.; Nenoi, M.; Onoda, M. Most hydrogen peroxide-induced histone H2AX phosphorylation is mediated by ATR and is not dependent on DNA double-strand breaks. *J. Biochem.* **2014**, *156*, 85–95. [CrossRef] [PubMed]

26. Berniak, K.; Rybak, P.; Bernas, T.; Zarębski, M.; Biela, E.; Zhao, H.; Darzynkiewicz, Z.; Dobrucki, J.W. Relationship between DNA damage response, initiated by camptothecin or oxidative stress, and DNA replication, analyzed by quantitative 3D image analysis. *Cytom. A* **2013**, *83*, 913–924. [CrossRef] [PubMed]

27. Zhao, H.; Dobrucki, J.; Rybak, P.; Traganos, F.; Halicka, D.H.; Darzynkiewicz, Z. Induction of DNA damage signaling by oxidative stress in relation to DNA replication as detected using "click chemistry". *Cytom. A* **2011**, *79*, 897–902. [CrossRef] [PubMed]

28. De Feraudy, S.; Revet, I.; Bezrookove, V.; Feeney, L.; Cleaver, J.E. A minority of foci or pan-nuclear apoptotic staining of gammaH2AX in the S phase after UV damage contain DNA double-strand breaks. *Proc. Natl. Acad. Sci. USA* **2010**, *107*, 6870–6875. [CrossRef] [PubMed]

29. Broadley, K.W.R.; Hunn, M.K.; Farrand, K.J.; Price, K.M.; Grasso, C.; Miller, R.J.; Hermans, I.F.; McConnell, M.J. Side population is not necessary or sufficient for a cancer stem cell phenotype in glioblastoma multiforme. *Stem Cells* **2011**, *29*, 452–461. [CrossRef] [PubMed]

30. Berrdige, M.; Herst, P.; Tan, A. Tetrazolium dyes as tools in cell biology: New insights into their cellular reduction. *Biotechnol. Annu. Rev.* **2005**, *11*, 127–152.

31. Limsirichaikul, S.; Niimi, A.; Fawcett, H.; Lehmann, A.; Yamashita, S.; Ogi, T. A rapid non-radioactive technique for measurement of repair synthesis in primary human fibroblasts by incorporation of ethynyl deoxyuridine (EdU). *Nucleic Acids Res.* **2009**, *37*, 1–10. [CrossRef] [PubMed]

32. Yan, L.J.; Sohal, R.S. Mitochondrial adenine nucleotide translocase is modified oxidatively during aging. *Proc. Natl. Acad. Sci. USA* **1998**, *95*, 12896–12901. [CrossRef]

33. Cerella, C.; Dicato, M.; Diederich, M. Modulatory roles of glycolytic enzymes in cell death. *Biochem. Pharmacol.* **2014**, *92*, 22–30. [CrossRef] [PubMed]

34. Quinlan, C.L.; Perevoshchikova, I.V.; Hey-Mogensen, M.; Orr, A.L.; Brand, M.D. Sites of reactive oxygen species generation by mitochondria oxidizing different substrates. *Redox Biol.* **2013**, *1*, 304–312. [CrossRef] [PubMed]

4

Vitamin C Status Correlates with Markers of Metabolic and Cognitive Health in 50-Year-Olds: Findings of the CHALICE Cohort Study

John F. Pearson [1], Juliet M. Pullar [2], Renee Wilson [3], Janet K. Spittlehouse [4], Margreet C. M. Vissers [2], Paula M. L. Skidmore [5], Jinny Willis [6], Vicky A. Cameron [3] and Anitra C. Carr [2,*]

[1] Biostatistics and Computational Biology Unit, University of Otago, Christchurch 8140, New Zealand; john.pearson@otago.ac.nz
[2] Department of Pathology, University of Otago, Christchurch 8140, New Zealand; juliet.pullar@otago.ac.nz (J.M.P.); margreet.vissers@otago.ac.nz (M.C.M.V.)
[3] Department of Medicine, University of Otago, Christchurch 8140, New Zealand; renee.wilson@postgrad.otago.ac.nz (R.W.); vicky.cameron@otago.ac.nz (V.A.C.)
[4] Department of Psychological Medicine, University of Otago, Christchurch 8140, New Zealand; janet.spittlehouse@otago.ac.nz
[5] Department of Human Nutrition, University of Otago, Dunedin 9054, New Zealand; paula.skidmore@otago.ac.nz
[6] Lipid & Diabetes Research Group, Canterbury District Health Board, Christchurch 8140, New Zealand; jinny.willis@cdhb.health.nz
*   Correspondence: anitra.carr@otago.ac.nz

Abstract: A cohort of 50-year-olds from Canterbury, New Zealand ($N = 404$), representative of midlife adults, undertook comprehensive health and dietary assessments. Fasting plasma vitamin C concentrations ($N = 369$) and dietary vitamin C intake ($N = 250$) were determined. The mean plasma vitamin C concentration was 44.2 μmol/L (95% CI 42.4, 46.0); 62% of the cohort had inadequate plasma vitamin C concentrations (i.e., <50 μmol/L), 13% of the cohort had hypovitaminosis C (i.e., <23 μmol/L), and 2.4% had plasma vitamin C concentrations indicating deficiency (i.e., <11 μmol/L). Men had a lower mean plasma vitamin C concentration than women, and a higher percentage of vitamin C inadequacy and deficiency. A higher prevalence of hypovitaminosis C and deficiency was observed in those of lower socio-economic status and in current smokers. Adults with higher vitamin C levels exhibited lower weight, BMI and waist circumference, and better measures of metabolic health, including HbA1c, insulin and triglycerides, all risk factors for type 2 diabetes. Lower levels of mild cognitive impairment were observed in those with the highest plasma vitamin C concentrations. Plasma vitamin C showed a stronger correlation with markers of metabolic health and cognitive impairment than dietary vitamin C.

Keywords: ascorbate; cognition; HbA1c; insulin; glucose; hypovitaminosis C

1. Introduction

The role of vitamin C in health and disease has been actively studied since its discovery over 80 years ago [1]. Vitamin C has a number of well-recognized biological functions, all of which depend upon its ability to act as an electron donor [2]. One of the most significant of these is its cofactor activity for a variety of enzymes with critical functions throughout the body. These include the copper-containing monoxygenases dopamine hydroxylase and peptidyl-glycine α-amidating monooxygenase [3] and the Fe (II) and 2-oxoglutarate-dependent family of dioxygenases [4]. The latter is a large and varied family, with a continually expanding membership that includes the collagen prolyl hydroxylases responsible for stabilization of the tertiary structure of collagen, the prolyl and asparaginyl hydroxylases which regulate hypoxia-inducible factors (HIF) activity, and DNA and histone demethylases involved in the epigenetic regulation of gene expression. Vitamin C also functions as a highly effective water-soluble antioxidant, protecting in vivo biomolecules from oxidation [5], and there is good evidence to suggest it is involved in the regeneration of vitamin E in vivo [6,7].

Because humans are unable to synthesize their own vitamin C, it must be obtained from the diet, principally through fruit and vegetable consumption. Inadequate dietary intake results in the potentially fatal deficiency disease, scurvy. As little as 10 mg/day vitamin C is sufficient to prevent overt scurvy [8] and, although scurvy is considered to be relatively rare in Western populations, vitamin C deficiency is the fourth most prevalent nutrient deficiency reported in the United States [9,10]. Hypovitaminosis C (defined as a plasma concentration ≤ 23 µmol/L) affects a significant proportion of the population, with estimates as large as 15–20% in the United States [9]. Similar data for the New Zealand population are lacking, although dietary vitamin C intake has been used to estimate the prevalence of inadequate intake, defined as not meeting the estimated average requirement (EAR) [11].

The classical symptoms of scurvy, such as joint pain, lassitude, bleeding and ulceration are thought to be due to the loss in activity of the vitamin C-cofactor enzymes, particularly the collagen hydroxylases. It is becoming increasingly acknowledged, however, that vitamin C is required at concentrations above those needed for the prevention of scurvy for the maintenance of good health [12,13]. For example, individuals with hypovitaminosis C are known to present with fatigue, depression and deficiencies in wound healing [14,15], suggesting a requirement for vitamin C status to be above 23 µmol/L in plasma to support these functions. There is also epidemiological evidence to support a role for vitamin C in the prevention of some chronic disease, with intakes >100 mg/day recommended [12]; these intakes will provide adequate plasma levels (i.e., >50 µmol/L) [14,16]. Although the Australasian Recommended Dietary Intake (RDI) for vitamin C is only 45 mg/day, the New Zealand Ministry of Health, in accord with other international bodies, has a suggested dietary target of ~200 mg/day vitamin C for the reduction of chronic disease risk [17]. As the many cofactor functions of vitamin C become more widely understood, epidemiological studies in areas in which its biological activity can be justified are required.

The CHALICE (Canterbury Health, Ageing and Lifecourse) study is a unique New Zealand study comprising a comprehensive database of determinants of health. It has prospectively recruited ~400 fifty-year-olds at random from the electoral roll within the Canterbury region. Participants have undergone extensive health, dietary and social assessments [18]. Here we report on the plasma vitamin C status and dietary vitamin C intake of the participants, and examine the relationships between these measures and a range of health indicators.

2. Materials and Methods

2.1. Study Population

Participants were from a random sample drawn from the New Zealand electoral roll, recruited to take part in a prospective longitudinal study of health and wellbeing (2010–2013), called the Canterbury Health, Ageing and Lifecourse (CHALICE) study (detailed in [18]). Participants had to be aged 49–51 years, intend to reside within the greater Christchurch area for at least 6 of the next 12 months, live in the community (i.e., not in a prison or a rest home) and be able to complete the assessment (e.g., speak English proficiently). Māori, the indigenous people of New Zealand, were over-sampled so that they represented 15% of the CHALICE study sample. Enrolment statistics estimate that, in 2012, 94.9% of the target population were registered to vote in the Christchurch City Council area [19]. Relative to the rest of New Zealand, the Canterbury area has a slightly higher proportion of people aged ≥ 40 years and a higher proportion of people living in the least economically deprived national quintile [20].

Ethical approval was obtained from the Upper South A Regional Ethics Committee (URA/10/03/021) and all participants provided written informed consent.

Data were collected during a 4–6 h interview, via self-completed questionnaires and lifestyle diaries, and from blood and urine tests. The full cohort was 404 participants, and the present analysis is based on the 369 participants for whom fasting plasma vitamin C measurements were obtained and a sample of 250 for whom dietary vitamin C intake was determined.

2.2. Blood Sample Collection

Fasting blood samples were collected into EDTA anticoagulant tubes and sent to Canterbury Health Laboratories, an International Accreditation New Zealand (IANZ) laboratory, for analysis of biomarkers. Additional fasting samples were centrifuged at 4000 rpm for 10 min at 4 °C to separate plasma, and the plasma stored at −80 °C for vitamin C analysis.

2.3. Sample Preparation for Vitamin C Analysis

Stored EDTA-plasma was rapidly thawed and a 500 μL aliquot was treated with an equal volume of ice-cold 0.54 M HPLC-grade perchloric acid solution (containing 100 μmol/L of the metal chelator DTPA) to precipitate protein and stabilize the vitamin C. Samples were mixed, incubated on ice for a few minutes, then centrifuged. A 100 μL aliquot of the deproteinated supernatant was treated with 10 μL of the reducing agent TCEP (100 mg/mL stock) for 2 h at 4 °C to recover any oxidized vitamin C [21]. Samples were further diluted with an equal volume of ice-cold 77 mM perchloric acid/DTPA solution for HPLC analysis.

2.4. Vitamin C HPLC Analysis

The total vitamin C content (ascorbic acid plus dehydroascorbic acid) of the samples was determined by HPLC with electrochemical detection as described previously [22]. Samples (20 μL) were separated on a Synergi 4 μ Hydro-RP 80A column 150 mm × 4.6 mm (Phenomenex NZ Ltd, Auckland, New Zealand) using a Dionex Ultimate 3000 HPLC unit (with autosampler chilled to 4 °C and column temperature set at 30 °C) and an ESA coulochem II detector (+200 mV electrode potential and 20 μA sensitivity). The mobile phase comprised 80 mM sodium acetate buffer, pH 4.8, containing DTPA (0.54 mmol/L) and freshly added ion pair reagent n-octylamine (1 μmol/L), delivered at a flow rate of 1.2 mL/min. A standard curve of sodium-L-ascorbate, standardized spectrophotometrically at 245 nm (ε = 9860), was freshly prepared for each HPLC run in 77 mmol/L HPLC-grade perchloric acid containing DTPA (100 μmol/L). Plasma vitamin C content is expressed as μmol/L.

Fasting plasma vitamin C concentrations were classified as follows; deficient <11 μmol/L, marginal 11–23 μmol/L, inadequate 23–50 μmol/L or adequate >50 μmol/L [13,15].

2.5. Metabolic and Heart Health Assessments

Metabolic health was assessed by body measurements and fasting blood tests. Participants' height, weight and waist circumference were taken by the study interviewer, and body mass index (BMI) calculated (kg/m^2). Fasting blood tests comprised triglycerides, high-density lipoprotein (HDL), glucose, HbA1c and insulin (Canterbury Health Laboratories).

Heart health was assessed by blood pressure and participants had their NZ cardiovascular risk score calculated. Blood pressure measurements were taken while seated. Five year cardiovascular risk (%) was derived according to the New Zealand adaptation of the Framingham risk score; the following variables are included in the calculation: age, gender, systolic blood pressure, diabetic status, smoking history, and total cholesterol to HDL ratio [23].

2.6. Dietary Intake Assessment

Participants were asked to complete the Four Day Estimated Food Diary (4DEFD) in the week after their interview; on one weekend day and three weekdays. The 4DEFD included detailed instructions on how to record portion sizes, using common household measures. The completed 4DEFD were checked by a trained nutritionist and additional information obtained from participants where necessary before the data were entered into the nutrient analysis program Kai-culator (version 1.08d, Department of Human Nutrition, University of Otago, Dunedin, New Zealand). Dietary analysis was performed on 250 of the CHALICE participants, who had dietary data entered and cleaned at the time of analysis, for whom the mean daily intake of vitamin C was calculated. Data entry was undertaken by experienced nutritionists and all diaries were further checked for accuracy by one person who also made any necessary changes, to ensure consistency of data entry.

2.7. Wellbeing, Depression and Cognition

2.7.1. Mental Wellbeing

The Warwick–Edinburgh Mental Wellbeing Scale (WEMWBS) was used to assess general wellbeing. The 14 item questionnaire aims to measure positive mental health by assessing both aspects of well-being: eudaimonic and hedonic [24].

2.7.2. Depression

During the assessment, trained interviewers used the Mini-International Neuropsychiatric Interview (MINI) for diagnosis of current and past depressive episodes using DSM IV criteria [25].

2.7.3. Cognition

Participants completed the Montreal Cognitive Assessment (MoCA) version 7.1 (original version) [26], a short screening test for mild cognitive impairment. It assesses the cognitive domains of attention and concentration, executive functions, memory, language, visuoconstructional skills, conceptual thinking, calculations, and orientation. A score of 26 or more indicates normal functioning, while a score less than 26 might indicate mild cognitive impairment. MoCA scores were excluded from the analysis if English was the second language or if a previous event (e.g., carbon monoxide poisoning) had affected cognitive ability.

2.8. Socio-Economic Status

The Economic Living Standard Index Short Form (ELSI$_{SF}$) was used to assess standard of living [27]. Developed in New Zealand, the ELSI$_{SF}$ assesses a person's consumption and personal possessions, calculating a total score by combining information from all items of the survey. The ELSI$_{SF}$ scores range from 0–31, with those who score 0–16 described as being in hardship, scores of 17–24 as comfortable and scores of 25 or above as socio-economically good or very good. The ELSI$_{SF}$ has excellent internal consistency (coefficient alpha of 0.88).

2.9. Statistical Analyses

Statistical analyses were performed using R 3.3.1 software (R Foundation for Statistical Computing, Vienna, Austria). Univariate tests on continuous variables were t-tests with Satterthwhaite's adjustment for unequal variances while Wald odds ratios and Fisher exact p-values were calculated for categorical variables. Sample characteristics were compared with census proportions using the chi squared goodness of fit test. All health measures were examined independently for association with vitamin C (plasma vitamin C concentration or dietary vitamin C intake) using linear or logistic regression models. The models fitted the dietary measure, gender (dichotomous), Māori ethnicity (dichotomous) and current smoking (dichotomous). Models were fitted on males and females separately and the whole cohort combined. Modeling assumptions were verified with no material departures observed. For each outcome, the p values were adjusted for multiple comparisons using the Benjamini and Yekutieli method. The nominal p value for statistical significance is the usual 0.05 or 5% type II error rate. All $p < 0.1$ are shown in the tables with $p > 0.1$ shown as NS (not significant). The odds of currently smoking for those in the lowest socio-economic strata was 3.8 times that of the highest strata (95% CI 1.7–9.0), $p = 0.002$. Similarly the odds of current smoking were 3.4 times higher in the least educated strata than the most educated (95% CI 1.75, 6.54), $p = 0.0006$. To prevent over fitting, socio-economic status and education were not fitted, however smoking acts as a reasonable proxy for population modeling.

3. Results

3.1. Characteristics of the Study Population

Of the full CHALICE cohort ($N = 404$), 46.8% (189) were male, with 83.7% (338) self-identifying as New Zealand European and 14.9% (60) as Māori (Table 1). The majority of the participants were in the highest ELSI$_{SF}$ category. There were 60 current smokers in the cohort.

Table 1. CHALICE participants compared with Census 2006 50–54-year-olds from same region.

		Chalice (*n*, %)		Census 2006 (%)	*p*
Gender	Female	215	53.2	50.9	NS
	Male	189	46.8	49.1	
Ethnicity	Māori	60	14.9	4.5	<0.0001
	NZ European	338	83.7	74.2	
Socio-Economic Status	Low (ELSI$_{SF}$ score 0–16)	30	7.4	8.2	NS
	Medium (ELSI$_{SF}$ score 17–24)	122	30.2	29.4	
	High (ELSI$_{SF}$ score 25–31)	252	62.4	62.5	
Education	No Qualification	53	13.1	23.9	<0.0001
	Secondary School Qualification	110	27.2	35.2	
	Post-secondary	168	41.6	25.6	
	University Degree	73	18.1	15.3	
Current Smoker		60	14.9	16.6	NS

$N = 404$; p (χ^2_{n-1}) > 0.1 shown as not significant, NS.

Table 1 compares the CHALICE participants to the New Zealand Census 2006 data for similar age and region. The CHALICE participants had higher rates of Māori ethnicity and higher qualifications than the Canterbury average (Table 1), whereas socio-economic status and smoking were within stochastic limits. This suggests the sample is reasonably representative of Canterbury 50-year-olds and hence the national cohort allowing for regional bias.

The CHALICE cohort also had typical levels of health for a community sample (Table 2). Anthropometric measures were close to those of the New Zealand population. Average metabolic and cardiac markers for the cohort were generally within the healthy range. However, the high prevalence of chronic conditions in the New Zealand population was also readily apparent.

Table 2. Health of CHALICE participants and normal ranges for the New Zealand population.

Body Measurements	Female Mean	Min	Max	NZ Female Mean	Male Mean	Min	Max	NZ Male Mean
Weight kg	78.6	49.1	149.9	74.8 (73.5–76.1)	88.4	50.8	143.8	88.0 (86.9–89.1)
BMI kg/m^2	29.1	17.4	63.4	28.1 (27.6–28.6)	28.1	19.2	48.6	28.6 (28.2–28.9)
Waist cm	92.0	63.0	144.0	86.6 (85.5–87.6)	98.3	72.5	148.0	98.4 (97.4–99.3)
Metabolism	**Mean**	**Min**	**Max**	**Healthy Range**	**Mean**	**Min**	**Max**	**Healthy Range**
Triglycerides mmol/L	1.3	0.4	11.7	<1.7	1.6	0.4	11.7	<1.7
HDL mmol/L	1.4	0.8	2.7	1.0–2.2	1.2	0.7	1.9	0.9–2.0
Glucose mmol/L	5.1	3.2	10.8	<6.1	5.4	3.7	17.9	<6.1
HbA1c mmol/L	38.2	27.0	74.0	<40	39.9	28.0	102.0	<40
Insulin pmol/L	60.9	10.0	277.0	10–80	61.2	4.0	480.0	10–80
Heart Health	**Mean**	**Min**	**Max**	**Healthy Range**	**Mean**	**Min**	**Max**	**Healthy Range**
BP (systolic) mmHg	131.1	104.0	183.7	120	134.2	97.7	185.7	120
BP (diastolic) mmHg	82.5	60.3	106.0	80	85.0	61.0	128.3	80
CVD risk score %	2.5–5	<2.5	20–25	<2.5	5–10	2.5–5	20–25	<2.5
Mental Health	**Mean**	**Min**	**Max**		**Mean**	**Min**	**Max**	
Wellbeing	53.0	16	70		52.7	30	70	
Cognition	27.1	19	30		26.6	16	30	
Current Depression n (%)	17 (7.9)				12 (6.3)			

BMI: body mass index, HDL: high-density lipoprotein, BP: blood pressure, CVD: Cardiovascular disease. Body measurements compared with New Zealand mean (95% confidence interval) for 45–55 age range [28]. Metabolic and heart health compared with normal healthy range [23,29,30]. Wellbeing measured by Warwick–Edinburgh scale, cognition by MoCA. Current depression is those currently clinically depressed excluding those diagnosed bipolar (N = 203 female, 179 male). One female has no waist measurement, three females no fasting metabolic measures, one male no fasting metabolic measures, one male glucose assay failed and two males HbA1c assay failed, otherwise data are for 215 females and 189 males.

3.2. Vitamin C Status of the Study Population

Fasting plasma vitamin C measurements were available for 369 of the CHALICE participants. The mean plasma vitamin C concentration was 44.2 μmol/L (95% CI 42.4, 46.0); 62% of the participants were below the adequate level (i.e., 50 μmol/L), and 93% of the participants were below the optimal saturating level (i.e., 70 μmol/L; Figure 1). Ten percent of the cohort had marginal vitamin C concentrations (i.e., 11–23 μmol/L), and vitamin C deficiency, defined as a plasma concentration of <11 μmol/L, was apparent in 2.4% of the cohort (Table 3).

Plasma vitamin C status was substantially lower in men than in women (p = 0.005), and it also varied by socio-economic status (p = 0.003). For example, 8% of those in the lowest socio-economic category were vitamin C deficient compared to 2.4% of the entire cohort (n = 369). Smoking status was also associated with plasma vitamin C status with current smokers having lower vitamin C levels (p < 0.001; Table 3).

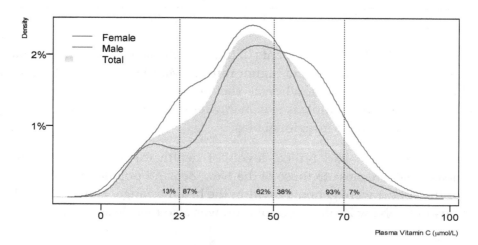

Figure 1. Density plot of plasma vitamin C. Proportion of sample at given vitamin C level; n = 369.

Table 3. Categories of vitamin C status.

		Plasma Vitamin C		Deficient		Marginal		Inadequate		Adequate		p
		Mean	95% CI	n	%	n	%	n	%	n	%	
Total		44.2	(42.4, 46.0)	9	2.4	39	10.6	183	49.6	138	37.4	
Gender	Female	47.4	(44.9, 49.9)	2	1.0	20	10.3	85	43.6	88	45.1	0.005
	Male	40.6	(38.2, 43.0)	7	4.0	19	10.9	98	56.3	50	28.7	
Ethnicity	Non Māori	44.5	(42.6, 46.4)	7	2.2	31	9.8	159	50.3	119	37.7	NS
	Māori	42.4	(37.2, 47.6)	2	3.8	8	15.1	24	45.3	19	35.8	
Socio-Economic Status	Low	36.8	(28.3, 45.3)	2	8.0	7	28.0	9	36.0	7	28.0	0.003
	Medium	43.7	(40.3, 47.1)	4	3.5	14	12.3	53	46.5	43	37.7	
	High	45.3	(43.2, 47.4)	3	1.3	18	7.8	121	52.6	88	38.3	
Education	None	38.7	(33.6, 43.9)	3	6.1	6	12.2	26	53.1	14	28.6	NS
	Secondary School	45.9	(42.1, 49.7)	1	1.0	13	12.6	49	47.6	40	38.8	
	Post-secondary	43.1	(40.6, 45.7)	5	3.3	16	10.6	75	49.7	55	36.4	
	University Degree	48.1	(44.4, 51.9)	0	0.0	4	6.1	33	50.0	29	43.9	
Tobacco	Not Current Smoker	45.9	(44.1, 47.8)	6	1.9	26	8.2	157	49.7	127	40.2	<0.001
	Current Smoker	34.1	(29.2, 38.9)	3	5.7	13	24.5	26	49.1	11	20.8	

Plasma vitamin C classified as deficient <11 µmol/L, marginal 11–23 µmol/L, inadequate 23–50 µmol/L or adequate >50 µmol/L; $n = 369$.

Study participants with and without vitamin C measurements do not differ significantly by gender, ethnicity, education, socio-economic status, smoking status, waist, weight or BMI (all $p > 0.13$), hence are treated as missing at random.

3.3. Associations of Vitamin C Status with Markers of Metabolic and Mental Health

The results of the statistical modeling with plasma vitamin C are summarized in Table 4. Higher plasma vitamin C status was associated with lower weight, BMI and waist circumference in the CHALICE cohort, even after adjustment for gender, ethnicity and current smoking. Of the other markers of metabolic health, plasma vitamin C was negatively associated with blood triglycerides, HbA1c and insulin, and positively associated with HDL levels. However, after multiple adjustment only triglycerides, HbA1c and insulin levels remained significant. No correlation was found between plasma vitamin C and the two indicators of heart health; blood pressure and cardiovascular risk score.

Table 4. Significant plasma vitamin C effects for body measures, metabolic health and mental health.

	Vitamin C <23 µmol/L (n = 47)		Vitamin C >23 µmol/L (n = 321)		p	p Adjusted
	Mean	95% CI	Mean	95% CI		
Body measurements						
Weight	90.3	(83.3, 97.4)	81.7	(79.8, 83.6)	0.024	0.004
BMI	31.4	(28.7, 34.0)	28.1	(27.5, 28.7)	0.021	<0.001
Waist	103.3	(97.6, 108.9)	93.3	(91.8, 94.8)	0.001	<0.001
Metabolism						
Triglycerides	1.8	(1.4, 2.3)	1.4	(1.3, 1.5)	0.061	0.029
HDL	1.3	(1.2, 1.3)	1.4	(1.3, 1.4)	0.033	NS
Glucose	5.6	(5.2, 6.0)	5.2	(5.0, 5.3)	0.072	0.073
HbA1c	42.2	(39.6, 44.8)	38.5	(37.7, 39.3)	0.009	0.015
Insulin	91.0	(68.4, 113.6)	56.3	(51.9, 60.8)	0.004	0.000
Heart health						
BP (systolic)	132.2	(128.0, 136.4)	132.5	(130.8, 134.2)	NS	NS
BP (diastolic)	83.6	(81.0, 86.3)	83.5	(82.4, 84.6)	NS	NS
CVD risk score	5–10%	(<2.5%, 20–25%)	2.5–5%	(3.5–5%, 5–10%)	0.057	NS
Mental Health						
Wellbeing	50.9	(48.4, 53.4)	53.0	(52.0, 53.9)	NS	NS
	n	%	n	%		
MCI	17	40.5	66	21.5	0.012	0.02
Current Depression	6	12.5	20	6.2	NS	NS

MCI: Mild Cognitive Impairment indicated by MoCA score <26 for those without excluding conditions. Current depression is for those without Bipolar Disorder. P values less than 0.1 shown otherwise NS: Not Significant. p values adjusted for gender, ethnicity and current smoking.

Mild cognitive impairment was assessed by the MoCA test. Higher plasma vitamin C status was correlated with lower mild cognitive impairment, which was maintained after adjustment for gender, ethnicity and current smoking (Table 4). A 1 μmol/L increase in plasma vitamin C was associated with 3% reduced odds of mild cognitive impairment (OR = 0.97, 95% CI = (0.96, 0.99), p = 0.004). Indeed, the odds of mild cognitive impairment were twice as high for those below 23 μmol/L plasma vitamin C (OR = 2.1, 95% CI = (1.2, 3.7), p = 0.01). Plasma vitamin C status was not associated with wellbeing or depression.

3.4. Dietary Vitamin C Intake

Dietary intake analysis was performed on 250 of the CHALICE participants. The average dietary vitamin C intake was 110 mg/day, with 12% falling below the New Zealand recommended dietary intake (RDI, Table 5). There was little effect of gender, ethnicity or socio-economic status on dietary intake. However, those with the lowest educational qualifications tended to have lower dietary vitamin C intake, although this was not quite significant. Current smokers also had a lower dietary intake of vitamin C (p < 0.001). Dietary vitamin C intake correlated somewhat less than expected with plasma levels of vitamin C, although the correlation was statistically significant (Pearson's correlation coefficient r = 0.27, p = 0.00002).

Table 5. Categories of dietary vitamin C intake.

		Dietary Vitamin C		Below RDI		RDI-Average		Above Average		p
		Mean	95% CI	n	%	n	%	n	%	
Total		109.8	(101.5, 118.1)	30	12	126	50.4	94	37.6	
Gender	Female	107.4	(96.6, 118.2)	13	9.7	73	54.5	48	35.8	NS
	Male	112.6	(99.7, 125.6)	17	14.7	53	45.7	46	39.7	
Ethnicity	Non Māori	112.0	(102.7, 121.2)	22	10.3	111	51.9	81	37.9	NS
	Māori	97.2	(79.6, 114.7)	8	22.2	15	41.7	13	36.1	
Socio-Economic Status	Low	78.8	(54.4, 103.1)	4	26.7	8	53.3	3	20.0	NS
	Medium	105.0	(90.7, 119.2)	12	15.2	36	45.6	31	39.2	
	High	115.3	(104.4, 126.1)	14	9.0	82	52.6	60	38.5	
Education	None	83.5	(64.2, 102.7)	8	28.6	13	46.4	7	25.0	0.1
	Secondary School	117.1	(98.4, 135.7)	6	10.0	32	53.3	22	36.7	
	Post-secondary	108.6	(97.1, 120.1)	11	9.9	59	53.2	41	36.9	
	University Degree	118.4	(97.6, 139.2)	5	9.8	22	43.1	24	47.1	
Tobacco	Not Current Smoker	114.1	(105.3, 122.8)	20	9.0	112	50.7	89	40.3	<0.001
	Current Smoker	77.5	(54.6, 100.5)	10	34.5	14	48.3	5	17.2	

The cut-off values for the vitamin C categories are as follows: New Zealand recommended dietary intake is 45 mg/day, the average New Zealand intake is 109 mg/day for men and 106 mg/day for women [11]; n = 250.

3.5. Associations of Dietary Vitamin C Intake with Markers of Metabolic and Mental Health

There was evidence that higher dietary intake of vitamin C was associated with lower waist circumference and insulin levels, after adjustment for gender, ethnicity and current smoking (Table 6). Glucose and HbA1c levels were inversely associated with dietary vitamin C intake in the initial models, however they did not remain so after correction for multiple comparisons. Higher dietary vitamin C intake was also associated with lower blood pressure, although there was no effect on cardiovascular risk score. There was little association between dietary vitamin C intake and mental health measures, although dietary intake was inversely associated with mild cognitive impairment in the unadjusted model.

Table 6. Significant dietary vitamin C effects based on average intake for body measures, metabolic health and heart health.

	Intake < Average (n = 147)		Intake > Average (n = 103)		p	p Adjusted
	Mean	95% CI	Mean	95% CI		
Body measurements						
Weight	82.2	(79.2, 85.3)	79.8	(76.4, 83.3)	NS	NS
BMI	28.5	(27.4, 29.6)	27.2	(26.2, 28.1)	0.08	0.063
Waist	94.6	(92.2, 97.0)	91.2	(88.5, 93.8)	0.06	0.047
Metabolism						
Triglycerides	1.4	(1.3, 1.5)	1.3	(1.1, 1.6)	NS	NS
HDL	1.4	(1.3, 1.4)	1.4	(1.3, 1.4)	NS	NS
Glucose	5.3	(5.1, 5.5)	5.0	(4.9, 5.2)	0.03	0.078
HbA1c	39.6	(38.3, 41.0)	37.8	(36.9, 38.7)	0.03	NS
Insulin	64.6	(55.5, 73.6)	52.3	(44.3, 60.3)	0.05	0.041
Heart health						
BP (systolic)	135.0	(132.5, 137.5)	130.6	(127.4, 133.8)	0.03	0.016
BP (diastolic)	85.2	(83.6, 86.7)	82.3	(80.4, 84.1)	0.02	0.007
CVD risk score	2.8	(2.6, 3.0)	2.6	(2.2, 2.9)	NS	NS
Mental Health						
Wellbeing	52.5	(51.1, 53.8)	52.9	(51.3, 54.4)	NS	NS
	n	%	n	%		
MCI	36	24.5	14	13.6	0.04	NS
Current Depression	13	8.8	4	3.9	NS	NS

MCI Mild Cognitive Impairment indicated by MoCA score <26 for those without excluding conditions. Current depression is for those without Bipolar Disorder. p values less than 0.1 shown otherwise NS: Not Significant. p values adjusted for gender, ethnicity and current smoking. Average is New Zealand average of 109 mg/day for men, 106 mg/day for women [11].

4. Discussion

These findings were drawn from the first phase of the CHALICE study, a longitudinal observational study of randomly selected 50-year-olds from the Canterbury region, New Zealand in 2010–2013. The comprehensive range of instruments used in the CHALICE study gives a broad picture of the cohort's health and the agreement between the study data and national demographics provides confidence that the study is representative of the health of 50-year-old New Zealanders in 2010. The cohort has typical levels of metabolic and cardiac markers, with indications of overweight/obesity and hypertension in some individuals. Our study provides new evidence that mid-life adults with higher vitamin C levels exhibited better measures of metabolic health and lower levels of mild cognitive impairment.

In New Zealand, dietary vitamin C intake has been estimated by several comprehensive national dietary surveys, including the 2008/2009 New Zealand Adult Nutrition Survey in which the mean usual adult daily intake was 108 mg based on 24 h dietary recall data [11]. This is close to the average dietary intake of 110 mg/day found in the current study. However, measuring vitamin C concentrations in the body has a number of advantages over dietary intake. It does not rely on participant's recall of their diet, and takes in all sources of the vitamin, including supplements, and the potential impact of vitamin C losses due to food processing and preparation. More particularly, it accounts for confounders of vitamin C status such as smoking, alcohol consumption, prescription medications and health conditions which may affect turnover of the vitamin [31]. The CHALICE study is the first representative study of plasma vitamin C status within the New Zealand population. Only smaller studies in specific, non-representative groups have measured plasma vitamin C concentrations within the New Zealand population [32,33].

In our study, we found that 2.4% of 50-year-olds were deficient in vitamin C (i.e., <11 μmol/L), putting them at higher risk of developing scurvy and other health effects that may be associated with very low vitamin C status. Men were at greater risk of being deficient than women, and having lower socio-economic status significantly increased risk. Smoking also increased the risk of deficiency, most likely due to increased oxidative stress causing faster turnover of the vitamin [31]. In addition, in our cohort, smokers had a lower dietary intake of vitamin C. Numerous studies have previously shown gender, socio-economic status and smoking to be important predictors of vitamin C status [9,33–37]. A recent study suggests the effect of gender on vitamin C status may be due to the differing fat free mass between men and women, meaning vitamin C is distributed throughout a higher volume in men, leading to lower vitamin C concentrations in the plasma [36].

Data from large international cohorts show similar levels of vitamin C deficiency and hypovitaminosis C to the CHALICE cohort [37,38], although the United States and lower socio-economic groups in the United Kingdom stand out as having higher rates of deficiency [9,34]. In the current study, hypovitaminosis C (i.e., <23 μmol/L) was apparent in 13% of participants, and this increased to 36% for those in the lowest socio-economic category. Symptoms such as decreased mood and energy levels may be observed with hypovitaminosis C, and are possibly related to the role of vitamin C as a cofactor in carnitine and catecholamine neurotransmitter synthesis [3,14]. A high proportion (63%) of our participants had inadequate plasma vitamin C concentrations (i.e., <50 μmol/L). Indeed, very few of our participants, only 7%, had saturating plasma vitamin C status (i.e., >70 μmol/L), implying that current Ministry of Health guidelines recommending consumption of at least five servings of vegetables and fruit per day are ineffective [39]. Since the vitamin C content of fruit and vegetables is quite variable, we suggest that it is important to highlight the consumption of high vitamin C-content fruit and/or vegetables to provide plasma saturation in this age group.

High vitamin C concentrations in the blood were associated with significantly lower weight, waist circumference and BMI, and the effect of plasma vitamin C status was significant enough to survive the correction for multiple comparisons. The association of low vitamin C with obesity in this study replicates results in the literature [35,40–44], and it is apparent that individuals with higher weight require higher intakes of vitamin C to reach adequate vitamin C status [45,46]. We also show that higher plasma vitamin C status is associated with lower circulating levels of blood triglycerides, insulin and HbA1c, associations which survive correction for gender, ethnicity and current smoking. These findings are in agreement with a number of smaller intervention studies that have found inverse relationships of vitamin C with various markers of metabolic health [47–49], although others have failed to observe an effect of intervention [50]. Dakhale and coworkers show a small decrease in HbA1c and fasting blood glucose in individuals with type 2 diabetes after vitamin C supplementation of 1 g/day for 12 weeks [51]. Observational studies also provide evidence that low vitamin C status is associated with increased risk of metabolic syndrome [52–54].

A role for vitamin C in the prevention or management of diabetes and/or metabolic syndrome has been suggested [47,51,53,54]. Obesity is a major risk factor for diabetes, and it may be that vitamin C has a role in moderating the inflammatory effect of adipose tissue. Vitamin C is thought to have anti-inflammatory activity, decreasing levels of inflammatory markers such as C-reactive protein and pro-inflammatory cytokines, although the exact mechanism(s) responsible for this are unknown [55,56]. Disorders of energy balance and metabolism are common worldwide. For example, in New Zealand, around 241,000 individuals have been diagnosed with diabetes, and significant numbers have undiagnosed diabetes, or pre-diabetes [57]. Further, among people aged over 15 years, 65% of individuals meet the criteria for overweight and obesity [58]. Diet and lifestyle factors are associated with these disorders and represent key modifiable determinants. Interestingly, in the CHALICE cohort there were no consistent significant effects identified between plasma vitamin C status and blood pressure or cardiovascular disease risk, although higher dietary vitamin C intake was associated with decreased blood pressure, an effect that has been observed previously [59].

In this study, we also demonstrate lower levels of mild cognitive impairment in those with high vitamin C status, even after adjustment for gender, ethnicity and smoking. Current smoking was a good proxy for socio-economic status and educational achievement in the model; thus, the relationship with vitamin C status survived correction for these important predictors of cognitive impairment. The odds of mild cognitive impairment were twice as high for those below 23 μmol/L plasma vitamin C concentration. Vitamin C is present at very high concentrations in the brain [60], and animal models have shown that the brain is the last organ to be depleted of the vitamin during prolonged deficiency [61], suggesting an important requirement for vitamin C in the central nervous system. A recent animal study has shown that moderate vitamin C deficiency may play a role in accelerating amyloid plaque accumulation in Alzheimer's disease, the most common form of dementia [62]. However, epidemiological studies have been inconclusive in regards to whether vitamin C status may affect cognitive decline [63,64] and Alzheimer's disease specifically [65,66]. Lu and co-workers investigated the relationship between dietary nutrients and mild cognitive impairment in 2892 elderly Chinese participants using the MoCA test, and found that vitamin C intake exhibited a significant protective effect [64]. Our study has the advantage over many in that plasma vitamin C concentrations have been measured; we were not reliant on dietary intake, which may be susceptible to problems with recall ability and the other confounders mentioned above.

In later life, dementia and disorders of cognition are highly prevalent. Even in the CHALICE sample of 50-year-olds, 15% of the sample scored below the recommended cut point on the MoCA. There is considerable interest in the effect of diet on maintaining cognitive function and delaying neuro-degenerative disease in old age. A 2015 study with 37 older healthy adults demonstrated reduced rates of cognitive decline following consumption of orange juice [67]. This was attributed to the high flavanone content of the orange juice, since flavonoids have been associated with reduced rates of cognitive decline [68,69]. However, it is possible that the vitamin C content of the orange juice may have contributed to the observed effect. In support of this premise, studies have shown that supplementation of older adults with the antioxidant vitamins C and E was able to preserve cognitive performance [70–72]. Another study, however, found no impact of antioxidant vitamin supplementation on cognition, despite improvements in markers of oxidative stress [73], demonstrating mixed results in the literature. Intervention studies often look for relatively short-term impacts on cognition instruments in response to different nutrient intakes. In contrast, the CHALICE study measured the association of plasma vitamin C status and dietary intake, more likely to be markers of longer-term lifestyle patterns, with a cognitive instrument (MoCA) as an assessment of current mild cognitive impairment.

There are several limitations to our study, notably the observational design, in which associations do not imply causation. Many factors impact on the health status of individuals and groups, including diet, exercise, temperament, behaviors, socio-economic status and genetics. These factors typically interact and correlate with each other, as they do in the CHALICE cohort, with the result that predictors of health outcomes are related (e.g., low blood pressure is associated with low BMI). We have addressed multiple testing issues with the use of corrected p values, and multi-collinearity does not affect individual models as each model only has one independent predictor, with the dichotomous covariates having limited capacity to induce collinearity. While we have focused on the associations of vitamin C with health outcomes, these associations could include the effects of unmeasured nutrients associated with vitamin C intake. Dietary vitamin C and plasma vitamin C status did not always correlate with the same health indicators. However, as detailed above, this is likely due to fasting plasma vitamin C concentration being a more accurate indicator of body status.

5. Conclusions

The CHALICE cohort of 404 individuals aged 50 years had an average vitamin C intake of ~110 mg/day, which should provide adequate plasma concentrations [14]. Despite this, a significant proportion of the participants had inadequate plasma vitamin C status. This indicates the likely effects of confounding factors, such as chronic disease, on plasma vitamin C status, and suggests that dietary interventions targeting increased consumption of fruit and vegetables, and increased vitamin C intake in particular, are required for this age group. Metabolic health markers were significantly better in participants with higher plasma vitamin C concentrations, even after correction for confounders. The association of high vitamin C concentrations with the reduction in risk of impaired cognition is intriguing and merits further investigation.

Acknowledgments: We would like to acknowledge the participants of the CHALICE study and the CHALICE study investigators. The CHALICE study was supported by grants awarded from the Department of Internal Affairs' Lotteries Health (grant number: AP265022), Canterbury Community Trust, Otago Thyroid Research Foundation and University of Otago Foundation Trust (grant number: TL1060). Funding for the vitamin C analyses was provided by Zespri International Ltd, Mt Maunganui, New Zealand. A.C. is the recipient of a Health Research Council of New Zealand Sir Charles Hercus Health Research Fellowship.

Author Contributions: J.S. coordinated study; A.C., J.M.P. and M.V. measured vitamin C status; R.W. and P.S. calculated dietary intakes; V.C. contributed to design of cardiovascular measures; A.C., P.S. and J.F.P. conceived paper; J.F.P. analyzed data; J.M.P., A.C. and J.F.P. interpreted data and wrote paper; and M.V., P.S., J.W., J.S. and V.C. edited paper. J.F.P., J.M.P. and A.C. contributed to the work equally.

References

1.   Svirbely, J.L.; Szent-Gyorgyi, A. The chemical nature of vitamin C. *Biochem. J.* **1933**, *27*, 279–285. [CrossRef] [PubMed]

2.   Du, J.; Cullen, J.J.; Buettner, G.R. Ascorbic acid: Chemistry, biology and the treatment of cancer. *Biochim. Biophys. Acta* **2012**, *1826*, 443–457. [CrossRef] [PubMed]

3.   Englard, S.; Seifter, S. The biochemical functions of ascorbic acid. *Annu. Rev. Nutr.* **1986**, *6*, 365–406. [CrossRef] [PubMed]

4.   Vissers, M.C.; Kuiper, C.; Dachs, G.U. Regulation of the 2-oxoglutarate-dependent dioxygenases and implications for cancer. *Biochem. Soc. Trans.* **2014**, *42*, 945–951. [CrossRef] [PubMed]

5.   Carr, A.; Frei, B. Does vitamin C act as a pro-oxidant under physiological conditions? *Faseb J.* **1999**, *13*, 1007–1024. [PubMed]

6.   Bruno, R.S.; Leonard, S.W.; Atkinson, J.; Montine, T.J.; Ramakrishnan, R.; Bray, T.M.; Traber, M.G. Faster plasma vitamin E disappearance in smokers is normalized by vitamin C supplementation. *Free. Radic. Biol. Med.* **2006**, *40*, 689–697. [CrossRef] [PubMed]

7.   Lin, J.Y.; Selim, M.A.; Shea, C.R.; Grichnik, J.M.; Omar, M.M.; Monteiro-Riviere, N.A.; Pinnell, S.R. UV photoprotection by combination topical antioxidants vitamin C and vitamin E. *J. Am. Acad. Dermatol.* **2003**, *48*, 866–874. [CrossRef] [PubMed]

8.   Krebs, H.A. The Sheffield Experiment on the vitamin C requirement of human adults. *Proc. Nutr. Soc.* **1953**, *12*, 237–246. [CrossRef]

9.   Schleicher, R.L.; Carroll, M.D.; Ford, E.S.; Lacher, D.A. Serum vitamin C and the prevalence of vitamin C deficiency in the United States: 2003–2004 National Health and Nutrition Examination Survey (NHANES). *Am. J. Clin. Nutr.* **2009**, *90*, 1252–1263. [CrossRef] [PubMed]

10.   CDC's Second Nutrition Report. Available online: https://www.cdc.gov/nutritionreport/report.html (accessed on 28 June 2017).

11.   A Focus on Nutrition: Key findings from the 2008/09 NZ Adult Nutrition Survey. Available online: http://www.health.govt.nz/publication/focus-nutrition-key-findings-2008-09-nz-adult-nutrition-survey (accessed on 8 June 2017).

12.   Carr, A.C.; Frei, B. Toward a new recommended dietary allowance for vitamin C based on antioxidant and health effects in humans. *Am. J. Clin. Nutr.* **1999**, *69*, 1086–1107. [PubMed]

13.   Lykkesfeldt, J.; Poulsen, H.E. Is vitamin C supplementation beneficial? Lessons learned from randomised controlled trials. *Br. J. Nutr.* **2010**, *103*, 1251–1259. [CrossRef] [PubMed]

14.   Levine, M.; Conry-Cantilena, C.; Wang, Y.; Welch, R.W.; Washko, P.W.; Dhariwal, K.R.; Park, J.B.; Lazarev, A.; Graumlich, J.F.; King, J.; et al. Vitamin C pharmacokinetics in healthy volunteers: Evidence for a recommended dietary allowance. *Proc. Natl. Acad. Sci. USA* **1996**, *93*, 3704–3709. [CrossRef] [PubMed]

15.   Jacob, R.A. Assessment of human vitamin C status. *J. Nutr.* **1990**, *120*, 1480–1485. [PubMed]

16.   Tetens, I. Scientific opinion on dietary reference values for vitamin C. *EFSA. J.* **2013**, *11*, 3418–3486.

17.   Nutrient Reference Values for Australia and New Zealand Executive Summary. Available online: https://www.nhmrc.gov.au/guidelines-publications/n35-n36-n37 (accessed on 7 June 2017).

18.   Schluter, P.J.; Spittlehouse, J.K.; Cameron, V.A.; Chambers, S.; Gearry, R.; Jamieson, H.A.; Kennedy, M.; Lacey, C.J.; Murdoch, D.R.; Pearson, J.; et al. Canterbury Health, Ageing and Life Course (CHALICE) study: Rationale, design and methodology. *N. Z. Med. J.* **2013**, *126*, 71–85. [PubMed]

19. Enrolment Statistics: Comparison of Estimated Eligible Voting Population to Enrolled Electors for Christchurch City. Available online: http://www.elections.org.nz/councils/ages/district_60_christchurch_city.html (accessed on 12 March 2013).

20. Population of Canterbury DHB. Available online: http://www.health.govt.nz/new-zealand-health-system/my-dhb/canterbury-dhb/population-canterbury-dhb (accessed on 12 March 2013).

21. Sato, Y.; Uchiki, T.; Iwama, M.; Kishimoto, Y.; Takahashi, R.; Ishigami, A. Determination of dehydroascorbic acid in mouse tissues and plasma by using tris(2-carboxyethyl)phosphine hydrochloride as reductant in metaphosphoric acid/ethylenediaminetetraacetic acid solution. *Biol. Pharm. Bull.* **2010**, *33*, 364–369. [CrossRef] [PubMed]

22. Carr, A.C.; Pullar, J.M.; Moran, S.; Vissers, M.C. Bioavailability of vitamin C from kiwifruit in non-smoking males: Determination of 'healthy' and 'optimal' intakes. *J. Nutr. Sci.* **2012**, *1*, e14. [CrossRef] [PubMed]

23. New Zealand Primary Care Handbook 2012. Available online: http://www.health.govt.nz/publication/new-zealand-primary-care-handbook-2012 (accessed on 9 July 2017).

24. Tennant, R.; Hiller, L.; Fishwick, R.; Platt, S.; Joseph, S.; Weich, S.; Parkinson, J.; Secker, J.; Stewart-Brown, S. The Warwick-Edinburgh mental well-being scale (WEMWBS): Development and UK validation. *Health Qual. Life Outcomes* **2007**, *5*, 63. [CrossRef] [PubMed]

25. Sheehan, D.V.; Lecrubier, Y.; Sheehan, K.H.; Janavs, J.; Weiller, E.; Keskiner, A.; Schinka, J.; Knapp, E.; Sheehan, M.F.; Dunbar, G.C. The validity of the Mini International Neuropsychiatric Interview (MINI) according to the SCID-P and its reliability. *Eur. Psychiatry* **1997**, *12*, 232–241. [CrossRef]

26. Nasreddine, Z.S.; Phillips, N.A.; Bedirian, V.; Charbonneau, S.; Whitehead, V.; Collin, I.; Cummings, J.L.; Chertkow, H. The Montreal Cognitive Assessment, MoCA: A brief screening tool for mild cognitive impairment. *J. Am. Geriatr. Soc.* **2005**, *53*, 695–699. [CrossRef] [PubMed]

27. ELSI Short Form: User Manual for a Direct Measure of Living Standards. Available online: https://www.msd.govt.nz/about-msd-and-our-work/publications-resources/monitoring/living-standards/elsi-short-form.html (accessed on 7 June 2017).

28. A Portrait of Health: Key results of the 2006/07 New Zealand Health Survey. Available online: http://www.health.govt.nz/publication/portrait-health-key-results-2006-07-new-zealand-health-survey (accessed on 15 May 2017).

29. The Royal College of Pathologists of Australasia: RCPA. Available online: https://www.rcpa.edu.au/ (accessed on 9 July 2017).

30. Definition and Diagnosis of Diabetes Mellitus and Intermediate Hyperglycaemia. Available online: http://www.who.int/diabetes/publications/diagnosis_diabetes2006/en/ (accessed on 15 May 2017).

31. Kallner, A.B.; Hartmann, D.; Hornig, D.H. On the requirements of ascorbic acid in man: Steady-state turnover and body pool in smokers. *Am. J. Clin. Nutr.* **1981**, *34*, 1347–1355. [PubMed]

32. McClean, H.E.; Stewart, A.W.; Riley, C.G.; Beaven, D.W. Vitamin C status of elderly men in a residential home. *N. Z. Med. J.* **1977**, *86*, 379–382. [PubMed]

33. McClean, H.E.; Dodds, P.M.; Abernethy, M.H.; Stewart, A.W.; Beaven, D.W. Vitamin C concentration in plasma and leucocytes of men related to age and smoking habit. *N. Z. Med. J.* **1976**, *83*, 226–229. [PubMed]

34. Mosdol, A.; Erens, B.; Brunner, E.J. Estimated prevalence and predictors of vitamin C deficiency within UK's low-income population. *J. Public Health (Oxf.)* **2008**, *30*, 456–460. [CrossRef] [PubMed]

35. Galan, P.; Viteri, F.E.; Bertrais, S.; Czernichow, S.; Faure, H.; Arnaud, J.; Ruffieux, D.; Chenal, S.; Arnault, N.; Favier, A.; et al. Serum concentrations of beta-carotene, vitamins C and E, zinc and selenium are influenced by sex, age, diet, smoking status, alcohol consumption and corpulence in a general French adult population. *Eur. J. Clin. Nutr.* **2005**, *59*, 1181–1190. [CrossRef] [PubMed]

36. Jungert, A.; Neuhauser-Berthold, M. The lower vitamin C plasma concentrations in elderly men compared with elderly women can partly be attributed to a volumetric dilution effect due to differences in fat-free mass. *Br. J. Nutr.* **2015**, *113*, 859–864. [CrossRef] [PubMed]

37. Langlois, K.; Cooper, M.; Colapinto, C.K. Vitamin C status of Canadian adults: Findings from the 2012/2013 Canadian Health Measures Survey. *Health Rep.* **2016**, *27*, 3–10. [PubMed]

38. Faure, H.; Preziosi, P.; Roussel, A.M.; Bertrais, S.; Galan, P.; Hercberg, S.; Favier, A. Factors influencing blood concentration of retinol, alpha-tocopherol, vitamin C, and beta-carotene in the French participants of the SU.VI.MAX trial. *Eur. J. Clin. Nutr.* **2006**, *60*, 706–717. [CrossRef] [PubMed]

39.   Eating and Activity Guidelines for New Zealand Adults. Available online: http://www.health.govt.nz/publication/eating-and-activity-guidelines-new-zealand-adults (accessed on 7 July 2017).

40.   Block, G.; Jensen, C.D.; Dalvi, T.B.; Norkus, E.P.; Hudes, M.; Crawford, P.B.; Holland, N.; Fung, E.B.; Schumacher, L.; Harmatz, P. Vitamin C treatment reduces elevated C-reactive protein. *Free Radic. Biol. Med.* **2009**, *46*, 70–77. [CrossRef] [PubMed]

41.   Canoy, D.; Wareham, N.; Welch, A.; Bingham, S.; Luben, R.; Day, N.; Khaw, K.T. Plasma ascorbic acid concentrations and fat distribution in 19,068 British men and women in the European Prospective Investigation into Cancer and Nutrition Norfolk cohort study. *Am. J. Clin. Nutr.* **2005**, *82*, 1203–1209. [PubMed]

42.   Garcia, O.P.; Ronquillo, D.; Caamano Mdel, C.; Camacho, M.; Long, K.Z.; Rosado, J.L. Zinc, vitamin A, and vitamin C status are associated with leptin concentrations and obesity in Mexican women: Results from a cross-sectional study. *Nutr. Metab. (Lond.)* **2012**, *9*, 59. [CrossRef] [PubMed]

43.   Johnston, C.S.; Beezhold, B.L.; Mostow, B.; Swan, P.D. Plasma vitamin C is inversely related to body mass index and waist circumference but not to plasma adiponectin in nonsmoking adults. *J. Nutr.* **2007**, *137*, 1757–1762. [PubMed]

44.   Moor de Burgos, A.; Wartanowicz, M.; Ziemlanski, S. Blood vitamin and lipid levels in overweight and obese women. *Eur. J. Clin. Nutr.* **1992**, *46*, 803–808. [PubMed]

45.   Block, G.; Mangels, A.R.; Patterson, B.H.; Levander, O.A.; Norkus, E.P.; Taylor, P.R. Body weight and prior depletion affect plasma ascorbate levels attained on identical vitamin C intake: A controlled-diet study. *J. Am. Coll. Nutr.* **1999**, *18*, 628–637. [CrossRef] [PubMed]

46.   Carr, A.C.; Pullar, J.M.; Bozonet, S.M.; Vissers, M.C. Marginal Ascorbate Status (Hypovitaminosis C) Results in an Attenuated Response to Vitamin C Supplementation. *Nutrients* **2016**, *8*, 341. [CrossRef] [PubMed]

47.   Ellulu, M.S.; Rahmat, A.; Patimah, I.; Khaza'ai, H.; Abed, Y. Effect of vitamin C on inflammation and metabolic markers in hypertensive and/or diabetic obese adults: A randomized controlled trial. *Drug Des. Dev. Ther.* **2015**, *9*, 3405–3412. [CrossRef] [PubMed]

48.   Chaudhari, H.V.; Dakhale, G.N.; Chaudhari, S.; Mahatme, M. The beneficial effect of vitamin C supplementation on serum lipids in type 2 diabetic patients: A randomised double blind study. *Int. J. Diabetes Metab.* **2012**, *20*, 53–58.

49.   Paolisso, G.; Balbi, V.; Volpe, C.; Varricchio, G.; Gambardella, A.; Saccomanno, F.; Ammendola, S.; Varricchio, M.; D'Onofrio, F. Metabolic benefits deriving from chronic vitamin C supplementation in aged non-insulin dependent diabetics. *J. Am. Coll. Nutr.* **1995**, *14*, 387–392. [CrossRef] [PubMed]

50.   Chen, H.; Karne, R.J.; Hall, G.; Campia, U.; Panza, J.A.; Cannon, R.O.; Wang, Y.; Katz, A.; Levine, M.; Quon, M.J. High-dose oral vitamin C partially replenishes vitamin C levels in patients with Type 2 diabetes and low vitamin C levels but does not improve endothelial dysfunction or insulin resistance. *Am. J. Physiol. Heart Circ. Physiol.* **2006**, *290*, H137–H145. [CrossRef] [PubMed]

51.   Dakhale, G.N.; Chaudhari, H.V.; Shrivastava, M. Supplementation of vitamin C reduces blood glucose and improves glycosylated hemoglobin in type 2 diabetes mellitus: A randomized, double-blind study. *Adv. Pharmacol. Sci.* **2011**, *2011*, 195271. [CrossRef] [PubMed]

52.   Godala, M.M.; Materek-Kusmierkiewicz, I.; Moczulski, D.; Rutkowski, M.; Szatko, F.; Gaszynska, E.; Tokarski, S.; Kowalski, J. Lower Plasma Levels of Antioxidant Vitamins in Patients with Metabolic Syndrome: A Case Control Study. *Adv. Clin. Exp. Med.* **2016**, *25*, 689–700. [CrossRef] [PubMed]

53.   Kim, J.; Choi, Y.H. Physical activity, dietary vitamin C, and metabolic syndrome in the Korean adults: The Korea National Health and Nutrition Examination Survey 2008 to 2012. *Public Health* **2016**, *135*, 30–37. [CrossRef] [PubMed]

54.   Wei, J.; Zeng, C.; Gong, Q.Y.; Li, X.X.; Lei, G.H.; Yang, T.B. Associations between Dietary Antioxidant Intake and Metabolic Syndrome. *PLoS ONE* **2015**, *10*, e0130876. [CrossRef] [PubMed]

55.   Mazidi, M.; Kengne, A.P.; Mikhailidis, D. P.; Cicero, A.F.; Banach, M. Effects of selected dietary constituents on high-sensitivity C-reactive protein levels in U.S. adults. *Ann. Med.* **2017**, 1–6. [CrossRef] [PubMed]

56.   Mikirova, N.; Casciari, J.; Rogers, A.; Taylor, P. Effect of high-dose intravenous vitamin C on inflammation in cancer patients. *J. Transl. Med.* **2012**, *10*, 189. [CrossRef] [PubMed]

57.   Ministry of Health: Virtual Diabetes Register. Available online: http://www.health.govt.nz/our-work/diseases-and-conditions/diabetes/about-diabetes/virtual-diabetes-register-vdr (accessed on 10 July 2017).

58.   Understanding Excess Body Weight: New Zealand Health Survey. Available online: http://www.health.govt.nz/publication/understanding-excess-body-weight-new-zealand-health-survey (accessed on 12 June 2017).

59. Juraschek, S.P.; Guallar, E.; Appel, L.J.; Miller, E.R. Effects of vitamin C supplementation on blood pressure: A meta-analysis of randomized controlled trials. *Am. J. Clin. Nutr.* **2012**, *95*, 1079–1088. [CrossRef] [PubMed]

60. Hornig, D. Distribution of ascorbic acid, metabolites and analogues in man and animals. *Ann. N. Y. Acad. Sci.* **1975**, *258*, 103–118. [CrossRef] [PubMed]

61. Vissers, M.C.; Bozonet, S.M.; Pearson, J.F.; Braithwaite, L.J. Dietary ascorbate intake affects steady state tissue concentrations in vitamin C-deficient mice: Tissue deficiency after suboptimal intake and superior bioavailability from a food source (kiwifruit). *Am. J. Clin. Nutr.* **2011**, *93*, 292–301. [CrossRef] [PubMed]

62. Dixit, S.; Bernardo, A.; Walker, J.M.; Kennard, J.A.; Kim, G.Y.; Kessler, E.S.; Harrison, F.E. Vitamin C deficiency in the brain impairs cognition, increases amyloid accumulation and deposition, and oxidative stress in APP/PSEN1 and normally aging mice. *ACS Chem. Neurosci.* **2015**, *6*, 570–581. [CrossRef] [PubMed]

63. Masaki, K.H.; Losonczy, K.G.; Izmirlian, G.; Foley, D.J.; Ross, G.W.; Petrovitch, H.; Havlik, R.; White, L.R. Association of vitamin E and C supplement use with cognitive function and dementia in elderly men. *Neurology* **2000**, *54*, 1265–1272. [CrossRef] [PubMed]

64. Lu, Y.; An, Y.; Guo, J.; Zhang, X.; Wang, H.; Rong, H.; Xiao, R. Dietary Intake of Nutrients and Lifestyle Affect the Risk of Mild Cognitive Impairment in the Chinese Elderly Population: A Cross-Sectional Study. *Front. Behav. Neurosci.* **2016**, *10*, 229. [CrossRef] [PubMed]

65. Morris, M.C.; Evans, D.A.; Bienias, J.L.; Tangney, C.C.; Bennett, D.A.; Aggarwal, N.; Wilson, R.S.; Scherr, P.A. Dietary intake of antioxidant nutrients and the risk of incident Alzheimer disease in a biracial community study. *JAMA* **2002**, *287*, 3230–3237. [CrossRef] [PubMed]

66. Zandi, P.P.; Anthony, J.C.; Khachaturian, A.S.; Stone, S.V.; Gustafson, D.; Tschanz, J.T.; Norton, M.C.; Welsh-Bohmer, K.A.; Breitner, J.C. Reduced risk of Alzheimer disease in users of antioxidant vitamin supplements: The Cache County Study. *Arch. Neurol.* **2004**, *61*, 82–88. [CrossRef] [PubMed]

67. Kean, R.J.; Lamport, D.J.; Dodd, G.F.; Freeman, J.E.; Williams, C.M.; Ellis, J.A.; Butler, L.T.; Spencer, J.P. Chronic consumption of flavanone-rich orange juice is associated with cognitive benefits: An 8-wk, randomized, double-blind, placebo-controlled trial in healthy older adults. *Am. J. Clin. Nutr.* **2015**, *101*, 506–514. [CrossRef] [PubMed]

68. Letenneur, L.; Proust-Lima, C.; Le Gouge, A.; Dartigues, J.F.; Barberger-Gateau, P. Flavonoid intake and cognitive decline over a 10-year period. *Am. J. Epidemiol.* **2007**, *165*, 1364–1371. [CrossRef] [PubMed]

69. Touvier, M.; Druesne-Pecollo, N.; Kesse-Guyot, E.; Andreeva, V.A.; Fezeu, L.; Galan, P.; Hercberg, S.; Latino-Martel, P. Dual association between polyphenol intake and breast cancer risk according to alcohol consumption level: A prospective cohort study. *Breast Cancer Res. Treat* **2013**, *137*, 225–236. [CrossRef] [PubMed]

70. Smith, A.P.; Clark, R.E.; Nutt, D.J.; Haller, J.; Hayward, S.G.; Perry, K. Vitamin C, Mood and Cognitive Functioning in the Elderly. *Nutr. Neurosci.* **1999**, *2*, 249–256. [CrossRef] [PubMed]

71. Kang, J.H.; Cook, N.R.; Manson, J.E.; Buring, J.E.; Albert, C.M.; Grodstein, F. Vitamin E, vitamin C, beta carotene, and cognitive function among women with or at risk of cardiovascular disease: The Women's Antioxidant and Cardiovascular Study. *Circulation* **2009**, *119*, 2772–2780. [CrossRef] [PubMed]

72. Kesse-Guyot, E.; Fezeu, L.; Jeandel, C.; Ferry, M.; Andreeva, V.; Amieva, H.; Hercberg, S.; Galan, P. French adults' cognitive performance after daily supplementation with antioxidant vitamins and minerals at nutritional doses: A post hoc analysis of the Supplementation in Vitamins and Mineral Antioxidants (SU.VI.MAX) trial. *Am. J. Clin. Nutr.* **2011**, *94*, 892–899. [CrossRef] [PubMed]

73. Naeini, A.M.; Elmadfa, I.; Djazayery, A.; Barekatain, M.; Ghazvini, M.R.; Djalali, M.; Feizi, A. The effect of antioxidant vitamins E and C on cognitive performance of the elderly with mild cognitive impairment in Isfahan, Iran: A double-blind, randomized, placebo-controlled trial. *Eur. J. Nutr.* **2014**, *53*, 1255–1262. [CrossRef] [PubMed]

5

Poor Vitamin C Status Late in Pregnancy is Associated with Increased Risk of Complications in Type 1 Diabetic Women

Bente Juhl [1], Finn Friis Lauszus [2] and Jens Lykkesfeldt [3],*

[1] Medical Department, Aarhus University Hospital, Nørrebrogade 44, 8000 Aarhus C, Denmark; bente311057@gmail.com

[2] Gynecology & Obstetrics Department, Herning Hospital, Gl. Landevej 61, 7400 Herning, Denmark; Finn.Friis.Lauszus@vest.rm.dk

[3] Faculty of Health and Medical Sciences, University of Copenhagen, Ridebanevej 9, Frederiksberg C, 1870 Copenhagen, Denmark

* Correspondence: jopl@sund.ku.dk

Abstract: Vitamin C (vitC) is essential for normal pregnancy and fetal development and poor vitC status has been related to complications of pregnancy. We have previously shown lower vitC status in diabetic women throughout pregnancy compared to that of non-diabetic controls. Here, we evaluate the relationship between vitC status late in diabetic pregnancy in relation to fetal outcome, complications of pregnancy, diabetic characteristics, and glycemic control based on data of 47 women from the same cohort. We found a significant relationship between the maternal vitC level > or $\leq$ the 50% percentile of 26.6 µmol/L, respectively, and the umbilical cord blood vitC level (mean (SD)): 101.0 µmol/L (16.6) versus 78.5 µmol/L (27.8), $p = 0.02$; $n = 12/16$), while no relation to birth weight or Apgar score was observed. Diabetic women with complications of pregnancy had significantly lower vitC levels compared to the women without complications (mean (SD): 24.2 µmol/L (10.6) vs. 34.6 µmol/L (14.4), $p = 0.01$; $n = 19$ and 28, respectively) and the subgroup of women (about 28%) characterized by hypovitaminosis C (<23 µmol/L) had an increased relative risk of complications of pregnancy that was 2.4 fold higher than the one found in the group of women with a vitC status above this level ($p = 0.02$, 95% confidence interval 1.2–4.4). No correlation between diabetic characteristics of the pregnant women and vitC status was observed, while a negative association of maternal vitC with HbA1c at delivery was found at regression analysis ($r = -0.39$, $p < 0.01$, $n = 46$). In conclusion, our results may suggest that hypovitaminosis C in diabetic women is associated with increased risk of complications of pregnancy.

Keywords: type 1 diabetes; pregnancy; vitamin C; pregnancy outcome; pregnancy complications; cross-sectional study

1. Introduction

The importance of an adequate supply of micronutrients for normal pregnancy and fetal development is well established, particularly in the last trimester due to the increasing needs during the growth spurt of the fetus [1,2]. As early as 1938, Teel and co-workers described the fetus as *acting as a parasite on the mother's vitamin C pool* based on the observed gradient between maternal plasma and umbilical cord vitamin C (vitC) concentration at term, and the fact that the fetus apparently was preferentially supplied with vitC at the expense of the mother [3–5]. Subsequently, several studies have reported that pregnancy in healthy women is associated with a significant decrease in maternal vitC status during pregnancy [4,6–8], perhaps partly due to increased blood volume in pregnancy.

In experimental studies in guinea pigs, which like humans depend on an adequate supply of vitC through their diet, the offspring of vitC deficient guinea pigs have shown abnormalities of fetal bone development, with atrophy of the osteoblasts and retarded osteoid formation [9]. Macroscopic fetal, uterine, and placental hemorrhages as well as poor attachment of the placenta to the uterus were also evident in vitC deficient animals [9]. Other experimental studies have shown an association of infertility, increased incidence of premature- and stillbirths, and increased frequency of abortion with vitC deficiency [10,11]. Intrauterine growth retardation was related to insufficient vitC status in guinea pigs [10]. More recently, experimental reports from animal studies demonstrated that CNS development in particular requires high amounts of vitC and may be impaired by an inadequate maternal supply [12–15].

In humans, abortion and premature rupture of the fetal membrane are related to low levels of vitC in plasma, leucocytes, and amniotic fluid [16–24]. Abnormalities of cardiotocography (CTG) and discolored/green amniotic fluid was also associated with low vitC status at the time of delivery [25]. Furthermore, vitC deficiency may play a leading role in placental abruption [26]. Human studies suggest that poor vitC status leads to fetal oxidative stress and impaired placental implantation due to oxidative stress is thought to increase risk of preeclampsia and miscarriages [27]. Epidemiological studies have also supported an association between vitC deficiency and preeclampsia [28,29]. However recently, human intervention studies using vitC in the prevention of preeclampsia have produced conflicting results [30–32]. Another study found no effect of vitamin C on prevention of spontaneous preterm birth [33]. A recent review concluded that a general recommendation of vitC supplementation to pregnant women was not warranted, but subpopulations such as women with vitC deficiency, smokers or diabetics were not discussed [34].

Thus in diabetic animals, experimental data support the amelioration of these risks by vitC supplementation [35–38]. In one human study, borderline gestational diabetes mellitus had an increased risk of adverse health outcomes compared with women no diabetes [39]. Another human controlled intervention study in type 1 diabetes mellitus (T1DM) pregnancy found a lower risk of premature birth in women receiving vitC and E supplementation and suggested regarding preeclampsia that vitC supplementation may be beneficial in women with a low antioxidant status at baseline; no effect on preeclampsia was observed in the T1DM cohort as a whole [40]. Another study also failed to prevent preeclampsia with vitC and E supplementation in women with T1DM and even a high risk pro-angiogenic haptoglobin genotype [41].

In T1DM, vitC levels are significantly lower than in non-diabetic subjects [42,43]. This seems to be the case in the diabetic pregnancy, too, as we recently reported in a prospective study [8]. We found that the level of vitC was lower throughout pregnancy compared to the control group, and hypovitaminosis C (vitC < 23 µmol/L [44]) was found in 51% of the diabetic women at some stage during pregnancy. Here, we report our evaluation of vitC status in the same cohort of pregnant T1DM women with regard to labor data and the outcome of pregnancies.

2. Materials and Methods

All T1DM women from June 1992 to August 1994 attending the Department of Obstetrics, Aarhus University Hospital (Aarhus, Denmark), were screened for participation in the prospective study on vitC during pregnancy and compared to controls as described previously [8]. The inclusion criteria were pregestational T1DM, age >18 years, no other systemic disease than diabetes, and singleton pregnancy. Blood samples for vitC were taken when the diabetic women attended the maternity ward and were taken in a non-fasting state to avoid hypoglycemic episodes. At delivery, an umbilical blood sample for vitC was taken from the newborn. In total, 76 women with T1DM consented to participate in the prospective study [8]. Of these, 47 women had vitC measurements taken in late pregnancy within four weeks of delivery and were included in the present cross-sectional evaluation of vitC status in relation to labor data and outcome of pregnancy. If more than one sample in the 4-week interval before labor were obtained, the mean concentration of the samples was used in the analysis.

Blood samples for plasma vitC measurements were stabilized in sodium EDTA-anticoagulated vacutainer tubes containing dithiothreitol. Tubes were centrifuged and plasma was removed and deproteinized by the addition of 6% perchloric acid. The samples were kept at minus 80 degrees Celsius until analysis and assayed by HPLC using 3,4-dihydroxybenzylamine hydrobromide as internal standard [45]. A plot of the ratio of vitC to internal standard versus the concentration of 6 aqueous standards resulted in a linear curve to at least 86 μmol/L (y = 0.16x − 0.028, R^2 = 0.99). The within-day and between-day coefficient of variation was 2.6% and 3.9%, respectively, of a mean concentration of 19 μmol/L. Limit of detection and limit of quantification were 0.525 μmol/L and 1.75 μmol/L, respectively. The analytical recoveries were 111%, 104%, 102%, and 101% at vitC concentrations of 5.75, 28.75, 43.125, and 57.5 μmol/L, respectively.

We carried out predefined plasma vitC subgroup analyses according to the 50% percentile of maternal vitC level and these subgroups were used for evaluating other quantitative and qualitative data on pregnancy, labor, and neonates. This 50% percentile was chosen as we a priori had calculated, that we thereby had sufficient data to minimize a type2 error (power > 80%) on expected SDs in relation to third trimester measurements of pregnancy and in relation to labor and fetus related features as we earlier have reported in T1DM pregnancy [8].

Twenty-eight blood samples from the umbilical cords were also obtained as a surrogate measure of the level of vitC of the fetus. However umbilical cord blood was in the same level as found in the heel blood of 200 newborns [25].

The following data were recorded: Age, duration of diabetes, presence of diabetic microangiopathy, glycemic control, diurnal blood pressure, albumin excretion rate, creatinine, creatinine clearance, pregnancy and labor data, and the neonate's Apgar score at one minute, birth weight, and presence of malformations. The study was part of an evaluation of morbidity in diabetic pregnancy with respect to nephropathy and retinopathy approved by the local Ethics Committee (jr.nr.1992/2523, 1998/4147, and 2026-99). It was performed in concordance with the Helsinki II declaration and all women had given their informed consent. The collection of samples for vitC was approved by the local Ethics Committee (jr.nr. 1992/2328). Hypovitaminosis C was defined as a plasma vitC <23 μmol/L [44].

Preeclampsia was defined as systolic/diastolic blood pressure >140/90 mmHg when normo-hypertensive before week 20 and, simultaneously, albuminuria >300 mg in previously normo-albuminuric women. Pregnancy-induced hypertension was defined as hypertension without signs of preeclampsia. Preterm delivery was defined as delivery following <37 weeks of gestation.

Statistics was performed with IBM SPSS Statistics 20. Difference between two means was tested with Student's t-test if data followed Gaussian distribution; otherwise, Mann-Whitney's test was used. Proportional data were analyzed by χ^2 test or Fisher's Exact test. Values are given as mean ± SD if not otherwise stated. Median (25%–75% interval) indicates variable of non-Gaussian distribution and values were subjected to non-parametric testing. A two-sided $p < 0.05$ was chosen as level of significance.

3. Results

Clinical data from the pregnant diabetic women are shown in Table 1 and are also presented in subgroups according to the median value (25%–75%) of maternal plasma vitC taken within four weeks of delivery. All comparisons of baseline data and diabetic characteristics in relation to the 50% percentile of vitC (26.6 (22.0–37.2) μmol/L) were non-significant (Table 1). The range (0%–100%) of plasma vitC in the cohort was 3.1–61.0 μmol/L.

Results regarding pregnancy and fetal related features are presented in Table 2. No relationship between maternal vitC level and birth weight or Apgar score was observed. Nor was the way of delivery (acute cesarean section, elective cesarean and induced delivery; 7/19/21) associated with vitC status. Moreover, no difference was observed in the level of HbA1c in relation of the median maternal vitC of 26.6 μmol/L, but a negative association of maternal vitC with HbA1c at delivery was found at regression analysis ($r = -0.39$, $p = 0.006$, $n = 46$). The vitC levels of the umbilical cord blood correlated positively with the obtained Apgar score of the newborn ($r = 0.45$, $p = 0.011$), also when corrected for maternal vitC, HbA1c and diabetes duration ($r = 0.52$, $p = 0.025$).

Table 1. Clinical data and characteristics of the diabetic status by maternal vitamin C (vitC) within the last four weeks of pregnancy ($n = 23/24$) and of the whole cohort ($n = 47$).

	VitC > Median >26.6 µmol/L	VitC ≤ Median ≤26.6 µmol/L	p Value	Characteristics of the Whole Cohort
Vit C (µmol/L), $n = 23/24/47$	37.1 (28.2–61.0) [1]	22.1 (3.1–28.2)		30.1 (13.6)
Age (yr), $n = 23/24/47$	28.8 (3.7) [2]	27.7 (3.5)	0.314	27 (26–31)
Maternal weight at delivery (kg) $n = 12/11/23$	78.5 (72.3–87.5)	74.0 (68.0–86.0)	0.32	78 (70–86)
Maternal height (cm), $n = 11/11/22$	166.2 (6.2)	164.4 (8.3)	0.569	165.3 (7.2)
Diabetes duration (year), $n = 23/24/47$	15.0 (8.9)	13.2 (9.0)	0.486	14.1 (8.9)
Parity, $n = 23/24/47$	1.8 (0.8)	1.8 (0.7)	0.876	2 (1.2)
Systolic blood pressure at entry (mmHg), $n = 15/14/29$	120.1 (10.3)	120.5 (9.9)	0.641	120.0 (9.9)
Diastolic blood pressure at entry (mmHg) $n = 15/14/29$	72.1 (6.6)	70.9 (6.7)	0.673	71.2 (6.9)
Retinopathy Non/Simplex/Proliferative, $n = N/S/P$	12/8/3	12/9/3	0.881	24/17/6
BMI (kg/m^2) at delivery, $n = 11/10/21$	29.2 (3.8)	27.6 (4.4)	0.607	28.6 (4.3)
Normo-/Micro-/Macro-albuminuria $n = N/Mi/Ma$	18/4/1	20/4/0	0.581	38/8/1
HbA1c (%) at entry, $n = 22/23/45$	7.7 (1.6)	7.9 (1.2)	0.0697	7.7 (1.4)
Creatinine clearance at entry (ml/min) $n = 15/15/30$	123.3 (22.1)	116.2 (32.3)	0.869	122.1 (27.1)
Smoking, $n = $ Yes/no/unknown	6/16/1	10/14/0	0.538	16/30/1

[1] VitC levels in each subgroup is reported given as median (range); [2] Other data are listed as mean (SD), median (25%–75%) or n-values.

Table 2. Labor and fetus related features in relation to above or below the median level of maternal vitC in late pregnancy.

	VitC > Median >26.6 µmol/L	VitC ≤ Median ≤26.6 µmol/L	p Value
VitC in umbilical cord (µmol/L), $n = 12/16$	101.0 (16.6) [1]	78.5 (27.8)	0.02
Umbilical cord/maternal vitC ratio, $n = 12/16$	2.6 (2.1–2.9)	4.1 (2.8–5.1)	0.007
Apgar score at one minute, $n = 19/23$	10 (9–10)	9 (9–10)	0.56
Birth weight (g), $n = 23/24$	3867 (649)	3533 (771)	0.12
Gestations age at labor (weeks), $n = 23/24$	37.4 (1.1)	37.2 (1.5)	0.64
Normal delivery (n)	0	0	
Induced delivery and elective section/acute section, (n/n)	20/3	20/4	1.0
HbA1c at delivery (%), $n = 23/23$	6.7 (1.1)	7.2 (1.0)	0.14

[1] Data are listed as mean (SD), median (25%–75%) or n-values.

Hypovitaminosis C was found in 13 out of 47 diabetic women (28%) and was associated with a risk of complications of 69%, while the risk of complications was 29% in case of higher levels of vitC (Table 3). The relative risk of having complications of pregnancy was 2.4 times in case of maternal hypovitaminosis C compared to higher levels of maternal vitC ($p = 0.02$). In accordance, the diabetic women with complications of pregnancy had a significantly lower vitC status in late pregnancy compared to those without complications (mean (SD) 24.2 µmol/L (95% CI: 19.4–30) vs. 34.6 µmol/L (95% CI: 29.6–40); $p = 0.011$, $n = 19$ and 28, respectively). The type and distribution of complications are given in Table 4.

Table 3. Women with complications in subgroups according to vitC status in late pregnancy.

Complications of Pregnancy	Hypovitaminosis C [1]	Above Hypovitaminosis C Level	All Women	Fisher's Exact Test
Yes (n)	9	10	19	
No (n)	4	24	28	
Total (n)	13	34	47	$p = 0.02$

[1] Plasma concentration <23 µmol/L.

Table 4. The type and distribution of complications in T1DM women ($n = 47$). Recorded complications were prematurity, gestational hypertension, asphyxia, malformation, still birth, placental abruption, preeclampsia.

Complication	Frequency	VitC µmol/L Mean (SD)
Women with/without complications	19/47 vs. 28/47	24.2 (10.6)/34.6 (14.4)
Fetal malformation	4/47 [1]	18.1 (9.0)
Asphyxia/abnormal CTG [2]	9/47	22.9 (12.8)
Preeclampsia	5/47	25.0 (10.6)
Prematurity	5/47	20.9 (6.0)
Placental abruption	2/47	18.6 (0.9)
Still birth	2/47	30.9 (0.4)
Pregnancy-induced hypertension	2/47	30.0 (7.1)

[1] The fetal malformations consisted of two neonates with cardiac malformations with transposition and atrium septum defect and two others were related to skeletal abnormalities; [2] CTG: Cardiotocography. Abnormal CTG was diagnosed in nine women at delivery and of these, seven ended in acute cesarean section and two in induced delivery. Women may have more than one complication.

4. Discussion

The present cross-sectional study of T1DM pregnancy found an inverse relationship between vitC status and risks of complications in pregnancy. Thus, poor vitC status within four weeks of delivery was a positive predictor (69%) for complications of pregnancy, while a maternal vitC >23 µmol/L was a negative predictor (71%) for complications of pregnancy, respectively. In support of the observed relationship between maternal vitC status in late pregnancy and complications, we found a low maternal plasma vitC in case of complications of pregnancy (power of test > 80%).

The mean level of vitC was 24.2 µmol/L in the group with complications in pregnancy, thus in this normally distributed group nearly the half of the women had a level of vitC characterized as hypovitaminosis C. Much of the literature showing associations between vitC status and complications in pregnancy was conducted in pregnant experimental animals with or without induced diabetes and related to severe vitC deficiency (<11 µmol/L). This level increases the risk of developing outright scurvy, the ultimately mortal manifestation of prolonged severe vitC deficiency. However, only about 4% of the present cohort (2 patients out of 47) had severe vitC deficiency within four weeks of delivery and no clinical symptoms of scurvy were recorded in the case records of the pregnant women in this study. Therefore, it appears that the complications in diabetic pregnancy are already present at suboptimal vitC levels. In agreement, previous human studies identified a range of complications of pregnancy in non-diabetic women, the risks of which were inversely correlated with plasma vitC; this was, indeed, found over a wide concentration range above the level critical for development of scorbutic manifestations [16–27]. Thus, although higher levels of vitC are not associated with scurvy, lack of scurvy does not preclude the presence of several other negative health effects of a suboptimal vitC status, and the optimal vitC intake in humans is still a matter of considerable debate [46].

In humans, a randomized placebo-controlled intervention study with vitamin C and E in T1DM pregnancies showed no overall effect of supplementation (1000 mg vitamin C and 400 IU vitamin E (α-tocopherol) daily until delivery) on the incidence of preeclampsia [40]. However, subgroup analysis did reveal a significant positive effect of supplementation vs placebo on preeclampsia among patients who were vitC deficient at baseline (<10 µmol/L). Thus, the authors suggested that the significant benefit of supplementation on preeclampsia may be limited to women with severe vitC deficiency [40]. VitC and E supplementation also resulted in fewer preterm deliveries compared to placebo in the cohort as a whole, but the potential correlation to vitC status at entry was not explored [40]. Another study has also reported lack of effects of supplementation with vitC on the incidence of preeclampsia in high-risk T1DM women [41]. The absence of effect of vitC supplementation on preeclampsia in humans with or without diabetes may arise from the variation in the degree of plasma saturation and subsequent differential outcomes of supplementation as discussed elsewhere [47].

Another interesting result of the present study is the difference in vitC level in umbilical cord blood of newborns reflects some of the difference in the mothers' vitC level. Combined with the observation that the ratio of umbilical cord/maternal vitC favors babies born by mothers with vitC level below the median, our data collectively support the notion that the fetus is preferentially supplied with vitC at the expense of the mother [5,48]. However, as the vitC level in these babies is significantly lower than that of those born by mothers with vitC level above the median, it also suggests that such a preferential supply cannot fully compensate for poor maternal vitC status. The maternal as well the umbilical vitC measurements were conducted with sufficient data to minimize a type 2 error on conclusions (power of t test > 80%). Thus in this study—in spite of the fetus acting as a "parasite" as described by Teel et al. [3]—the newborns of mothers with low maternal vitC seem not to be able to obtain the same level of vitC in the umbilical cord as newborns of mothers with a higher vitC level, although their ratio is larger. This is in line with experimental data from guinea pigs showing that the preferential fetal transport may be overridden by increased needs of the mother during situations of deficiency, thereby potentially influencing the health of the offspring [13,49]. In accordance, the vitC levels of the umbilical cord blood correlated positively with the obtained Apgar score of the newborn.

Finally, no correlation between diabetic characteristics of the pregnant women and vitC status was observed, although glycemic control measured as HbA1c showed an inverse correlation with maternal vitC level. VitC is thought to be actively transported by SVCT transporters in the placenta [50]; however, it also shares the same transporters as glucose via the GLUT-mediated transport of dehydroascorbic acid (DHA; the oxidized form of vitC) [51]. Thus, it may be speculated that the degree of glycemic control and, consequently, the level of oxidative stress and ascorbate oxidation rate may affect the bioavailability of vitC in T1DM pregnant women through competitive inhibition of DHA transport as proposed by Mann and Newton already in 1975 [52] and supported by the NHANES study 2003–2006 data [53]; here an inverse relationship between vitC and HbA1c was reported in 7697 non-diabetic participants. Moreover, Tu et al. have recently proposed that impaired red cell recycling of DHA may be a key link in diabetes [54].

Limitations of the present study include the small number of participants and that the registration of complications of pregnancy was done retrospectively on the case report forms, which in some cases may be imprecise. The included T1DM patients with diabetic complications, i.e., retino- and nephropathy, could potentially influence the outcome of pregnancy. However, we did not find any relationship of these variables with vitC probably due to the small number of participants. Finally, the samples for vitC were taken in a non-fasting state to avoid hypoglycemic episodes, which may have increased the SD of the vitC measurements and, thus, the risk of type 2 error.

5. Conclusions

In conclusion, the results from this small study of a pregnant T1DM cohort suggest that hypovitaminosis C in late pregnancy may be associated with an increased risk of developing complications in pregnancy and may also, to some extent, limit the obtainable level of vitC of the fetus as measured by umbilical values in the newborn. Further investigations are needed to disclose the possible clinical significance of vitC in the diabetic pregnancy and to confirm in larger studies that a benefit of vitC supplementation exists in pregnancies characterized by hypovitaminosis C.

Acknowledgments: Jens Lykkesfeldt is partly supported by the Lifepharm Centre for In Vivo Pharmacology.

Author Contributions: Bente Juhl designed and performed the experiments; Bente Juhl, Finn Friis Lauszus, and Jens Lykkesfeldt analyzed and interpreted the data; Bente Juhl, Finn Friis Lauszus, and Jens Lykkesfeldt wrote the paper.

References

1.   Christian, P. Micronutrients, birth weight, and survival. *Annu. Rev. Nutr.* **2010**, *30*, 83–104. [CrossRef] [PubMed]
2.   World Health Organization (WHO). *Vitamin and Minerals Requirements in Human Nutrition*, 2nd ed.; WHO: Geneva, Switzerland, 2004; p. 341.
3.   Teel, H.M.; Burke, B.S.; Draper, R. Vitamin C in human pregnancy and lactation: I Studies During pregnancy. *Am. J. Dis. Child* **1938**, *56*, 1004–1010. [CrossRef]
4.   Scaife, A.R.; McNeill, G.; Campbell, D.M.; Martindale, S.; Devereux, G.; Seaton, A. Maternal intake of antioxidant vitamins in pregnancy in relation to and fetal levels at delivery. *Br. J. Nutr.* **2006**, *95*, 771–778. [CrossRef]
5.   Wang, Y.Z.; Ren, W.H.; Liao, W.Q.; Zhang, G.Y. Concentrations of antioxidant vitamins in maternal and cord serum and their effect on birth outcomes. *J. Nutr. Sci. Vitam.* **2009**, *55*, 1–8. [CrossRef]
6.   Mason, M.; Rivers, J.M. Plasma ascorbic levels in pregnancy. *Am. J. Obstst. Gynecol.* **1971**, *109*, 960–961. [CrossRef]
7.   Vobecky, J.S.; Vobecky, J.; Shapcoot, D.; Munan, L. Vitamin C and outcome of pregnancy. *Lancet* **1974**, *303*, 630–631. [CrossRef]
8.   Juhl, B.; Lauszus, F.F.; Lykkesfeldt, J. Ascorbic acid is lower during pregnancy in diabetic women compared to controls: A prospective study. *Int. J. Vit. Nutr. Res.* **2017**, *87*, 1–6. [CrossRef] [PubMed]
9.   Rivers, J.M.; Lennart, K.; Cormier, A. Biochemimical and histological study of guinea pig fetal and uterine tissue in ascorbic acid deficiency. *J. Nutr.* **1970**, *100*, 217–227. [PubMed]
10. Pye, O.F.; Tayler, C.M.; Fontanares, E. The effect of different levels of ascorbic acid in the diet of guinea pigs on health, reproduction and survival. *J. Nutr.* **1961**, *73*, 236–242.
11. Kramer, M.M.; Harman, M.T.; Brill, A.K. Disturbances of reproduction and ovarian changes in the guinea pig in relation to vitamin deficiency. *Am. J. Physiol.* **1933**, *106*, 611–622.
12. Paidi, M.D.; Schjoldager, J.G.; Lykkesfeldt, J.; Tveden-Nyborg, P. Prenatal vitamin C deficiency results in differential expression of oxidative stress during late gestation in foetal guinea pig brains. *Redox Biol.* **2014**, *2*, 361–367. [CrossRef] [PubMed]
13. Schjoldager, J.G.; Tveden-Nyborg, P.; Lykkesfeldt, J. Prolonged maternal vitamin C deficiency overrides preferential fetal ascorbate transport but does not influence perinatal survival in guinea pigs. *Br. J. Nutr.* **2013**, *110*, 1573–1579. [CrossRef] [PubMed]
14. Tveden-Nyborg, P.; Vogt, L.; Schjoldager, J.G.; Jeannet, N.; Hasselholt, S.; Paidi, M.; Christen, S.; Lykkesfeldt, J. Maternal vitamin C deficiency during pregnancy persistently impairs hippocampal neurogenesis in offspring of guinea pigs. *PLoS ONE* **2012**, *7*, e48488. [CrossRef] [PubMed]
15. Tveden-Nyborg, P.; Johansen, L.K.; Hansen, Z.L.; Villumsen, C.K.; Larsen, J.O.; Lykkesfeldt, J. Vitamin C deficiency induces impaired neuronal and cognitive development in neonatal guinea pigs. *Am. J. Clin. Nutr.* **2009**, *90*, 540–546. [CrossRef] [PubMed]
16. Wideman, G.L.; Baird, G.H.; Bolding, O.T. Ascorbic acid deficiency and premature rupture of fetal membranes. *Am. J. Obstet. Gynecol.* **1964**, *88*, 592–595. [CrossRef]
17. Aplin, J.D.; Campbell, S.; Donnai, P.; Bard, J.B.L.; Allen, T.D. Importance of vitamin C in maintenance of the normal amnion: An experimental study. *Placenta* **1986**, *7*, 377–389. [CrossRef]
18. Casanueva, E.; Magana, L.; Pfeffer, F.; Baez, A. Incidence of premature rupture of membranes in pregnant women with low leucocyte levels of vitamin, C. *Eur. J. Clin. Nutr.* **1991**, *45*, 401–405. [PubMed]
19. Casanueva, E.; Polo, E.; Tejero, E.; Meza, C. Premature rupture of amniotic membranes as functional assessment of vitamin C status during pregnancy. *Ann. N. Y. Acad. Sci.* **1993**, *678*, 369–370. [CrossRef] [PubMed]
20. Barret, B.; Gunter, E.; Jenkins, J.; Wang, M. Ascorbic acid concentration in amniotic fluid in late pregnancy. *Biol. Neonate* **1991**, *60*, 333–335. [CrossRef]
21. Barret, B.M.; Sowell, A.; Gunter, E.; Wang, M. Potential role of ascorbic acid and β-carotene in the prevention of preterm rupture of fetal membranes. *Int. J. Vit. Nutr. Res.* **1994**, *64*, 192–197. [CrossRef]
22. Javert, C.T.; Stander, H.J. Plasma vitamin C and prothrombin concentrations in pregnancy and in threatened, spontaneous and habitual abortions. *J. Surg. Gynec. Obstet.* **1943**, *76*, 115–122.

23. Parry, S.; Strauss, J.F. Premature rupture of the fetal membranes. *N. Engl. J. Med.* **1998**, *338*, 663–670. [PubMed]

24. Casanueva, E.; Ripoll, C.; Tolentino, M.; Morales, R.M.; Pfeffer, F.; Vilchis, P.; Vadillo-ortega, F. Vitamin C supplementation to prevent premature rupture of the chorioamniotic membranes: A randomized trial. *Am. J. Clin. Nutr.* **2005**, *81*, 859–863. [PubMed]

25. Heinz-Erian, P.; Achmuller, M.; Berger, H.; Brabec, W.; Nirk, S.; Rufer, R. Vitamin C concentrations in maternal plasma, amniotic fluid, cord blood, in the plasma of the newborn and in colostrum, transitorial and mature breastmilk. *Padiatrie Padol.* **1987**, *22*, 163–178.

26. Clemetson, C.A.B.; Cafaro, V. Abruptio placentae. *Int. J. Gynaecol. Obstet.* **1981**, *19*, 453–460. [CrossRef]

27. Jauniaux, E.; Poston, L.; Burton, G.J. Placental-related diseases of pregnancy: Involvement of oxidative stress and implications in human evolution. *Hum. Reprod. Update* **2006**, *12*, 747–755. [CrossRef] [PubMed]

28. Mikhail, M.S.; Anyaegbunam, A.; Garfinkel, D.; Palan, P.R.; Basu, J.; Romney, S.L. Preeclampsia and antioxidant nutrients- decreased plasma levels of reduces ascorbic acid, alfa tocopherol and beta-caroten in women with preeclampsia. *Am. J. Obstet. Gynecol.* **1994**, *171*, 150–157. [CrossRef]

29. Zhang, C.; Williams, M.A.; King, I.B. Vitamin C and risk of preeclapsia—Results from dietary questionnaire and plasma assay. *Epidemiology* **2002**, *13*, 409–416. [CrossRef] [PubMed]

30. Chappell, L.C.; Seed, P.T.; Kelly, F.J.; Briley, A.; Hunt, B.J.; Charnock-Jones, D.S.; Mallet, A.; Poston, L. Vitamin C and E supplementation in women at risk of preeclampsia is associated with changes in indices of oxidative stress and placental function. *Am. J. Obstet. Gynecol.* **2002**, *187*, 777–784. [CrossRef] [PubMed]

31. Rumbold, A.R.; Crowther, C.A.; Haslan, R.R.; Dekker, G.A.; Robinson, J.S.; ACTS Study Group. Vitamin C and E and the risk of preeclampsia and perinatal complications. *N. Engl. J. Med.* **2006**, *354*, 1796–1806. [CrossRef] [PubMed]

32. Roberts, J.M.; Myatt, L.; Spongy, C.Y.; Thom, E.A.; Hauth, J.C.; Leveno, K.J.; Pearson, G.D.; Wapner, R.J.; Varner, M.W.; Mercer, B.M.; et al. Eunice Kennedy Shriver National Institute of Child Health and Human Development (NICHD) Maternal-Fetal Medicine Unit Network (MFMU) Vitamin C and E to prevent complications of pregnancy-associated hypertension. *N. Engl. J. Med.* **2010**, *362*, 1282–1291. [CrossRef] [PubMed]

33. Hauth, J.C.; Clifton, R.G.; Roberts, J.M.; Spongy, C.Y.; Myatt, L.; Leveno, K.J.; Pearson, G.D.; Varner, M.W.; Mercer, B.M.; Peaceman, A.M.; et al. Eunice Kennedy Shriver National Institute of Child Health and Human Development (NICHD) Maternal-Fetal Medicine Unit Network (MFMU). Vitamin C and E to prevent spontaneous preterm birth: A randomized controlled trial. *Obstet. Gynecol.* **2010**, *116*, 653–658. [CrossRef] [PubMed]

34. Duerbeck, N.B.; Dowling, D.D.; Duerbeck, J.M. Vitamin, C. promises not kept. *Obstet. Gynecol. Surv.* **2016**, *71*, 187–193. [CrossRef] [PubMed]

35. Dheen, S.T.; Tay, S.S.; Boran, J.; Ting, L.W.; Kumar, S.D.; Fu, J.; Ling, E.A. Recent studies on neural tube defects in embryos of diabetic pregnancy: An overview. *Curr. Med. Chem.* **2009**, *16*, 2345–2354. [CrossRef] [PubMed]

36. Cederberg, J.; Eriksson, U.K. Antioxidative treatment of pregnant diabetic rats diminished embryonic dysmorphogenesis. *Birth Defect. Res. A Clin. Mol. Teratol.* **2005**, *3*, 498–505. [CrossRef] [PubMed]

37. Cederberg, J.; Siman, C.M.; Eriksson, U.J. Combined treatment with vitamin E and C decreases oxidative stress and improves fetal outcome in experimental diabetic pregnancy. *Pediatr. Res.* **2001**, *49*, 755–762. [CrossRef] [PubMed]

38. Siman, C.M.; Eriksson, U.J. Vitamin C supplementation of the maternal diet reduces the rate of malformations in the offspring of diabetic rats. *Diabetologia* **1997**, *40*, 1416–1424. [CrossRef] [PubMed]

39. Ju, H.; Rumbold, A.R.; Willson, K.J.; Crowther, C.A. Borderline gestational diabetes mellitus and pregnancy outcomes. *BMC Pregnancy Childbirth* **2008**, *30*, 8–31. [CrossRef] [PubMed]

40. McCance, D.R.; Holmes, V.A.; Maresh, M.J.; Patterson, C.C.; Walker, J.D.; Pearson, D.W.; Young, I.S. Diabetes and Pre-eclampsia Intervention Trial (DAPIT) Study Group. Vitamins C and E for prevention of pre-eclampsia in women with type 1 diabetes (DAPIT): A randomised placebo-controlled trial. *Lancet* **2010**, *376*, 259–266. [CrossRef]

41. Weissgerber, T.L.; Gandley, R.E.; Roberts, J.M.; Patterson, C.C.; Holmes, V.A.; Young, I.S.; McCance, D.R. Diabetes and preeclampsia interventions Trial (DAPIT) study group. *BJOG* **2013**, *120*, 1192–1199. [CrossRef] [PubMed]

42. Brownlee, M. The Pathobiology of Diabetic Complications: A Unifying Mechanism. *Diabetes* **2006**, *54*, 1615–1625. [CrossRef]

43. Sinclair, A.J.; Girling, A.J.; Gray, L.; Le Guen, C.; Lunec, J.; Barnett, A.H. Disturbed handling of ascorbic acid in diabetic patients with and without microangiopathy during high dose ascorbate supplementation. *Diabetologia* **1991**, *34*, 171–175. [CrossRef] [PubMed]

44. Jacob, R.A.; Otradovec, C.L.; Russell, R.M.; Munro, H.N.; Hartz, S.C.; McGandy, R.B.; Morrow, F.D.; Sadowski, J.A. Vitamin C status and nutrient interactions in a healthy elderly population. *Am. J. Clin. Nutr.* **1988**, *48*, 1436–1442. [PubMed]

45. Lee, W.; Hamernyik, P.; Hutchinson, M.; Raisys, V.A.; Labbé, R.F. Ascorbic acid in lymphocytes: Cell preparation and liquid-chromatographic assay. *Clin. Chem.* **1982**, *28*, 2165–2169. [PubMed]

46. Frei, B.; Birlouez-Aragon, I.; Lykkesfeldt, J. Author's perspective: What is the optimum intake of vitamin C in humans? *Crit. Rev. Food Sci. Nutr.* **2012**, *52*, 815–829. [CrossRef] [PubMed]

47. Tveden-Nyborg, P.; Lykkesfeldt, J. Does vitamin C deficiency increase lifestyle-associated vascular disease progression?—Evidence based on experimental and clinical studies. *Antioxid. Redox Sign.* **2013**, *19*, 2084–2104. [CrossRef] [PubMed]

48. Jain, S.; Wise, R.; Yanamandra, K.; Dhanireddy, R.; Bocchini, J. The effect of maternal and cord-blood vitamin C, vitamin E and lipid peroxide levels on newborn birth weight. *Mol. Cell. Biochem.* **2008**, *309*, 217–221. [CrossRef] [PubMed]

49. Schjoldager, J.G.; Paidi, M.D.; Lindblad, M.M.; Birck, M.M.; Kjærgaard, A.B.; Dantzer, V.; Lykkesfeldt, J.; Tveden-Nyborg, P. Maternal vitamin C deficiency during pregnancy results in transient fetal and placental growth retardation in guinea pigs but does not affect prenatal survival. *Eur. J. Nutr.* **2015**, *54*, 667–676. [CrossRef] [PubMed]

50. Takanaga, H.; Mackenzie, B.; Hediger, M.A. Sodium-dependent ascorbic acid transporter family SLC23. *Pflug. Arch.* **2004**, *447*, 677–682. [CrossRef] [PubMed]

51. Lindblad, M.M.; Tveden-Nyborg, P.; Lykkesfeldt, J. Regulation of vitamin C homeostasis during deficiency. *Nutrients* **2013**, *5*, 2860–2879. [CrossRef] [PubMed]

52. Mann, G.V.; Newton, P. The membrane transport of ascorbic acid. *Ann. N. Y. Acad. Sci.* **1975**, *258*, 243–252. [CrossRef] [PubMed]

53. Kositsawat, J.; Freeman, V.L. Vitamin C and A1c relationship in the national health and nutrition examination Survey (NHANES) 2003–2006. *J. Am. Coll. Nutr.* **2011**, *30*, 477–483. [CrossRef] [PubMed]

54. Tu, H.; Li, H.; Wang, Y.; Niyyati, M.; Wang, Y.; Leshin, J.; Levine, M. Low red blood cell vitamin C concentrations induce red blood cell fragility: A link to diabetes via glucose, glucose transporters and dehydrascorbic acid. *EBiomedicine* **2015**, *2*, 1735–1750. [CrossRef] [PubMed]

6

Influence of Vitamin C on Lymphocytes

Gwendolyn N. Y. van Gorkom [1,*], Roel G. J. Klein Wolterink [1], Catharina H. M. J. Van Elssen [1], Lotte Wieten [2], Wilfred T. V. Germeraad [1] and Gerard M. J. Bos [1]

[1]   Division of Hematology, Department of Internal Medicine,
      GROW-School for Oncology and Developmental Biology, Maastricht University Medical Center,
      6202AZ Maastricht, The Netherlands; r.kleinwolterink@maastrichtuniversity.nl (R.G.J.K.W.);
      janine.van.elssen@mumc.nl (C.H.M.J.V.E.); w.germeraad@maastrichtuniversity.nl (W.T.V.G.);
      gerard.bos@mumc.nl (G.M.J.B.)
[2]   Department of Transplantation Immunology, Maastricht University Medical Center, 6202 AZ Maastricht,
      The Netherlands; Lotte.wieten@maastrichtuniversity.nl
[*]   Correspondence: gwendolyn.van.gorkom@mumc.nl

Abstract: Vitamin C or ascorbic acid (AA) is implicated in many biological processes and has been proposed as a supplement for various conditions, including cancer. In this review, we discuss the effects of AA on the development and function of lymphocytes. This is important in the light of cancer treatment, as the immune system needs to regenerate following chemotherapy or stem cell transplantation, while cancer patients are often AA-deficient. We focus on lymphocytes, as these white blood cells are the slowest to restore, rendering patients susceptible to often lethal infections. T lymphocytes mediate cellular immunity and have been most extensively studied in the context of AA biology. In vitro studies demonstrate that T cell development requires AA, while AA also enhances T cell proliferation and may influence T cell function. There are limited and opposing data on the effects of AA on B lymphocytes that mediate humoral immunity. However, AA enhances the proliferation of NK cells, a group of cytotoxic innate lymphocytes. The influence of AA on natural killer (NK) cell function is less clear. In summary, an increasing body of evidence indicates that AA positively influences lymphocyte development and function. Since AA is a safe and cheap nutritional supplement, it is worthwhile to further explore its potential benefits for immune reconstitution of cancer patients treated with immunotoxic drugs.

Keywords: vitamin C; ascorbic acid; lymphocytes; natural killer cells; NK cells; B cells; T cells

1. Introduction

Vitamin C or ascorbic acid (AA) has often been linked to cancer treatment. Already in the 1970s, Cameron and Pauling reported that high doses of AA intravenously increased the survival time of terminal cancer patients more than four times [1] but this finding could not be repeated in other studies where AA supplementation was given orally [2,3]. However, subsequent studies show that AA has a wide variety of effects on cancer cells and the immune system. In this review, we discuss the effects of AA on lymphocytes in the light of cancer treatment.

AA is an essential micronutrient for humans with many functions in the human body. It is an antioxidant and a free radical scavenger and serves as an essential cofactor for many enzymatic reactions through iron-, copper- and 2-oxoglutarate-dependent dioxygenases. Among many other functions, these dioxygenases are important in epigenetic regulation by catalysing the hydroxylation of methylated nucleic acids (DNA and RNA) and histones [4]. While most mammals use the enzyme gulono-gamma-lactone oxidase to synthesize AA in the liver, many primates and humans carry a non-functional copy of the *GULO*-gene and consequently depend on dietary sources of AA. When studying the effects of AA and AA deficiency in vivo in animal models, this is a complicating factor. Guinea pigs, like humans, also have a defect in the GULO-gene and are thereby often chosen for AA deficiency studies. Alternatively, there are two knockout mouse models, a *Gulo* knockout ($Gulo^-/^-$) and a senescence marker protein-30 knockout (*SMP30KO*), in which biosynthesis of AA in the liver is blocked [5,6].

AA has an extensive role in the immune system. Its role in phagocytic cells like neutrophils, has been investigated thoroughly and was recently reviewed [7]. In summary, AA enhances chemotaxis and phagocytosis of phagocytes and thereby promotes microbial killing. In contrast, the role of AA in different subsets of lymphocytes is less clear. Since lymphocytes actively acquire AA via sodium-dependent vitamin C transporters (SVCT) and sodium independent glucose transporters (GLUT) (reviewed in [8] and have intracellular AA concentrations that are 10–100-fold higher than plasma levels [9,10], it is likely that AA has an essential function in these cells. There are three main subsets of lymphocytes, namely T cells, B cells and natural killer (NK cells). T cells are involved in cell-mediated, cytotoxic adaptive immunity, B cells are responsible for the adaptive, humoral immunity and NK cells are part of the innate, antigen-independent immunity.

In our laboratory, we are interested in lymphocytes in cancer treatment, because these cells are often destroyed by anticancer treatment and take time to recover. During this phase, patients are highly susceptible to possibly lethal infections. Depending on the intensity of the chemotherapy used, this period may be relatively short, for example in breast cancer, or long, for example in leukaemia. After so-called myeloablative chemotherapy, hematopoietic stem cells (HSC) that are located in the bone marrow have to be replaced in order to restore all types of blood cells, including leukocytes. In particular, the regeneration of T-lymphocytes, a subset of lymphocytes that are especially important to fight against viral infections, is slow as a consequence of age-dependent involution of the thymus, the organ that is required for their development [11,12]. Looking at ways to improve T cell recovery after cancer therapy, we investigated factors that influence human T-lymphocyte development and found that AA acts as a factor that promotes maturation of T cells. AA is also indispensable for T cell development in vitro [13]. Additionally, we showed that NK cells regenerate faster under the influence of AA [14].

We also found that haematological cancer patients often have severely decreased serum AA levels compared to healthy controls (20.5 ± 12 μM versus 65 ± 4 μM, respectively). Serum AA levels were even undetectable in 19% of patients with a haematological malignancy, irrespective of the choice of treatment [15]. Since AA is a cheap and readily available supplement with a safe profile, it is attractive to speculate that cancer patients who need to regenerate their immune system after chemotherapy with or without hematopoietic stem cell transplantation (HSCT) may benefit from the effects of AA on immune reconstitution. In this way, we hypothesize that mortality and morbidity resulting from opportunistic infections could be reduced. It could also be that NK cells regenerate faster and are able to kill cancer cells sooner. AA supplementation could also be used in cellular therapies, where in vitro proliferated and adapted subtypes of lymphocytes are used to eliminate tumour cells in vivo. However, before using AA in clinical applications, it is important to have a better understanding of the role of AA in these lymphocytes.

In this article, we highlight the effects of AA on different subsets of lymphocytes as far as they are known for this moment. We will focus on the effects on the physiology of these cells and on the role of AA on lymphocytes in health and disease and not on the potential mechanisms behind these effects, since this was extensively reviewed before [4].

2. AA and T Lymphocytes

T lymphocytes are a major component of the human immune system and are involved in cell-mediated, cytotoxic adaptive immunity. On their surface, T cells express the T cell receptor (TCR) that is responsible for recognizing and binding specific antigens bound to major histocompatibility complex (MHC) molecules. There are different types of T lymphocytes, including cytotoxic T cells, T helper cells, memory T cells and regulatory T cells. Cytotoxic T cells are characterized by a MHC class I binding CD8 protein on their cell surface. The TCR and CD8 receptor bind infected cells and tumour cells. After binding, the cytotoxic T cells mature and, upon activation by an infected cell, secrete perforin and granzymes, that kill the infected cells. T helper cells are CD4 positive cells that regulate immune responses. Their TCR binds to MHC class II on antigen presenting cells (APCs). After binding, T-helper cells secrete cytokines that activate other immune cells, including cytotoxic T cells. Memory T cells are long-living cells that recognize previously encountered pathogens and provide lifelong immunity. Regulatory T cells shut down T cell mediated immunity toward the end of an immune reaction and help to maintain tolerance to self-antigens.

Here we describe the effects on AA on general T cell development and summarize what is known about the influence of AA on these most important subsets of T cells. We will not discuss cytotoxic T cells since we found no studies examining the effects of AA on this specific subset.

2.1. T Cell Development and AA

T cell development is a tightly controlled process that takes place in the thymus, which can be simulated in vitro using foetal thymic organ cultures [16], stromal cells [17] or in feeder-free conditions [13]. While mature T lymphocytes express either CD4 or CD8 for helper and cytotoxic subsets respectively, immature T cells are called "double negative" (DN) because they lack CD4 and CD8 expression. Traveling through the highly-organized thymus, the developing T cells undergo numerous rounds of proliferation. The thymic stromal cells provide the structural support and cytokines necessary for selection of a functional TCR that does not recognize self-antigens. This process of "education" is required to generate a diverse repertoire of TCRs to ensure immunity against a wide variety of antigens. The various stages of human T cell development are characterized by sequential acquisition of CD7, CD5, intracellular CD3, CD1a, CD4 and CD8, TCR$\alpha\beta$ and surface CD3 [18].

In search for factors that enhance T cell differentiation after stem cell transplantation, we discovered that AA enhances human T cell proliferation in vitro [13]. Beside this effect on T cell proliferation, we also found multiple effects on early T cell development. Most importantly, we showed that AA is required in vitro for the transition of DN precursors to the next, so-called "double positive" (DP, CD4$^+$ CD8$^+$) stage in feeder-free cultures as well as in cultures with stromal cells when culturing T cells from cord blood or G-CSF stimulated hematopoietic stem cells. Furthermore, we found that in a feeder-free system, early maturation of T cells after 3 weeks was improved under the influence of AA in a dose dependent way with an optimum at 95 µM [13]. These results are in line with a murine study in which the investigators cultured adult bone marrow-derived hematopoietic progenitor cells on stromal cells and showed that these cells only differentiate to the DP stage in the presence of AA. To determine the effect of AA in vivo, foetal liver chimeric mice were generated by transfer of Slc23a2-deficient HCS into recipient mice. In the absence of Slc23a2, hematopoietic cells are unable to concentrate AA. Consequently, in animals with a Slc23a2-deficient hematopoietic system, T cell maturation was virtually absent compared to control mice [19].

Since AA functions as an antioxidant, we tested if other antioxidants could restore T cell development. As this was not the case, the effect of AA on developing human T cells cannot be attributed to its antioxidant properties [11]. This finding is supported by Manning et al. [19] who showed that induction and maintenance of Cd8a gene expression is dependent on AA-dependent removal of repressive histone modifications, rather than on its function as an antioxidant.

In summary, in humans and mice, AA is required in vitro for the early development of T cells as it overcomes a development block from DN to DP. Furthermore, AA speeds up the maturation process of T lymphocytes. In mice, at least part of this effect is due to AA-dependent epigenetic regulation.

2.2. T Cell Proliferation and AA

Multiple researchers studied the effect of vitamin C on the proliferation and survival of T cells, in vitro as well as in vivo.

One study describes the effect of AA on in vitro culture of in vivo activated mouse T cells. While more than 70% apoptotic cells were found in cultures without AA, the addition of AA (450 μM) decreased apoptosis by one-third and induced more proliferation was seen compared to cultures without AA [20]. In another study, evaluating the effects of AA on murine T cells during in vitro activation, it was found that that low concentrations (62.5 μM and 125 μM) of AA do not change proliferation or viability of T cells, while higher concentrations (250 μM and 500 μM) do decrease both [21]. In a third study, researchers examined how AA prevents oxidative damage using purified human T cells. They report similar effects: medium-high concentrations of AA (57–142 μM) decrease T cell proliferation, while at higher concentrations (284 μM), AA decreases cell viability and IL-2 secretion more than 90% [22]. In another study studying the expression of SVCT on T cells, the investigators show a similar effect. Peripheral blood T cells of healthy human volunteers were activated in vitro in the absence or presence of different doses AA, before and after activation. AA did not have any effect on proliferation or apoptosis in low doses (62.5–250 μM). At high doses (500–1000 μM), the proliferation was inhibited and there was an increase in apoptosis when AA was added before activation [23].

In a study on the effect of AA-deficiency on lymphocyte numbers in guinea pigs, the investigators found that in animals with an 4-week AA-free diet, the number of T-lymphocytes decreased continuously while T cell number slightly increased in AA-supplemented animals (25 and 250 mg intraperitoneally/day) [24]. Plasma and tissue concentrations of AA were significantly lower in animals without AA compared to AA-treated animals. In another in vivo study using AA-deficient $SMP30KO^{-/-}$ mice, the researchers determined the long-term effect of AA on immune cells using a diet with an increased AA level (200 mg/kg vs. 20 mg/kg). During the one-year study, T-lymphocytes in the peripheral blood increased in number. More specifically, the number of naive T cells, memory T cells in the spleen and mature T cells in the thymus [6] increased. Plasma concentrations of AA in mice with a low-dose AA diet were similar to wildtype mice, while plasma concentrations in the high-dose diet were significantly higher.

Badr et al., examined if the impaired T cell function in type I diabetes can be improved by AA supplementation using a streptozotocin-induced diabetes type I rat model. These animals have diminished T cell cytokine production, less proliferation and lower surface expression of CD28, a protein that is important for T cell activation and survival. AA supplementation (100 mg/kg/day for 2 months) restored the CD28 expression, cytokine secretion and proliferation [25].

Studies in humans are limited. Because elderly people often have lower serum levels of AA and are more prone to infections, a placebo-controlled trial was performed in which elderly people received either an intramuscular injection of AA (500 mg/day) or placebo for 1 month. Compared to the placebo group, an increase in T cell proliferation was seen in the AA-supplemented group [26]. The only other study in humans could not recapitulate this effect [27]. Healthy volunteers were kept on an AA-free diet during a 5-week period to induce AA deficiency. This did not lead to any changes in T cell numbers or function, while the induction of AA deficiency was confirmed in plasma and leukocytes.

In summary, both animal and human studies show that physiological AA concentrations have a beneficial effect on T cell proliferation, while supraphysiological concentrations are toxic for T cells. In vivo, restoration of AA in deficient patients positively influences T cell proliferation as well, while this observation could not be reproduced in induced AA-deficiency.

2.3. T Helper Cells (Th) and AA

There are several subsets of Th cells, the most important ones being Th1, Th2 and Th17. Th1 cells are part of the defence against intracellular bacteria and protozoa. Using their main effector cytokines IFN-γ and TNF-α, they activate cytotoxic T cells and macrophages. Th2 cells are effective against extracellular parasites and produce mainly IL-4, IL-5 and IL-13. They stimulate eosinophils, basophils, mast cells and B-cells. Th2 cells are important mediators of allergy and hypersensitivity. For this reason, Th2 cells are often investigated in animal models for asthma. Th17 cells have an important role in pathogen clearance of mucosal surfaces and produce IL-17, a cytokine that stimulates B-cells. The various Th subsets differentiate from naïve CD4$^+$ T cells in a process called "polarization". In vivo, dendritic cells (DC) are the most important antigen-presenting cells (APC) that steer Th polarization via the production of cytokines.

Several researchers report that AA induces a shift of immune responses from Th2 to Th1. In one of these studies, a mouse model was used to examine the effect of AA (5 mg/day) on delayed-type hypersensitivity response against 2,4,-dinitro-I-fluorobenzene (DNFB). In this study, mice were intraperitoneally injected with AA before, during or after sensitization with DNFB. If T cells of mice supplemented with AA during the sensitization were later stimulated ex vivo, higher levels of Th1 cytokines (TNF-α and IFN-γ) and lower levels of Th2 cytokines (IL-4) were observed. This effect was not observed when mice were supplemented with AA before or after sensitization [28]. This modulation of immune balance from Th2 to Th1 was also seen in another study, in which the effects of AA supplementation on asthma was studied. Here, AA supplementation (130 mg/kg/day for 5 weeks) of ovalbumin-sensitized mice significantly increased the IFN-γ/IL-5 secretion ratio in bronchoalveolar lavage fluid compared to control mice, confirming a shift from Th2 to Th1 [29]. The mechanism underpinning this effect has not been elucidated yet but it was suggested to be mediated by DCs. In an in vitro study, murine bone marrow-derived DCs were pre-treated with different doses of AA before being activated with lipopolysaccharide (LPS). The DCs that were treated with AA secreted more IL-12, a polarizing cytokine for Th1 cells. It also showed that naïve murine T cells, when co-cultured with these activated and AA treated murine DCs, produced more IFN-γ and less IL-5 verifying this effect [30].

While most studies focus on the Th1/Th2 balance, we found only one study that describes that Th17 polarization of sorted murine naïve CD4$^+$ cells is more effective in the presence of AA [31]. Interestingly, the investigators demonstrate that this effect is probably due to AA-mediated effects on histone demethylation that enhances the expression of the IL-17 locus.

In summary, multiple animal studies show that AA promotes Th1 differentiation at the expense of Th2 polarization. There is limited data showing that Th17 polarization is promoted by AA acting as an epigenetic regulator.

2.4. Memory T Cells and AA

Memory T cells constitute a small subset of lymphocytes but provide life-long immunity to previously encountered antigens. At this moment, the effects of AA on memory T cells is hardly investigated. Jeong et al. examined the effect of DCs pre-treated with AA on CD8$^+$ T cell differentiation. In vitro, murine bone marrow-derived DCs were pre-treated with AA before activation with LPS and, like in the earlier study from the same research group [30], secreted more IL12p70 but also more IL-15, a cytokine that is linked to memory T cell generation. These DCs in co-culture with murine T cells led to an enhanced CD8$^+$ memory T cell production. The effect was also seen in a mouse model for melanoma, in which the immune response and anti-melanoma effect of melanoma-primed DCs was enhanced if pre-treated with AA: the investigators observed increased generation of tumour-specific CD8$^+$ memory T cells and an increased protective effect for inoculated melanoma cells [32].

In summary, in vitro and in a mouse model AA increased the generation of CD8$^+$ memory T cells through increased production of stimulating cytokines by DCs.

2.5. Regulatory T Cells (Tregs) and AA

Tregs are important for the maintenance of immune-balance and self-tolerance. They are characterized by the expression of the transcription factor Foxp3, required for their immunosuppressive capacity. Stable expression of Foxp3 is dependent on DNA demethylation of a region in the first intron. Two recent in vivo and in vitro studies on murine Tregs found that AA stabilizes expression of

Foxp3 by promoting active Ten Eleven Translocation (TET) 2-mediated DNA methylation of this region. Thus, AA is required for the development and function of Tregs [33,34]. Concordantly, AA is a known co-factor for Ten Eleven Translocation (TET) family proteins that catalyse the first step of DNA demethylation: the conversion of 5-methyl-cytosine (5 mC) to 5-hydroxy-methyl-cytosine (5 hmC) [35,36]. For instance, in embryonic stem cells, AA was shown to be an important epigenetic regulator through this pathway [37]. The addition of AA to embryonic stem cell cultures induced demethylation of over 2000 genes within one hour [38].

In another study, the influence of AA on skin graft rejection in mice after treatment with ex vivo cultured and alloantigen-induced Tregs was investigated. The in vivo alloantigen-induced murine Tregs showed more DNA demethylation and stability of Foxp3 expression when cultured in the presence of AA. These Tregs also showed better suppressive capacity in vivo, thereby promoting skin allograft acceptance [39]. In a mouse model for graft-versus-host-disease (GVHD), the effects of AA on these ex vivo alloantigen-induced Tregs was determined [40]. GVHD is a serious and sometimes lethal complication following allogeneic hematopoietic stem cell transplantation caused by alloreactive donor T cells that induce tissue injury in the recipient. In this model, in vitro murine alloantigen-induced Tregs pre-treated with AA showed more stable Foxp3 expression when transferred into mice with acute GVHD and were clinically effective to diminish GVHD symptoms. Moreover, cultured human alloantigen-induced Tregs also had a higher Foxp3 expression if cultured with AA.

In contrast, in a mouse model for sepsis, AA was found to decrease the inhibition of Tregs [41]. Here, sepsis was induced in AA-deficient $Gulo^-/^-$ mice that were supplemented with AA (200 mg/kg twice) or not. AA administration improved survival in both wild type and $Gulo^-/^-$ mice and diminished the negative inhibition of Tregs by decreasing the expression of Foxp-3, CTLA-4, a protein that functions as an immune checkpoint and downregulates immune responses and the inhibitory cytokine TGF-β.

In summary, AA directly regulates Treg function via epigenetic regulation of the master transcription factor Foxp3. In most studies employing more chronic situations (transplantation, GVHD), Foxp3 expression is increased. In this way, AA can be useful in generating ex vivo allo-antigen-induced Tregs that can be used for clinical applications in transplantation and autoimmune disorders. In one model of acute sepsis in mice, AA administration decreased Foxp3 expression but was still beneficial for the outcome.

3. AA and B Lymphocytes

B lymphocytes are at the centre of the adaptive, humoral immune system. They are responsible for the production of antigen-specific immunoglobulin (Ig) directed against invasive pathogens (antibodies). Similar to other leukocytes, AA accumulated in B lymphocytes but there is only limited data on the function of AA in these cells.

3.1. B Lymphocyte Numbers and AA

In an early study investigating the effect of AA deficiency on numbers of lymphocytes in guinea pigs, animals on a 4-week AA-free diet showed a continuous increase in the percentage of B-lymphocytes while the percentage of T-lymphocytes decreased. The opposite effect was seen in animals on AA supplementation (25 and 250 mg intraperitoneally/day) [24]. In a more recent and extensive study, the effect of AA-2G, a stable vitamin C derivate, was investigated on mouse B cells in vitro. Mouse spleen B cells were cultured for 2 days with an anti-μ antibody in the presence of stimulating cytokines and then washed and recultured with and without AA-2G. In these cultures, the number of viable cells decreased much quicker without AA, resulting in about 70% more viable cells in cultures with AA than without AA. AA-2G also increased the production of IgM dose-dependently [42]. Another group that studied the effect of AA on mouse spleen B cells in vitro published contradictive results. They showed a slight dose-dependent increase of apoptosis (16% at a concentration of 1 mM) in murine IgM/CD40-activated B cells pre-treated with AA [43]. Tanaka et al. investigated the effect of AA on immune responses in human peripheral blood lymphocytes cultured for 7 days with and without AA-2G before stimulating them with pokeweed mitogen (PWM), a T cell dependent B cell stimulus. The cultures treated with AAS-2G showed an increased number of IgM and IgG-secreting cells after stimulation [44].

3.2. B Lymphocyte Function and AA

We only found limited and conflicting data on the effect of vitamin C on the production of antibodies by B lymphocytes. Two early studies in guinea pigs show that high-dose AA supplementation increases immunoglobulin levels after immunization with sheep red blood cells (SRBC) and bovine serum albumin (BSA) [45,46]. However, in two other animal models, AA supplementation did not have an effect on antigen-induced immunoglobulin levels after immunization [47,48]. One study determined the effect of high dose AA (2500 mg/day for 4 weeks) in mice sensitized by topical application of di-nitro-chlorobenzene (DNCB) and re-challenged 2 weeks later. They found no effect of AA on immunoglobulin levels [47]. In the other study, the effect of different low doses of AA (0, 30 and 60 mg) on the immune functions of dogs immunized with PWM was studied but no differences in PWM-specific IgG and IgA levels were observed [48]. However, the latter two studies were performed in animals that are able to synthetize AA, while guinea pigs cannot. In AA-synthetizing calves, AA supplementation (1.75 g/day) led to lower plasma IgG levels against keyhole limpet haemocyanin (KLH), a T cell dependent antigen that is often used in immunological studies in animals [49]. Two studies were performed in AA-sufficient chickens to investigate if AA supplementation is beneficial for vaccination against infectious bursal disease (IBD). Chickens with AA supplementation (1 g/mL) showed higher immunoglobulin levels compared to chickens without extra AA [50,51]. Furthermore, non-vaccinated chickens receiving AA supplementation did not show any symptoms or mortality after challenge with IBD while non-vaccinated chickens without AA all experienced clinical symptoms and only 70% survived [50].

In one study in healthy human volunteers, researchers found a correlation between serum IgG and plasma and leukocyte AA concentration and serum IgM and leukocyte AA concentration. After daily supplementation of 1 g AA during one week, serum IgG significantly rose in those healthy volunteers as did plasma and leukocyte AA concentration [52]. Likewise, another study in healthy human volunteers showed an increase in serum levels of IgM and IgA after 1 g/day supplementation of AA for 75 days [53]. These findings were contradicted in two other studies. In one study, the investigators examined the effect of 2–3 g AA supplementation per day on the production of all immunoglobins in healthy volunteers and did not find any change [54]. The other study is an earlier described placebo-controlled trial in elderly people where they received either an intramuscular injection of AA (500 mg/day) or a placebo for 1 month. Also in this trial, AA supplementation did not have any influence on serum IgA, IgM and IgG levels [26].

In conclusion, it is possible that vitamin C has an effect on the proliferation and function of B lymphocytes but the results until now are inconclusive. When conducting an intervention study of AA in cancer patients it would be interesting to also examine B cell levels and immunoglobulin changes.

4. AA and Natural Killer Cells

Next to B and T lymphocytes, NK cells are the most prominent lymphocyte subset as they make up to 20% of the blood lymphocyte population and are important for the immunity against pathogens (especially viruses) and for tumour surveillance. They are large granular lymphocytes arising from the same lymphoid progenitors as T and B lymphocytes and are primarily formed in the bone marrow. NK cells are innate lymphoid cells (ILCs) that provide fast, antigen-independent immunity. They exhibit direct cytotoxic effects, secrete cytokines and chemokines and regulate other immune cells. NK cell cytotoxicity is based on the absence of self MHC class I to discriminate between normal and diseased cells. Killing of these MHC class I missing target cells can only be initiated after simultaneous detection of activating signals, like stress signals, on the surface of tumour or infected cells.

Our knowledge about the effects of AA on NK cell development is limited. We previously described that AA (95 μM) enhances proliferation of mature NK cells from peripheral blood mononuclear cells (PBMCs) in vitro in a cytokine-stimulated culture [14]. AA also improved the generation and expansion of NK cell progenitors from hematopoietic stem cells and from T/NK cell progenitors in vitro in a cytokine-stimulated culture.

Other studies investigated the role of AA on the function of NK cells. In our previously described study, we tested functionality of the mature NK cells that were expanded in vitro in a cytotoxicity assay on K562 cells, a chronic myeloid leukaemia cell line that is often used to assess NK cell function in vitro. There was no difference in killing capacity between NK cells that were cultured with or without AA. [14]. In contrast, an earlier study on the cytotoxicity of fresh human NK cells isolated from peripheral blood that had different doses of AA (10 μM to 2.5 mM) present during the killing showed a dose-dependent decrease of NK cell mediated killing of K562 cells in vitro [55]. A similar experiment was repeated in another study but with different results. A presence of 3 mM AA increased the cytotoxicity of NK cells 105% in average, while no change was found using lower concentrations (10 μM, 0.1 mM and 1 mM) [56].

Another group also investigated the effect of AA on peripheral blood NK cell function using a cytotoxicity assay on K562 with NK cells from healthy volunteers that were supplemented with a single high dose of vitamin C. The study showed a biphasic effect on NK cell cytotoxicity: a slight decrease 1 to 2 h after supplementation followed by a significant enhancement at 8 h with a maximum effect after 24 h and return to normal after 48 h [57]. Plasma and leukocyte concentration of AA increased after 1 h and maximized after 2 to 4 h. After that, the levels declined but were still elevated up to 24 h after supplementation. Since NK cell function is often decreased after exposure to toxic chemicals, these researchers also performed a similar experiment in 55 patients that where accidently exposed to various toxic chemicals (for instance pesticides, metals and organic solvents). Almost half of these patients showed a very low baseline NK cell activity and in 78% of the patients there was significantly enhancement of cytotoxicity compared to baseline 24 h after ingestion of 60 mg/kg AA [58]. It is difficult to interpret these findings, since the patients were very diverse and there was no control group.

A comparable study was performed with NK cells isolated from peripheral blood of patients with β-thalassemia major. NK cells of these patients show a severe reduction in their cytotoxic function compared to healthy controls, possibly due to oxidative stress caused by iron overload after multiple blood transfusions [59]. AA (200 μg/mL) almost normalized the cytotoxic capacity of these NK cells, while the NK cell function of healthy controls did not change [60]. Remarkably, AA and iron are connected in many biological processes. For example, AA enhances the absorption of nonheme iron from the intestines [61] and AA is an essential cofactor in many enzymatic reaction by iron-dependent dioxygenases. The positive effect of AA on the NK cell function in this case is probably related to its antioxidant properties, since NK cells in patients with iron overload are known to have more intracellular reactive oxygen species (ROS) [62].

The effects of vitamin C on NK cell cytotoxicity against ovarian cancer cells was also studied in vivo in AA deficient mice. Gulo⁻/⁻ mice that are dependent on dietary AA were not supplemented for 2 weeks and sub sequentially inoculated with MOSECs (murine ovarian surface epithelial cells) and compared with Gulo⁻/⁻ mice that received normal AA supplementation. After the inoculation of tumour cells, all animals received normal AA supplementation. Gulo⁻/⁻ mice that were AA-depleted during this period survived shorter than supplemented mice. NK cells isolated from these AA-depleted mice showed a significant decrease in killing capacity in vitro compared to AA-supplemented mice and wildtype mice. In concordance, their NK cells showed reduced expression of the activating receptors CD69 and NKG2D. Furthermore, these NK cells produced less IFN-γ and displayed reduced production of the cytolytic proteins perforin and granzyme B [63].

In conclusion, AA might have different effects on NK cells during different stages. Early and late human NK cell development is enhanced by AA in vitro, however the effect in vivo remains to be shown. It is likely that the effect of AA at this time point is caused by its role as an epigenetic regulator, since this is also observed in T cells that share various developmental steps.

The influence of AA on NK cell function is not fully determined yet. In most in vitro studies in which NK cells of healthy volunteers (that probably have normal AA levels) were used, no effect of AA was observed. However, in AA-deficient mice, NK cell function was decreased compared to mice with normal levels of AA. Furthermore, in two human studies employing NK cells with an impaired function AA was able to restore NK cell function to almost normal. These results suggest that at least physiological levels of AA are necessary for normal NK cell function and AA is probably not able to increase the cytotoxicity of NK cells that function normally but can help to restore the function in NK cells that are impaired.

It is unknown whether next to NK cells, the development and function of recently identified other members of the ILC family are also enhanced by AA. This may be important, because other ILC subsets may also provide immunity while T cell immunity has not yet recovered. Furthermore, it has been shown that, in allogeneic HSCT higher ILC 3 numbers are associated with less GVHD [64].

5. Conclusions

AA has multiple effects on the development, proliferation and function of lymphocytes. An overview of these effects and the relationship between different cell types can be seen in Figure 1. T-lymphocytes have been most extensively studied in this context: AA positively influences T cell development and maturation, especially in case of AA deficiency. There is very limited and conflicting data on the effects of AA on B-lymphocyte biology. As for NK cells, AA positively influences NK cell proliferation but its role in NK cell function is less clear. A limited number of studies suggest that NK cell function required normal AA levels, while supraphysiological levels do not enhance NK cell function. Overall, most conclusions are based on in vitro studies, that are difficult to interpret and compare since there are many differences in experimental setups (multiple derivates of AA used in various concentrations and different incubation times). AA is also known to oxidate easily to dehydroascorbate in cell-cultures. The in vivo studies require careful interpretation as well: little data is available on local (intracellular) AA levels, while it is known that intracellular AA levels can be more than 1000-fold higher compared to plasma levels.

The studies discussed in the present review provide some insight in the mechanisms that underpin the effect on AA on lymphocytes. There are important indications that AA acts as an epigenetic regulator/cofactor in TET-mediated DNA and histone demethylation. Plausibly, AA's epigenetic functions are mostly seen in cells that undergo change (e.g., early T cell development, T helper cell differentiation). In situations of cells under stress (e.g., thalassemia, sepsis), the antioxidant properties of AA are probably more important.

Since AA is a cheap supplement with limited side-effects, it is worthwhile to speculate on its potential for cancer patients that are proven to have lower serum AA levels. Here, AA could enhance immune reconstitution after treatments that give long immunosuppression (for instance, patients receiving intensive chemotherapy for leukaemia or autologous HSCT) as most studies indicate a positive effect of AA supplementation on lymphocyte development. In this case, AA's effect on NK cells may be most significant, because NK cell reconstitution after myeloablative chemotherapy and HSCT is much faster than T cell reconstitution and could provide temporary immunity against infections [65]. Furthermore, NK cells are capable of recognizing and eliminating cancer cells. Currently, several clinical trials already study the anti-cancer potential of ex vivo generated NK cells. AA supplementation can be used to generate these NK cells in vitro but could also have an effect in vivo in the proliferation and survival of these cells. Furthermore, AA supplementation could may also positively influence T cell reconstitution after myeloablative therapy. It is possible that slow T cell regeneration is (partly) due to the AA-deficient state in these patients.

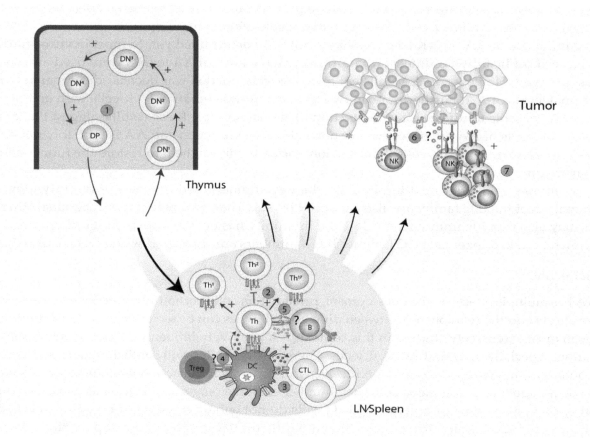

Figure 1. Effects of AA on Immune cells. **1.** T cell development: Enhanced T cell development due to fast transition from DN to DD stage. **2.** Th cell differentiation: skewing towards Th1 and Th17, with inhibition of Th2 polarization. **3.** CTL induction: Increased induction of CTLs due to production of IL-15 and IL-12 by DCs. **4.** Treg induction: Current data are conflicting. **5.** B cell: No conclusive data. **6.** NK cell function: No conclusive data. **7.** NK cell proliferation: increased NK cell proliferation.

On the other hand, AA supplementation in cancer patients may also have negative effects. Most of the curative effect of an allogeneic hematopoietic stem cell transplantation is attributed to the graft versus tumour effect mediated by the donor T cells that recognize cancer cells. This effect could potentially be diminished by increasing the amount and function of Tregs by vitamin C, as seen in some studies [33,34]. On the other hand, another study shows decreased Treg activity following AA administration [41]. In addition, stimulation of Tregs may also protect against GVHD.

Thus, AA plays a multitude of roles in lymphocyte development and function. However, its exact mechanism(s) of action and its effects in human health and disease are currently unknown. Given its safe profile and the fact that most animal studies have important limitations, we currently prepare a single arm phase II study to test the safety (GVHD) and efficacy of AA supplementation after allogeneic stem cell transplantation. This study is likely to provide important insights in how this vitamin functions in a complex, diseased organism and what groups of patients may benefit from this safe supplement.

Author Contributions: Gwendolyn N. Y. van Gorkom wrote the paper, Roel G. J. Klein Wolterink, Catharina H. M. J. Van Elssen, Lotte Wieten, Wilfred T. V. Germeraad and Gerard M. J. Bos were involved in the previous work on this topic in our group and/or substantively revised it.

References

1. Cameron, E.; Pauling, L. Supplemental ascorbate in the supportive treatment of cancer: Prolongation of survival times in terminal human cancer. *Proc. Natl. Acad. Sci. USA* **1976**, *73*, 3685–3689. [CrossRef] [PubMed]

2. Creagan, E.T.; Moertel, C.G.; O'Fallon, J.R.; Schutt, A.J.; O'Connell, M.J.; Rubin, J.; Frytak, S. Failure of high-dose vitamin C (ascorbic acid) therapy to benefit patients with advanced cancer. A controlled trial. *N. Engl. J. Med.* **1979**, *301*, 687–690. [CrossRef] [PubMed]

3. Moertel, C.G.; Fleming, T.R.; Creagan, E.T.; Rubin, J.; O'Connell, M.J.; Ames, M.M. High-dose vitamin C versus placebo in the treatment of patients with advanced cancer who have had no prior chemotherapy. A randomized double-blind comparison. *N. Engl. J. Med.* **1985**, *312*, 137–141. [CrossRef] [PubMed]

4. Young, J.I.; Zuchner, S.; Wang, G. Regulation of the Epigenome by Vitamin C. *Annu. Rev. Nutr.* **2015**, *35*, 545–564. [CrossRef] [PubMed]

5. Harrison, F.E.; Meredith, M.E.; Dawes, S.M.; Saskowski, J.L.; May, J.M. Low ascorbic acid and increased oxidative stress in gulo($^-$/$^-$) mice during development. *Brain Res.* **2010**, *1349*, 143–152. [CrossRef] [PubMed]

6. Uchio, R.; Hirose, Y.; Murosaki, S.; Yamamoto, Y.; Ishigami, A. High dietary intake of vitamin C suppresses age-related thymic atrophy and contributes to the maintenance of immune cells in vitamin C-deficient senescence marker protein-30 knockout mice. *Br. J. Nutr.* **2015**, *113*, 603–609. [CrossRef] [PubMed]

7. Carr, A.C.; Maggini, S. Vitamin C and Immune Function. *Nutrients* **2017**, *9*, 1211. [CrossRef] [PubMed]

8. Wilson, J.X. Regulation of vitamin C transport. *Annu. Rev. Nutr.* **2005**, *25*, 105–125. [CrossRef] [PubMed]

9. Omaye, S.T.; Schaus, E.E.; Kutnink, M.A.; Hawkes, W.C. Measurement of vitamin C in blood components by high-performance liquid chromatography. Implication in assessing vitamin C status. *Ann. N. Y. Acad. Sci.* **1987**, *498*, 389–401. [CrossRef] [PubMed]

10. Evans, R.M.; Currie, L.; Campbell, A. The distribution of ascorbic acid between various cellular components of blood, in normal individuals, and its relation to the plasma concentration. *Br. J. Nutr.* **1982**, *47*, 473–482. [CrossRef] [PubMed]

11. Roux, E.; Dumont-Girard, F.; Starobinski, M.; Siegrist, C.A.; Helg, C.; Chapuis, B.; Roosnek, E. Recovery of immune reactivity after T-cell-depleted bone marrow transplantation depends on thymic activity. *Blood* **2000**, *96*, 2299–2303. [PubMed]

12. Bosch, M.; Khan, F.M.; Storek, J. Immune reconstitution after hematopoietic cell transplantation. *Curr. Opin. Hematol.* **2012**, *19*, 324–335. [CrossRef] [PubMed]

13. Huijskens, M.J.; Walczak, M.; Koller, N.; Briede, J.J.; Senden-Gijsbers, B.L.; Schnijderberg, M.C.; Bos, G.M.; Germeraad, W.T. Technical advance: Ascorbic acid induces development of double-positive T cells from human hematopoietic stem cells in the absence of stromal cells. *J. Leukoc. Biol.* **2014**, *96*, 1165–1175. [CrossRef] [PubMed]

14. Huijskens, M.J.; Walczak, M.; Sarkar, S.; Atrafi, F.; Senden-Gijsbers, B.L.; Tilanus, M.G.; Bos, G.M.; Wieten, L.; Germeraad, W.T. Ascorbic acid promotes proliferation of natural killer cell populations in culture systems applicable for natural killer cell therapy. *Cytotherapy* **2015**, *17*, 613–620. [CrossRef] [PubMed]

15. Huijskens, M.J.; Wodzig, W.K.; Walczak, M.; Germeraad, W.T.; Bos, G.M. Ascorbic acid serum levels are reduced in patients with hematological malignancies. *Results Immunol.* **2016**, *6*, 8–10. [CrossRef] [PubMed]

16. Jenkinson, E.J.; Anderson, G.; Owen, J.J. Studies on T cell maturation on defined thymic stromal cell populations in vitro. *J. Exp. Med.* **1992**, *176*, 845–853. [CrossRef] [PubMed]

17. Schmitt, T.M.; Zuniga-Pflucker, J.C. Induction of T cell development from hematopoietic progenitor cells by delta-like-1 in vitro. *Immunity* **2002**, *17*, 749–756. [CrossRef]

18. Meek, B.; Cloosen, S.; Borsotti, C.; Van Elssen, C.H.; Vanderlocht, J.; Schnijderberg, M.C.; van der Poel, M.W.; Leewis, B.; Hesselink, R.; Manz, M.G.; et al. In vitro-differentiated T/natural killer-cell progenitors derived from human CD34$^+$ cells mature in the thymus. *Blood* **2010**, *115*, 261–264. [CrossRef] [PubMed]

19. Manning, J.; Mitchell, B.; Appadurai, D.A.; Shakya, A.; Pierce, L.J.; Wang, H.; Nganga, V.; Swanson, P.C.; May, J.M.; Tantin, D.; et al. Vitamin C promotes maturation of T-cells. *Antioxid. Redox Signal.* **2013**, *19*, 2054–2067. [CrossRef] [PubMed]

20. Campbell, J.D.; Cole, M.; Bunditrutavorn, B.; Vella, A.T. Ascorbic acid is a potent inhibitor of various forms of T cell apoptosis. *Cell. Immunol.* **1999**, *194*, 1–5. [CrossRef] [PubMed]

21. Maeng, H.G.; Lim, H.; Jeong, Y.J.; Woo, A.; Kang, J.S.; Lee, W.J.; Hwang, Y.I. Vitamin C enters mouse T cells as dehydroascorbic acid in vitro and does not recapitulate in vivo vitamin C effects. *Immunobiology* **2009**, *214*, 311–320. [CrossRef] [PubMed]

22. Eylar, E.; Baez, I.; Navas, J.; Mercado, C. Sustained levels of ascorbic acid are toxic and immunosuppressive for human T cells. *P. R. Health Sci. J.* **1996**, *15*, 21–26. [PubMed]

23. Hong, J.M.; Kim, J.H.; Kang, J.S.; Lee, W.J.; Hwang, Y.I. Vitamin C is taken up by human T cells via sodium-dependent vitamin C transporter 2 (SVCT2) and exerts inhibitory effects on the activation of these cells in vitro. *Anat. Cell Biol.* **2016**, *49*, 88–98. [CrossRef] [PubMed]

24. Fraser, R.C.; Pavlovic, S.; Kurahara, C.G.; Murata, A.; Peterson, N.S.; Taylor, K.B.; Feigen, G.A. The effect of variations in vitamin C intake on the cellular immune response of guinea pigs. *Am. J. Clin. Nutr.* **1980**, *33*, 839–847. [CrossRef] [PubMed]

25. Badr, G.; Bashandy, S.; Ebaid, H.; Mohany, M.; Sayed, D. Vitamin C supplementation reconstitutes polyfunctional T cells in streptozotocin-induced diabetic rats. *Eur. J. Nutr.* **2012**, *51*, 623–633. [CrossRef] [PubMed]

26. Kennes, B.; Dumont, I.; Brohee, D.; Hubert, C.; Neve, P. Effect of vitamin C supplements on cell-mediated immunity in old people. *Gerontology* **1983**, *29*, 305–310. [CrossRef] [PubMed]

27. Kay, N.E.; Holloway, D.E.; Hutton, S.W.; Bone, N.D.; Duane, W.C. Human T-cell function in experimental ascorbic acid deficiency and spontaneous scurvy. *Am. J. Clin. Nutr.* **1982**, *36*, 127–130. [CrossRef] [PubMed]

28. Noh, K.; Lim, H.; Moon, S.K.; Kang, J.S.; Lee, W.J.; Lee, D.; Hwang, Y.I. Mega-dose Vitamin C modulates T cell functions in Balb/c mice only when administered during T cell activation. *Immunol. Lett.* **2005**, *98*, 63–72. [CrossRef] [PubMed]

29. Chang, H.-H.; Chen, C.; Lin, J.-Y. High dose vitamin C supplementation increases the Th1/Th2 cytokine secretion ratio, but decreases eosinophilic infiltration in bronchoalveolar lavage fluid of ovalbumin-sensitized and challenged mice. *J. Agric. Food Chem.* **2009**, *57*, 10471–10476. [CrossRef] [PubMed]

30. Jeong, Y.J.; Hong, S.W.; Kim, J.H.; Jin, D.H.; Kang, J.S.; Lee, W.J.; Hwang, Y.I. Vitamin C-treated murine bone marrow-derived dendritic cells preferentially drive naive T cells into Th1 cells by increased IL-12 secretions. *Cell. Immunol.* **2011**, *266*, 192–199. [CrossRef] [PubMed]

31. Song, M.H.; Nair, V.S.; Oh, K.I. Vitamin C enhances the expression of IL17 in a Jmjd2-dependent manner. *BMB Rep.* **2017**, *50*, 49–54. [CrossRef] [PubMed]

32. Jeong, Y.J.; Kim, J.H.; Hong, J.M.; Kang, J.S.; Kim, H.R.; Lee, W.J.; Hwang, Y.I. Vitamin C treatment of mouse bone marrow-derived dendritic cells enhanced CD8(+) memory T cell production capacity of these cells in vivo. *Immunobiology* **2014**, *219*, 554–564. [CrossRef] [PubMed]

33. Sasidharan Nair, V.; Song, M.H.; Oh, K.I. Vitamin C Facilitates Demethylation of the Foxp3 Enhancer in a Tet-Dependent Manner. *J. Immunol.* **2016**, *196*, 2119–2131. [CrossRef] [PubMed]

34. Yue, X.; Trifari, S.; Aijo, T.; Tsagaratou, A.; Pastor, W.A.; Zepeda-Martinez, J.A.; Lio, C.W.; Li, X.; Huang, Y.; Vijayanand, P.; et al. Control of Foxp3 stability through modulation of TET activity. *J. Exp. Med.* **2016**, *213*, 377–397. [CrossRef] [PubMed]

35. Tahiliani, M.; Koh, K.P.; Shen, Y.; Pastor, W.A.; Bandukwala, H.; Brudno, Y.; Agarwal, S.; Iyer, L.M.; Liu, D.R.; Aravind, L.; et al. Conversion of 5-methylcytosine to 5-hydroxymethylcytosine in mammalian DNA by MLL partner TET1. *Science* **2009**, *324*, 930–935. [CrossRef] [PubMed]

36. Ito, S.; D'Alessio, A.C.; Taranova, O.V.; Hong, K.; Sowers, L.C.; Zhang, Y. Role of Tet proteins in 5mC to 5hmC conversion, ES-cell self-renewal and inner cell mass specification. *Nature* **2010**, *466*, 1129–1133. [CrossRef] [PubMed]

37. Blaschke, K.; Ebata, K.T.; Karimi, M.M.; Zepeda-Martinez, J.A.; Goyal, P.; Mahapatra, S.; Tam, A.; Laird, D.J.; Hirst, M.; Rao, A.; et al. Vitamin C induces Tet-dependent DNA demethylation and a blastocyst-like state in ES cells. *Nature* **2013**, *500*, 222–226. [CrossRef] [PubMed]

38. Chung, T.L.; Brena, R.M.; Kolle, G.; Grimmond, S.M.; Berman, B.P.; Laird, P.W.; Pera, M.F.; Wolvetang, E.J. Vitamin C promotes widespread yet specific DNA demethylation of the epigenome in human embryonic stem cells. *Stem Cells* **2010**, *28*, 1848–1855. [CrossRef] [PubMed]

39. Nikolouli, E.; Hardtke-Wolenski, M.; Hapke, M.; Beckstette, M.; Geffers, R.; Floess, S.; Jaeckel, E.; Huehn, J. Alloantigen-Induced Regulatory T Cells Generated in Presence of Vitamin C Display Enhanced Stability of Foxp3 Expression and Promote Skin Allograft Acceptance. *Front. Immunol.* **2017**, *8*, 748. [CrossRef] [PubMed]

40. Kasahara, H.; Kondo, T.; Nakatsukasa, H.; Chikuma, S.; Ito, M.; Ando, M.; Kurebayashi, Y.; Sekiya, T.; Yamada, T.; Okamoto, S.; et al. Generation of allo-antigen-specific induced Treg stabilized by vitamin C treatment and its application for prevention of acute graft versus host disease model. *Int. Immunol.* **2017**, *29*, 457–469. [CrossRef] [PubMed]

41. Gao, Y.; Lu, B.; Zhai, J.; Liu, Y.; Qi, H.; Yao, Y.; Chai, Y.; Shou, S. The Parenteral Vitamin C Improves Sepsis and Sepsis-Induced Multiple Organ Dysfunction Syndrome via Preventing Cellular Immunosuppression. *Mediat. Inflamm.* **2017**, *2017*, 4024672. [CrossRef] [PubMed]

42. Ichiyama, K.; Mitsuzumi, H.; Zhong, M.; Tai, A.; Tsuchioka, A.; Kawai, S.; Yamamoto, I.; Gohda, E. Promotion of IL-4- and IL-5-dependent differentiation of anti-µ-primed B cells by ascorbic acid 2-glucoside. *Immunol. Lett.* **2009**, *122*, 219–226. [CrossRef] [PubMed]

43. Woo, A.; Kim, J.H.; Jeong, Y.J.; Maeng, H.G.; Lee, Y.T.; Kang, J.S.; Lee, W.J.; Hwang, Y.I. Vitamin C acts indirectly to modulate isotype switching in mouse B cells. *Anat. Cell Biol.* **2010**, *43*, 25–35. [CrossRef] [PubMed]

44. Tanaka, M.; Muto, N.; Gohda, E.; Yamamoto, I. Enhancement by ascorbic acid 2-glucoside or repeated additions of ascorbate of mitogen-induced IgM and IgG productions by human peripheral blood lymphocytes. *Jpn. J. Pharmacol.* **1994**, *66*, 451–456. [CrossRef] [PubMed]

45. Prinz, W.; Bloch, J.; Gilich, G.; Mitchell, G. A systematic study of the effect of vitamin C supplementation on the humoral immune response in ascorbate-dependent mammals. I. The antibody response to sheep red blood cells (a T-dependent antigen) in guinea pigs. *Int. J. Vitam. Nutr. Res.* **1980**, *50*, 294–300. [PubMed]

46. Feigen, G.A.; Smith, B.H.; Dix, C.E.; Flynn, C.J.; Peterson, N.S.; Rosenberg, L.T.; Pavlovic, S.; Leibovitz, B. Enhancement of antibody production and protection against systemic anaphylaxis by large doses of vitamin C. *Res. Commun. Chem. Pathol. Pharmacol.* **1982**, *38*, 313–333. [CrossRef]

47. Albers, R.; Bol, M.; Bleumink, R.; Willems, A.A.; Pieters, R.H. Effects of supplementation with vitamins A, C, and E, selenium, and zinc on immune function in a murine sensitization model. *Nutrition* **2003**, *19*, 940–946. [CrossRef]

48. Hesta, M.; Ottermans, C.; Krammer-Lukas, S.; Zentek, J.; Hellweg, P.; Buyse, J.; Janssens, G.P. The effect of vitamin C supplementation in healthy dogs on antioxidative capacity and immune parameters. *J. Anim. Physiol. Anim. Nutr.* **2009**, *93*, 26–34. [CrossRef] [PubMed]

49. Goodwin, J.S.; Garry, P.J. Relationship between megadose vitamin supplementation and immunological function in a healthy elderly population. *Clin. Exp. Immunol.* **1983**, *51*, 647–653. [PubMed]

50. Amakye-Anim, J.; Lin, T.L.; Hester, P.Y.; Thiagarajan, D.; Watkins, B.A.; Wu, C.C. Ascorbic acid supplementation improved antibody response to infectious bursal disease vaccination in chickens. *Poult. Sci.* **2000**, *79*, 680–688. [CrossRef] [PubMed]

51. Wu, C.C.; Dorairajan, T.; Lin, T.L. Effect of ascorbic acid supplementation on the immune response of chickens vaccinated and challenged with infectious bursal disease virus. *Vet. Immunol. Immunopathol.* **2000**, *74*, 145–152. [CrossRef]

52. Vallance, S. Relationships between ascorbic acid and serum proteins of the immune system. *Br. Med. J.* **1977**, *2*, 437–438. [CrossRef] [PubMed]

53. Prinz, W.; Bortz, R.; Bregin, B.; Hersch, M. The effect of ascorbic acid supplementation on some parameters of the human immunological defence system. *Int. J. Vitam. Nutr. Res.* **1977**, *47*, 248–257. [PubMed]

54. Anderson, R.; Oosthuizen, R.; Maritz, R.; Theron, A.; Van Rensburg, A.J. The effects of increasing weekly doses of ascorbate on certain cellular and humoral immune functions in normal volunteers. *Am. J. Clin. Nutr.* **1980**, *33*, 71–76. [CrossRef] [PubMed]

55. Huwyler, T.; Hirt, A.; Morell, A. Effect of ascorbic acid on human natural killer cells. *Immunol. Lett.* **1985**, *10*, 173–176. [CrossRef]

56. Toliopoulos, I.K.; Simos, Y.V.; Daskalou, T.A.; Verginadis, I.I.; Evangelou, A.M.; Karkabounas, S.C. Inhibition of platelet aggregation and immunomodulation of NK lymphocytes by administration of ascorbic acid. *Indian J. Exp. Biol.* **2011**, *49*, 904–908. [PubMed]

57. Vojdani, A.; Ghoneum, M. In vivo effect of ascorbic acid on enhancement of natural killer cell activity. *Nutr. Res.* **1993**, *13*, 753–764. [CrossRef]

58. Heuser, G.; Vojdani, A. Enhancement of natural killer cell activity and T and B cell function by buffered vitamin C in patients exposed to toxic chemicals: The role of protein kinase-C. *Immunopharmacol. Immunotoxicol.* **1997**, *19*, 291–312. [CrossRef] [PubMed]

59. Farmakis, D.; Giakoumis, A.; Polymeropoulos, E.; Aessopos, A. Pathogenetic aspects of immune deficiency associated with beta-thalassemia. *Med. Sci. Monit.* **2003**, *9*, Ra19–R22. [PubMed]

60. Atasever, B.; Ertan, N.Z.; Erdem-Kuruca, S.; Karakas, Z. In vitro effects of vitamin C and selenium on NK activity of patients with beta-thalassemia major. *Pediatr. Hematol. Oncol.* **2006**, *23*, 187–197. [CrossRef] [PubMed]

61. Lynch, S.R.; Cook, J.D. Interaction of vitamin C and iron. *Ann. N. Y. Acad. Sci.* **1980**, *355*, 32–44. [CrossRef] [PubMed]

62. Hua, Y.; Wang, C.; Jiang, H.; Wang, Y.; Liu, C.; Li, L.; Liu, H.; Shao, Z.; Fu, R. Iron overload may promote alteration of NK cells and hematopoietic stem/progenitor cells by JNK and P38 pathway in myelodysplastic syndromes. *Int. J. Hematol.* **2017**, *106*, 248–257. [CrossRef] [PubMed]

63. Kim, J.E.; Cho, H.S.; Yang, H.S.; Jung, D.J.; Hong, S.W.; Hung, C.F.; Lee, W.J.; Kim, D. Depletion of ascorbic acid impairs NK cell activity against ovarian cancer in a mouse model. *Immunobiology* **2012**, *217*, 873–881. [CrossRef] [PubMed]

64. Munneke, J.M.; Bjorklund, A.T.; Mjosberg, J.M.; Garming-Legert, K.; Bernink, J.H.; Blom, B.; Huisman, C.; van Oers, M.H.; Spits, H.; Malmberg, K.J.; et al. Activated innate lymphoid cells are associated with a reduced susceptibility to graft-versus-host disease. *Blood* **2014**, *124*, 812–821. [CrossRef] [PubMed]

65. Vacca, P.; Montaldo, E.; Croxatto, D.; Moretta, F.; Bertaina, A.; Vitale, C.; Locatelli, F.; Mingari, M.C.; Moretta, L. NK Cells and Other Innate Lymphoid Cells in Hematopoietic Stem Cell Transplantation. *Front. Immunol.* **2016**, *7*, 188. [CrossRef] [PubMed]

7

Vitamin C Intake is Inversely Associated with Cardiovascular Mortality in a Cohort of Spanish Graduates: The SUN Project

Nerea Martín-Calvo [1,2,3] 🆔 and Miguel Ángel Martínez-González [1,2,3,4,*]

[1] Department of Preventive Medicine and Public Health, University of Navarra,
    31008 Pamplona, Navarra, Spain; nmartincalvo@unav.es
[2] IdiSNA, Navarra Institute for Health Research, 31008 Pamplona, Navarra, Spain
[3] CIBER Physiopathology of Obesity and Nutrition (CIBERobn), Carlos III Institute of Health,
    28029 Madrid, Spain
[4] Department of Nutrition, Harvard T.H. Chan School of Public Health, Boston, MA 02115, USA
[*] Correspondence: mamartinez@unav.es

Abstract: Observational studies have found a protective effect of vitamin C on cardiovascular health. However, results are inconsistent, and residual confounding by fiber might be present. The aim of this study was to assess the association of vitamin C with the incidence of cardiovascular disease (CVD) and cardiovascular mortality (CVM) while accounting for fiber intake and adherence to the Mediterranean dietary pattern. We followed up 13,421 participants in the Seguimiento Universidad de Navarra (University of Navarra follow-up) (SUN) cohort for a mean time of 11 years. Information was collected at baseline and every two years through mailed questionnaires. Diet was assessed with a validated semi-quantitative food frequency questionnaire. Incident CVD was defined as incident fatal or non-fatal myocardial infarction, fatal or non-fatal stroke, or death due to any cardiovascular cause. CVM was defined as death due to cardiovascular causes. Events were confirmed by physicians in the study team after revision of medical records. Cox proportional hazard models were fitted to assess the associations of (a) energy-adjusted and (b) fiber-adjusted vitamin C intake with CVD and CVM. We found energy-adjusted vitamin C was inversely associated with CVD and CVM after adjusting for several confounding factors, including fiber from foods other than fruits and vegetables, and adherence to the Mediterranean dietary pattern. On the other hand, when vitamin C was adjusted for total fiber intake using the residuals method, we found a significant inverse association with CVM (HR (95% confidence interval (CI)) for the third tertile compared to the first tertile, 0.30 (0.12–0.72), but not with CVD in the fully adjusted model.

Keywords: vitamin C; cardiovascular disease; cardiovascular mortality; fiber

---

1. Introduction

Vitamin C, also known as L-ascorbic acid, is a water-soluble vitamin naturally present in some foods, added to others, and available as dietary supplement. Vitamin C is an essential dietary component, since humans, unlike most animals, are unable to synthetize it. Vitamin C is required for the synthesis of collagen, L-carnitine and some neurotransmitters. Based on vitamin C's antioxidant capacity, there is growing interest in assessing whether vitamin C intake might help prevent or delay some type of cancer, cardiovascular disease (CVD) or other diseases in which oxidative stress plays an important role.

Recommended dietary allowances (RDA) for vitamin C—75 mg/day for women and 90 mg/day for men [1]—are based on its known physiological and antioxidant functions in white blood cells and are higher than the amount required to prevent deficiency. Nevertheless, given that vitamin C may relate to cancer, CVD, or other diseases through different mechanisms, whether classical RDAs are optimal to obtain maximum benefits is unclear [2].

The belief that vitamin C relates to cardiovascular health stemmed from the benefits observed from fruit and vegetable consumption [3–5]. Observational studies have found an inverse association of dietary vitamin C [6] and ascorbic acid plasma levels [6–8] with cardiovascular risk factors, CVD, and cardiovascular mortality (CVM). Nevertheless, those studies showed some limitations, including suboptimal adjustment for potential confounders such as fiber intake.

Vitamin C from foods and supplements seemed to be equally bioavailable [9]. However, observational studies [6] and clinical trials [10–13] concluded that supplementation with vitamin C (500 to 1000 mg/day) had no effect on different cardiovascular endpoints. Moreover, higher CVM and total mortality has been reported among participants under vitamin C supplementation in both observational [14] and interventional studies [15]. On the other hand, two meta-analyses reported that high dose supplementation with vitamin C ((500 to 2000 mg/day) and (500 to 4000 mg/day) respectively) was associated to endothelial function improvements [16] and reduced blood pressure [17].

The aim of this study was to assess whether vitamin C intake was independently associated with lower CVD and CVM risk among participants in the Seguimiento Universidad de Navarra (University of Navarra follow-up) (SUN) cohort.

2. Materials and Methods

2.1. Study Population

The SUN project is an ongoing, prospective and multipurpose cohort of Spanish university graduates. As a dynamic cohort, enrolment is permanently open, and follow-up information is gathered by mailed questionnaires every two years. Regarding the obtention of informed consent of potential participants, we duly informed these potential candidates of their right to refuse to participate in the SUN study or to withdraw their consent to participate at any time without reprisal, according to the principles of the Declaration of Helsinki. Special attention was given to the specific information needs of individual potential candidates as well as to the methods used to deliver their information and the feedback that may receive in the future from the research team. After ensuring that the candidate had understood the information, we sought their potential freely-given informed consent, and their voluntary completion of the baseline questionnaire. These methods were accepted by our Institutional Review Board as to imply an appropriately-obtained informed consent. A more detailed description of the SUN methodology can be found elsewhere [18]. The study protocol was approved by the Institutional Review Board of the University of Navarra (approval code 010830).

We assessed 22,280 participants recruited before March 2014 to ensure they completed at least the two-year follow-up questionnaire. We excluded 308 participants due to prevalent cardiovascular disease, 7384 participants younger than 40 years old who were considered too young to present a cardiovascular event during the follow-up, 290 participants with energy intake out of the sex-specific limits (under p1 or above p99), and 284 participants with vitamin C intake out of the sex-specific limits (under p1 or above p99). Out of the rest of the participants, 593 were lost to follow-up (retention in the cohort: 96%), leading to a final sample of 13,421 participants (Figure 1).

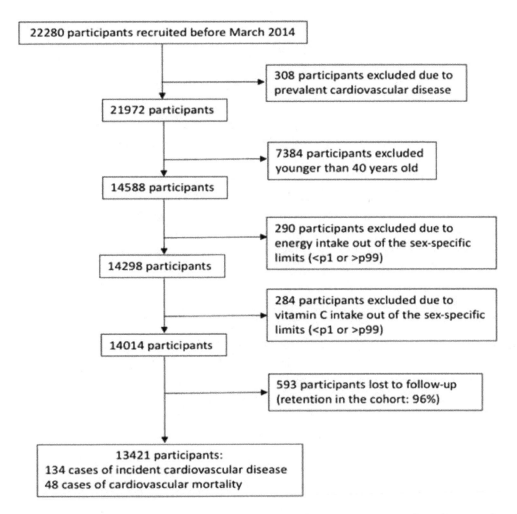

Figure 1. Flow chart of participants for the assessment of the association of cardiovascular disease and cardiovascular mortality with vitamin C intake in the Seguimiento Universidad de Navarra (University of Navarra follow-up) (SUN) cohort (follow-up 1999–2016).

2.2. Exposure Assessment

Participants were asked to complete a previously validated semi-quantitative food frequency questionnaire (FFQ) [19,20] and report how often on average they had consumed 136 foods and beverages during the past year. The FFQ had nine categories for intake frequency, from never to two or more servings per day. Multivitamin and supplements users were asked to specify the brand of multivitamin or supplement, the dose, and frequency of use. The nutritional content of each food was obtained from Spanish food composition guides [21,22] and supplemented with information from food and supplement manufacturers when needed. The nutrient contribution of each food item was calculated by multiplying the frequency of food consumption by the nutrient composition of the specified portion size. Dietary vitamin C intake was adjusted for energy intake using the residuals method, and categorized into tertiles. Total vitamin C intake was estimated by summing the vitamin C contribution of food items and supplements. In ancillary analyses, we assessed the independent effect of vitamin C from foods additionally adjusted for supplement intake (dichotomous variable).

In further analyses, to nullify the correlation between vitamin C and fiber, dietary vitamin C was alternatively adjusted for total fiber intake using the residuals method.

2.3. Outcome Assessment

Incident CVD was defined as either incident fatal or non-fatal myocardial infarction (with or without ST elevation), or fatal or non-fatal stroke and death due to other cardiovascular causes. CVM was defined as death due to cardiovascular causes.

Information about the events was initially gathered from follow-up questionnaires. When participants reported any of the previously mentioned events, they were asked for their medical reports, which were evaluated by physicians in the study team who were blinded to the nutritional information. Myocardial infarction was diagnosed using universal criteria. Non-fatal stroke was defined as sudden onset focal-neurological lack with a vascular mechanism that last more than 24 h. Confirmed events were classified according to the International Classification of Diseases (ICD-10). I21 and I63 codes were considered to define cardiovascular events [23]. The National Death Index is checked at least once a year to confirm the vital status of participants during follow-up. Deaths were reported by either participant's next of kin, work associates, or postal authorities.

Participants were followed-up from enrollment until December 2016, the diagnosis of the event, or death, whichever came first.

2.4. Covariates

Information about socio-demographic and anthropometric characteristics, lifestyle (physical activity, television watching, smoking status), classical cardiovascular risk factors (hypertension, hypercholesterolemia, hypertriglyceridemia and diabetes), prevalent diseases (cancer and cardiovascular related diseases), and family history of stroke and cardiovascular-related medication was collected at baseline.

Age was calculated as the difference between the date of recruitment and the date of birth. Body mass index (BMI) was calculated by dividing participants' weight (kg) by their squared height (m). A validation study in a subset of the SUN cohort showed that self-reported weight and height were highly reproducible and specific [24].

Dietary information was obtained from the baseline FFQ. Energy (kcal/day) and fiber (mg/day) intakes were calculated by multiplying the frequency of each food item consumed by the energy and fiber contribution of its specified portion size. Total energy and fiber intakes were calculated as the sum of energy and fiber provided by each food item. We also calculated the adherence to the Mediterranean dietary pattern based on the information from the FFQ using the classical Mediterranean Dietary Score (MDS) [25] without the fruit- and vegetable-related items (total seven items). We defined three categories of adherence to the MDS: Low (from 0 to 2 points), medium (from 3 to 4 points), and high (from 5 to 7 points).

Physical activity was collected at baseline with a previously validated questionnaire [26] that included 17 activities and 10 categories of response, from never to eleven or more hours per week. METs-h/week for each activity were calculated by multiplying the number of Metabolic Equivalent of Task (METs) of each activity [27] by the weekly participation in that activity, weighted according to the number of months dedicated to each activity. Total physical activity was quantified by summing the METs-h/week dedicated to all activities performed during leisure time. Time spent watching television was used as a proxy of sedentary behavior [28]. Hours per week of television watching were calculated as the mean of hours spent watching television during weekdays and hours spent watching television during weekends. Missing data were imputed based on the values of other covariates.

Cardiovascular-related diseases at baseline (coronary heart disease, tachycardia, atrial fibrillation, aortic aneurism, heart failure, venous thrombosis, and claudication) were grouped in a single quantitative variable (number of cardiovascular-related diseases) included in the multivariable adjustment. Validation studies in the SUN cohort showed self-reported information about cardiovascular risk factors was valid as to be used in epidemiological studies [29,30].

2.5. Statistical Analysis

Baseline characteristics of participants were presented by tertiles of total vitamin C intake as mean (standard deviation) for quantitative variables, and as proportions for qualitative variables. A *p* value for trend across tertiles was calculated using simple linear or logistic regressions.

We fitted Cox proportional hazard models to assess the association of energy-adjusted vitamin C intake with CVD and CVM. We estimated the hazard ratios (HR) and their 95% confidence intervals (CI) for second and third tertile of vitamin C intake compare to the lowest tertile (category of reference). Age was used as the underlying time variable in all the models. We fitted five multivariable adjusted models: (1) adjusted for age and sex; (2) additionally adjusted for body mass index (continuous), total energy intake (continuous), physical activity (continuous), television watching (continuous), smoking (never, current, or former), family history of stroke (dichotomus) and treatment with aspirin (dichotomus); (3) additionally adjusted for number of cardiovascular-related diseases at baseline (discrete), prevalent cancer (dichotomus), prevalent hypertension (dichotomus), prevalent diabetes (dichotomus), prevalent hypercholesterolemia (dichotomus) and prevalent hypertriglyceridemia (dichotomus); (4) additionally adjusted for dietary fiber (fiber from foods other than fruits and vegetables) (continuous); and (5) additionally adjusted for adherence to the MDS (without the fruit- and vegetable-related items (low, medium or high).

Interactions with vitamin C supplements intake, total fiber intake and age at the end of follow-up were assessed for both CVD and CVM by adding an interaction product term to the model and calculating the maximum likelihood ratio test.

In ancillary analyses, we evaluated the association of tertiles of dietary vitamin C with CVD and CVM fitting a model additionally adjusted for vitamin C supplements intake (dichotomus).

In further analyses, we re-ran the multivariable adjusted models for fiber-adjusted vitamin C intake categorized into tertiles.

Analyses were performed with STATA version 12.0 (StataCorp, College Station, TX, USA).

3. Results

We followed-up 13,421 participants for a mean time of 10.9 years (the standard deviation (SD) = 3.82). Baseline characteristics of participants by tertiles of vitamin C intake are described in Table 1. Participants in the highest tertile of vitamin C intake (from 320 to 1110 mg/day) were older, more likely to be women, and less likely to be current smokers. They were also more physically active and spent less time watching television. Moreover, they reported higher fiber intake and greater adherence to the Mediterranean dietary patter (MDP). We found total vitamin C intake showed a modest correlation with energy intake ($r = 0.33$), but it was highly correlated with total fiber intake ($r = 0.72$). Similar results were found for dietary vitamin C.

Aortic aneurism, heart failure, and hypertriglyceridemia at baseline were less prevalent among participants with higher vitamin C intake. However, cancer, venous thrombosis, diabetes, hypertension, and family history of stroke at baseline were more prevalent, probably due to the older age of participants with higher intake of vitamin C. Participants in the highest tertile of vitamin C intake were more likely to be under treatment with diuretics, antihypertensives, aspirin, and other cardiovascular treatment drugs.

Table 1. Baseline characteristics of participants over 40 years old in the SUN cohort by tertiles of total vitamin C intake. Numbers are means (SD) or percentages.

Baseline Characteristics	Tertiles of Vitamin C Intake			
	Q1	Q2	Q3	p
N	4474	4474	4473	
Vitamin C intake (mg/day)	148 (44.2)	257 (33.0)	445 (114)	<0.001
Fiber intake (g/day)	23.0 (10.0)	27.8 (9.8)	38.3 (14.1)	<0.001
Vittamin C range (mg/day)	0–205	206–319	320–1110	
Vittamin C from supplements (mg/day)	0.56 (4.2)	2.0 (10.0)	9.6 (33.4)	<0.001
Sex (female)	41.6	55.8	67.9	<0.001
Age (years)	41.2 (10.3)	42.8 (10.7)	43.7 (10.8)	<0.001
BMI (kg/m^2)	24.3 (3.6)	24.1 (3.5)	23.8 (3.5)	<0.001
Mediterranean Dietary Score [§]				<0.001
Low (0–2 points)	39.0	29.6	21.4	
Medium (3–4 points)	47.3	50.9	51.1	
High (5–7 points)	13.7	19.5	27.5	
Energy intake (kcal/day)	2548 (804)	2346 (710)	2530 (755)	0.26
Physical activity (MET-h/week)	23.4 (20.6)	25.8 (21.6)	29.2 (25.3)	<0.001
Television time (h/week)	1.63 (1.1)	1.57 (1.1)	1.51 (1.1)	<0.001
Family history of myocardial infarction	15.8	18.3	17.1	0.09
Smoking				0.03
Never	43	44	44	
Current	29	23	22	
Former	28	33	34	
Prevalent diseases				
Cancer	3.7	4.6	5.6	<0.001
Coronary heart disease	0.38	0.47	0.27	0.39
Tachycardia	1.9	1.6	2.3	0.12
Atrial fibrillation	0.65	0.72	0.69	0.80
Aortic aneurism	0.25	0.11	0.02	0.01
Heart failure	0.42	0.56	0.38	0.75
Pulmonary embolism	0.13	0.09	0.11	0.75
Venous thrombosis	0.51	0.92	0.92	0.03
Claudication	0.31	0.31	0.56	0.07
Diabetes	1.4	2.2	3.0	<0.001
Hypertension	9.7	11.3	10.9	0.07
Hypercholesterolemia	20.0	21.9	20.7	0.42
Hypertriglyceridemia	8.5	8.9	7.3	0.04
Drugs				
Digoxin	0.11	0.13	0.13	0.77
Diuretics	1.0	1.6	1.7	0.01
Beta blockers	1.7	2.3	1.9	0.40
Calcium antagonists	0.40	0.45	0.63	0.13
Nitrite	0.13	0.11	0.18	0.57
Antihypertensives	2.8	4.1	3.7	0.03
Aspirin	3.4	5.2	4.9	0.001
Other CV treatment drug	5.2	6.9	6.6	0.01

[§] Mediterranean Diet Score without the fruit- and vegetable-related items. N = 13,421.

Multivariable-adjusted associations of total vitamin C intake with both CVD and CVM are showed in Figure 2.

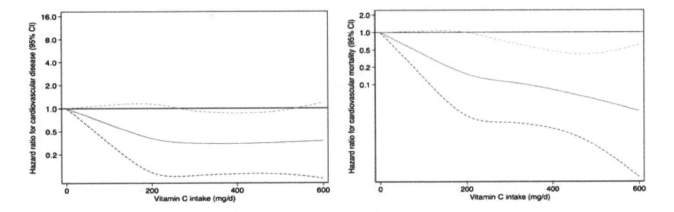

Figure 2. Restricted Cubic Splines for the Hazard Ratio (HR) and 95% Confidence Interval (CI) for cardiovascular disease and cardiovascular mortality associated with total vitamin C intake in the SUN cohort (follow-up 1999–2016). Age strata as underlying time variable. Multivariable model adjusted for sex, body mass index (continuous), total energy intake (continuous), physical activity (continuous), television watching (continuous), smoking (never, current or former), family history of stroke, treatment with aspirin, number of cardiovascular-related diseases at baseline, prevalent cancer, prevalent hypertension, prevalent diabetes, prevalent hypercholesterolemia, prevalent hypertriglyceridemia, fiber (from foods other than fruits and vegetables) (continuous), and Mediterranean Dietary Score (MDS) without fruit- and vegetable-related items (low, medium, high).

3.1. Cardiovascular Disease

A total of 134 cases of CVD were identified over 146,973 person-years at risk. The cumulative risk of a cardiovascular event was 0.07% in the highest tertile versus 0.12% in the lowest tertile of vitamin C intake.

We found that higher vitamin C intake was associated with a lower risk of CVD in the age-adjusted analysis (Table 2). Moreover, this association remained significant in the age and sex-adjusted model, in the model adjusted for demographic, metabolic, and lifestyle risk factors (multivariable adjusted model 1), and in the model additionally adjusted for prevalent diseases at baseline (multivariable adjusted model 2). Further adjustment for fiber intake (multivariable adjusted model 3) did not change the results. In the fully adjusted model (multivariable adjusted model 4), we found that, compared with participants in the first tertile of vitamin C intake, those in the second and third tertiles showed significant lower risk of CVD (HR (95% CI): 0.60 (0.40–0.91) and 0.62 (0.40–0.97), respectively).

High vitamin C intake showed no significant association with CVD when fiber from fruits and vegetables was also considered. HRs (95% CI) for the third tertile in models 3 and 4 were 0.66 (0.39–1.10) and 0.68 (0.40–1.13), respectively. Nevertheless, the association was still significant when the second and third tertiles were considered together (HR (95% CI): 0.63 (0.41–0.94) for model 3 and 0.64 (0.43–0.88) for model 4).

Neither age at the end of follow-up ($p = 0.79$) nor fiber intake ($p = 0.15$) resulted in effect modification. Marginally significant interaction was found between total vitamin C and vitamin C supplementation ($p = 0.05$).

Table 2. Hazard Ratio (HR) and 95% Confidence Interval (CI) for cardiovascular disease (CVD) associated with total vitamin C intake for participants over 40 years old in the SUN cohort (follow-up 1999–2016).

Main Analyses [§]	Tertiles of Vitamin C Intake		
	Q1 (N = 4474)	Q2 (N = 4474)	Q3 (N = 4473)
Incident CVD (person-years at risk)	61 (50,792)	38 (48,765)	35 (47,415)
Age-adjusted	1.00 (Ref.)	0.52 (0.35–0.78)	0.44 (0.29–0.67)
Sex- and age-adjusted	1.00 (Ref.)	0.59 (0.39–0.89)	0.56 (0.37–0.86)
Multivariable adjusted model 1	1.00 (Ref.)	0.59 (0.39–0.90)	0.60 (0.39–0.93)
T2 + T3 vs. T1	1.00 (Ref.)	0.60 (0.42–0.85)	
Multivariable adjusted model 2	1.00 (Ref.)	0.58 (0.38–0.88)	0.58 (0.37–0.90)
T2 + T3 vs. T1	1.00 (Ref.)	0.58 (0.41–0.83)	
Multivariable adjusted model 3	1.00 (Ref.)	0.58 (0.38–0.88)	0.58 (0.37–0.90)
T2 + T3 vs. T1	1.00 (Ref.)	0.58 (0.41–0.83)	
Multivariable adjusted model 4	1.00 (Ref.)	0.60 (0.40–0.91)	0.62 (0.40–0.97)
T2 + T3 vs. T1	1.00 (Ref.)	0.61 (0.43–0.88)	

[§] Age strata as underlying time variable in all the models; N = 13,421; Ref: reference category. Multivariable adjusted **model 1**: Additionally adjusted for sex, body mass index (continuous), total energy intake (continuous), physical activity (continuous), television watching (continuous), smoking (never, current or former), family history of stroke, and treatment with aspirin. Multivariable adjusted **model 2**: Additionally adjusted for the number of cardiovascular-related diseases at baseline, prevalent cancer, prevalent hypertension, prevalent diabetes, prevalent hypercholesterolemia and prevalent hypertrygliceridemia. Multivariable adjusted **model 3**: Additionally adjusted for dietary fiber (fiber from foods other than fruits and vegetables) (continuous). Multivariable adjusted **model 4**: Additionally adjusted for the MDS without fruit and vegetable intake related items (low, medium, or high).

3.2. Cardiovascular Mortality

A total of 48 cases of CVM occurred over 147,495 person-years at risk during the follow up. The cumulative risk was 0.02% in the third tertile versus 0.04% in the first tertile of vitamin C intake.

Compare to the category of reference, we found a significant inverse association for the highest tertile of vitamin C intake and CVM in the age-adjusted analysis (Table 3). Results were similar in the age and sex-adjusted model; the models adjusted for demographic, metabolic and lifestyle risk factors; (multivariable adjusted model 1); and in the model additionally adjusted for prevalent diseases at baseline (multivariable adjusted model 2). Additional adjustment for fiber from foods other than fruits and vegetables did not change the results, but they became non-significant when total fiber intake was considered (HR (95% CI): 0.48 (0.19–1.20)). No significant results were found in the fully-adjusted model that included the MDS.

Neither age at the end of follow-up ($p = 0.70$), fiber intake ($p = 0.42$), nor vitamin C supplements intake ($p = 0.12$) modified the association between total vitamin C intake and CVM.

Table 3. Hazard Ratios (HR) and 95% Confidence Intervals (CI) for cardiovascular mortality associated with total vitamin C intake for participants over 40 years old in the SUN cohort (follow-up 1999–2016).

Main Analyses §	Tertiles of Vitamin C Intake		
	Q1 (N = 4474)	Q2 (N = 4474)	Q3 (N = 4473)
Cardiovascular deaths (person-years at risk)	22 (51,016)	15 (48,901)	11 (47,577)
Age-adjusted	1.00 (Ref.)	0.55 (0.28–1.06)	0.34 (0.17–0.73)
Sex- and age-adjusted	1.00 (Ref.)	0.56 (0.29–1.10)	0.37 (0.17–0.79)
Multivariable adjusted model 1	1.00 (Ref.)	0.57 (0.29–1.12)	0.39 (0.18–0.86)
Multivariable adjusted model 2	1.00 (Ref.)	0.54 (0.27–1.08)	0.40 (0.18–0.89)
Multivariable adjusted model 3	1.00 (Ref.)	0.54 (0.27–1.09)	0.41 (0.19–0.92)
Multivariable adjusted model 4	1.00 (Ref.)	0.56 (0.28–1.12)	0.45 (0.20–1.01)

§ Age strata as underlying time variable in all the models; $N = 13,421$; Ref: reference category. Multivariable adjusted **model 1**: Additionally adjusted for sex, body mass index (continuous), total energy intake (continuous), physical activity (continuous), television watching (continuous), smoking (never, current or former), family history of stroke, and treatment with aspirin. Multivariable adjusted **model 2**: Additionally adjusted for the number of cardiovascular-related diseases at baseline, prevalent cancer, prevalent hypertension, prevalent diabetes, prevalent hypercholesterolemia, and prevalent hypertrygliceridemia. Multivariable adjusted **model 3**: Additionally adjusted for dietary fiber (fiber from foods other than fruits and vegetables) (continuous). Multivariable adjusted **model 4**: Additionally adjusted for the MDS without fruit and vegetable intake related items (low, medium, or high).

3.3. Fiber-Adjusted Vitamin C Intake

In further analyses, dietary vitamin C was adjusted for total fiber intake using the residuals method to nullify the correlation between vitamin C and fiber (Table 4). We found a cumulative risk for CVD of 0.07% in the third versus 0.12% in the first tertile. However, no significant association was found for vitamin C intake and CVD.

On the other hand, the cumulative risk for CVM was 0.01% in the third tertile versus 0.05% in the first one. Compared with participants in the first tertile, those in the highest tertile of vitamin C intake showed significant lower risk of CVM in multivariable adjusted analyses (HR (95% CI): 0.30 (0.13–0.73)). Further adjustment for the MDS did not change the results.

Neither CVD nor CVM were significantly associated with dietary vitamin C, independently of vitamin C supplement intake (Figure S1).

Table 4. Hazard Ratio (HR) and 95% Confidence Interval (CI) for the association of total vitamin C intake, adjusted for fiber intake using the residuals method with both cardiovascular disease (CVD) and cardiovascular mortality (CVM) for participants over 40 years old in the SUN cohort (follow-up 1999–2016).

Main Analyses §	Tertiles of Vitamin C Intake		
	Q1 (N = 4474)	Q2 (N = 4474)	Q3 (N = 4473)
Incident CVD (person-time-1 at risk)	58 (49,706)	44 (49,080)	32 (48,186)
Multivariable adjusted §‡	1.00 (Ref.)	0.86 (0.57–1.29)	0.74 (0.47–1.15)
Additionally adjusted for MDS	1.00 (Ref.)	0.86 (0.57–1.29)	0.74 (0.47–1.15)
Cardiovascular deaths (person-years at risk)	27 (49,879)	14 (49,247)	7 (48,368)
Multivariable adjusted §‡	1.00 (Ref.)	0.52 (0.26–1.02)	0.30 (0.13–0.73)
Additionally adjusted for MDS	1.00 (Ref.)	0.52 (0.26–1.04)	0.30 (0.12–0.72)

MDS: Mediterranean Dietary Score without fruit and vegetable intake related items (low, medium, or high); § Age as underlying time variable in all the models; ‡ Adjusted for sex, body mass index (continuous), total energy intake (continuous), total fiber intake (continuous), physical activity (continuous), television watching (continuous), smoking (never, current or former), number of cardiovascular-related diseases at baseline, prevalent cancer, prevalent hypertension, prevalent diabetes, prevalent hypercholesterolemia, prevalent hypertrigliceridemia, family history of stroke, and treatment with aspirin. $N = 13,421$; Ref: reference category.

4. Discussion

In this large cohort of Spanish university graduates followed-up over a mean time of 11 years, we found that, compared with the lowest category, the third tertile of total vitamin C intake was associated with 70% (95% CI 18%–88%) lower risk of CVM, but not with CVD. This analysis was based on a multivariable adjusted model that thoroughly controlled potential confounding by fiber and accounted for the adherence to the Mediterranean dietary pattern.

The belief that vitamin C benefits cardiovascular health is based on its antioxidant capability. Vitamin C may prevent oxidative changes to low-density lipoprotein (LDL)-cholesterol [31] and reduce monocyte adhesion [32], which are key in reducing the risk of atherosclerosis. Moreover, vitamin C prevents vascular smooth muscle cells apoptosis, which keeps atheroma plaques stables [33]. In addition, vitamin C improves the nitric oxide production of the endothelium [34], which in turn contributes to reduced blood pressure. This evidence, when added to the results found in the analyses to account for confounding by fiber and dietary variables included in the MDS, suggests that the associations of vitamin C intake with CVM may not be due to confounding factors, but may instead represent a true biological effect.

Observational studies had reported inverse associations of vitamin C with cardiovascular outcomes, particularly on hypertension [6] and heart failure [7]. However, those studies did not account for fiber intake. Due to the high correlation between vitamin C and fiber intakes found in this study, it was difficult to assess the effect of vitamin C on cardiovascular health independently of fiber intake in a multivariable adjusted model. In order to nullify that correlation, dietary vitamin C was adjusted for total fiber intake using the residuals method. On the other hand, reduced CVM risk associated to vitamin C intake had been previously reported in observational studies [8]. However, this association has not been confirmed in randomized controlled trials [10,11].

We found that energy-adjusted total vitamin C intake was associated with a lower risk of CVD. We obtained similar estimates in the comparisons of the second and the third tertiles, which suggests a threshold effect or L-shaped association between total vitamin C and CVD. However, in further analyses, we found the association of fiber-adjusted vitamin C with CVD was not significant.

We also found that high energy-adjusted total vitamin C intake was associated with lower risk of CVM after multivariable adjustment for demographic, metabolic, and lifestyle risk factors, prevalent diseases at baseline, and fiber from foods other than fruits and vegetables. However, results became non-significant when the model was additionally adjusted for the MDS. Nevertheless, further analyses showed that, compared to the first tertile, the highest category of fiber-adjusted vitamin C intake was associated with lower CVM risk in the fully adjusted model (HR: 0.30, 95% CI (0.12–0.72)).

These results suggest that most of the confounding effect by fiber was due to fiber from fruits and vegetables. Since vitamin C and fiber were highly correlated ($r = 0.72$) it was difficult to assess the effect of one of them while keeping the other one constant (Tables 2 and 3). When vitamin C was adjusted for fiber using the residuals method (Table 4), the correlation was nullified ($r = 0$), which allowed for the assessment of the effect of vitamin C on cardiovascular health independently of fiber. Nevertheless, given that vitamin C is a single nutrient and may not represent the whole dietary pattern, these results must be taken with caution. Several reasons support the hypothesis that attributing all of the observed effect to a single nutrient or food may be too simplistic and that when assessing the association of dietary variables with non-communicable diseases, the whole dietary pattern should be considered [35].

None significant associations with either CVD or CVM were found when vitamin C from food was considered alone. Importantly, means (SD) (mg/day) of fiber-adjusted dietary vitamin C intake across successive tertiles were 184 (57), 266.7 (20.5), and 387.7 (75.6) respectively. Therefore, the absence of significant results might be explained by the low variability in the exposure.

Regarding vitamin C supplements, our results parallel previous intervention studies that reported no effect of vitamin C supplementation on cardiovascular health [10–13]. It must be acknowledged that some clinical trials permitted the control group to an intake of vitamin C and multivitamin supplements, which made it harder to find significant differences between groups. Vitamin C supplementation in our study ranged from 3.4 to 440 mg/day, which is much lower than the doses assessed in the available clinical trials. We found the effect of total vitamin C on CVD may depend on vitamin C supplementation (p for interaction 0.05). However, among the 1055 participants undertaking vitamin C supplementation (8%), we found two cases of CVD and one single case of CVM; thus, stratified analyses were not possible.

Some limitations of this study must be acknowledged. First, because information about exposure was self-reported, some degree of misclassification is possible. Nevertheless, information bias would more likely be non-differential with respect to the outcomes, resulting in an attenuation of the observed associations. Moreover, little variability observed in the exposure might have reduced the possibility of significant findings. Second, the SUN cohort is not a representative sample of the general population, and therefore generalization of these results must be based on biological mechanisms rather than on statistical representativeness. Third, given the observational design of the study, the possibility of residual confounding for factors that were not considered (such as vitamin E) must be taken into account. Thus, before causality is implied, these results must be confirmed in well-designed randomized controlled trials. Finally, because participants in the SUN cohort are relatively young and health conscious, few incident cases of CVM were observed during follow-up. Further studies are need to determine if the magnitude of the association we observed represents the upper bound of the association between vitamin C and CVM. Despite these limitations, our study has several strengths. The sample size is large, the follow-up period is long, and the retention rate is high. Dietary information was collected with a validated FFQ, and outcomes were confirmed by physicians checking participant's medical records. Finally, participants in the SUN cohort are highly educated, and more than half are health professionals themselves, which reduces potential confounding by educational level, leads to better quality in self-reported data, and increases the internal validity of the study.

5. Conclusions

Energy-adjusted analyses suggest a threshold effect in the association of vitamin C intake with CVD, but not with CVM. Nevertheless, the model fitted to thoroughly control potential confounding for fiber showed that compared with the category of reference, the highest tertile of total vitamin C intake was associated with a significantly lower risk of CVM, but not CVD, after adjusting for several confounding factors, including adherence to the Mediterranean dietary pattern. Further research is needed in order to fully understand the biological mechanisms explaining these associations. Moreover, these results must be reproduced in different populations before clinical implications can be assessed.

Acknowledgments: The SUN project received funding from the Spanish Government-Instituto de Salud Carlos III and the European Regional Development Fund (FEDER) (RD 06/0045, CIBER-Obn Grants PI10/02658, PI10/02293, PI13/00615, PI14/01668, PI14/01798, PI14/01764 AND G03/140), the Navarra Regional Government (45/2011, 122/2014), and the University of Navarra. We also thank all the researchers in the SUN project, and all the participants for their collaboration.

Author Contributions: Miguel Ángel Martínez-González designed and started the SUN cohort. Miguel Ángel Martínez-González and Nerea Martín-Calvo designed the present study. Nerea Martín-Calvo conducted the statistical analyses and wrote the first version of the manuscript. Miguel Ángel Martínez Gonzalez helped in the interpretation of the results and critically review the manuscript. All the authors approved the final version of the paper.

References

1. Chun, O.K.; Floegel, A.; Chung, S.J.; Chung, CE.; Song, W.O.; Koo, S.I. Estimation of Antioxidant Intakes from Diet and Supplements in U.S. Adults. *J. Nutr.* **2010**, *140*, 317–324. [CrossRef] [PubMed]

2. Moser, M.; Chun, O. Vitamin C and Heart Health: A Review Based on Findings from Epidemiologic Studies. *Int. J. Mol. Sci.* **2016**, *17*, 1328. [CrossRef] [PubMed]

3. Joshipura, K.J.; Hu, F.B.; Manson, J.E.; Stampfer, M.J.; Rimm, E.B.; Speizer, F.E.; Colditz, G.; Ascherio, A.; Rosner, B.; Spiegelman, D.; et al. The effect of fruit and vegetable intake on risk for coronary heart disease. *Ann. Intern. Med.* **2001**, *134*, 1106–1114. [CrossRef] [PubMed]

4. Holmberg, S.; Thelin, A.; Stiernström, E.L. Food Choices and Coronary Heart Disease: A Population Based Cohort Study of Rural Swedish Men with 12 Years of Follow-up. *Int. J. Environ. Res. Public Health* **2009**, *6*, 2626–2638. [CrossRef] [PubMed]

5. Martínez-González, M.A.; de la Fuente-Arrillaga, C.; López-Del-Burgo, C.; Vázquez-Ruiz, Z.; Benito, S.; Ruiz-Canela, M. Low consumption of fruit and vegetables and risk of chronic disease: A review of the epidemiological evidence and temporal trends among Spanish graduates. *Public Health Nutr.* **2011**, *14*, 2309–2315. [CrossRef] [PubMed]

6. Buijsse, B.; Jacobs, D.R.; Steffen, L.M.; Kromhout, D.; Gross, M.D.; Abbott, R. Plasma Ascorbic Acid, A Priori Diet Quality Score, and Incident Hypertension: A Prospective Cohort Study. *PLoS ONE* **2015**, *10*, e0144920. [CrossRef] [PubMed]

7. Pfister, R.; Sharp, S.J.; Luben, R.; Wareham, N.J.; Khaw, K.T. Plasma vitamin C predicts incident heart failure in men and women in European Prospective Investigation into Cancer and Nutrition-Norfolk prospective study. *Am. Heart J.* **2011**, *162*, 246–253. [CrossRef] [PubMed]

8. Khaw, K.T.; Bingham, S.; Welch, A.; Luben, R.; Wareham, N.; Oakes, S.; Day, N. Relation between plasma ascorbic acid and mortality in men and women in EPIC-Norfolk prospective study: A prospective population study. European Prospective Investigation into Cancer and Nutrition. *Lancet* **2001**, *357*, 657–663. [CrossRef]

9. Mangels, A.R.; Block, G.; Frey, C.M.; Patterson, B.H.; Taylor, P.R.; Norkus, E.P.; Levander, O.A. The bioavailability to humans of ascorbic acid from oranges, orange juice and cooked broccoli is similar to that of synthetic ascorbic acid. *J. Nutr.* **1993**, *123*, 1054–1061. [PubMed]

10. Sesso, H.D.; Buring, J.E.; Christen, W.G.; Kurth, T.; Belanger, C.; MacFadyen, J.; Bubes, V.; Manson, J.E.; Glynn, R.J.; Gaziano, J.M. Vitamins E and C in the Prevention of Cardiovascular Disease in Men. *JAMA* **2008**, *300*, 2123–2133. [CrossRef] [PubMed]

11. Cook, N.R.; Albert, C.M.; Gaziano, J.M.; Zaharris, E.; MacFadyen, J.; Danielson, E; Buring, J.E.; Manson, J.E. A Randomized Factorial Trial of Vitamins C and E and Beta Carotene in the Secondary Prevention of Cardiovascular Events in Women. *Arch. Intern. Med.* **2007**, *167*, 1610–1618. [CrossRef] [PubMed]

12. Ellulu, M.S.; Rahmat, A.; Ismail, P.; Khaza' ai, H.; Abed, Y. Effect of vitamin C on inflammation and metabolic markers in hypertensive and/or diabetic obese adults: A randomized controlled trial. *Drug Des. Devel. Ther.* **2015**, *9*, 3405–3412. [CrossRef] [PubMed]

13. Brown, B.G.; Zhao, X.Q.; Chait, A.; Fisher, L.D.; Cheung, M.C.; Morse, J.S.; Dowdy, A.A.; Marino, E.K.; Bolson, E.L.; Alaupovic, P. Simvastatin and Niacin, Antioxidant Vitamins, or the Combination for the Prevention of Coronary Disease. *N. Engl. J. Med.* **2001**, *345*, 1583–1592. [CrossRef] [PubMed]

14. Lee, D.H.; Folsom, A.R.; Harnack, L.; Halliwell, B.; Jacobs, D.R. Does supplemental vitamin C increase cardiovascular disease risk in women with diabetes? *Am. J. Clin. Nutr.* **2004**, *80*, 1194–1200. [PubMed]

15. Waters, D.D.; Alderman, E.L.; Hsia, J.; Howard, B.V.; Cobb, F.R.; Rogers, W.J.; Ouyang, P.; Thompsom, P.; Tardif, J.C.; Higginson, L. Effects of hormone replacement therapy and antioxidant vitamin supplements on coronary atherosclerosis in postmenopausal women: a randomized controlled trial. *JAMA* **2002**, *288*, 2432–2440. [CrossRef] [PubMed]

16. Ashor, A.W.; Lara, J.; Mathers, J.C.; Siervo, M. Effect of vitamin C on endothelial function in health and disease: A systematic review and meta-analysis of randomised controlled trials. *Atherosclerosis* **2014**, *235*, 9–20. [CrossRef] [PubMed]

17. Juraschek, S.P.; Guallar, E.; Appel, L.J.; Miller, E.R. Effects of vitamin C supplementation on blood pressure: A meta-analysis of randomized controlled trials. *Am. J. Clin. Nutr.* **2012**, *95*, 1079–1088. [CrossRef] [PubMed]

18. Seguí-Gómez, M.; de la Fuente, C.; Vázquez, Z.; de Irala, J.; Martínez-González, M.A. Cohort profile: The "Seguimiento Universidad de Navarra" (SUN) study. *Int. J. Epidemiol.* **2006**, *35*, 1417–1422. [CrossRef] [PubMed]

19. Martin-Moreno, J.M.; Boyle, P.; Gorgojo, L.; Maisonneuve, P.; Fernandez-Rodriguez, J.C.; Salvini, S.; Willett, W.C. Development and validation of a food frequency questionnaire in Spain. *Int. J. Epidemiol.* **1993**, *22*, 512–519. [CrossRef] [PubMed]

20. De la Fuente-Arrillaga, C.; Vázquez-Ruiz, Z.; Bes-Rastrollo, M.; Sampson, L.; Martínez-Gonzlez, M.A. Reproducibility of an FFQ validated in Spain. *Public Health Nutr.* **2010**, *13*, 1364–1372. [CrossRef] [PubMed]

21. Mataix-Verdu, J.; Manas, M.; Martinez-Victoria, E.; Sanchez, J.J.; Borregon, A. *Tabla de Composición de Alimentos Españoles (Spanish Food Composition Tables)*, 4th ed.; Universidad de Granada Press: Granada, Spain, 2003.

22. Moreiras, O.; Carbajal, A.; Cabrera, L. *Tablas de Composición de Alimentos (Food Composition Tables)*, 9th ed.; Pirámide: Madrid, Spain, 2005.

23. World Health Organization. *International Classification of Diseases*; 10th Revision (ICD-10); World Health Organization: Geneva, Switzerland, 2010.

24. Bes-Rastrollo, M.; Valdivieso, J.R.; Sánchez-Villegas, A.; Alonso, Á.; Martínez-González, M.A. Validación del peso e índice de masa corporal auto-declarados de los participantes de una cohorte de graduados universitarios. *Rev. Española. Obes.* **2005**, *3*, 183–189.

25. Trichopoulou, A.; Costacou, T.; Bamia, C.; Trichopoulos, D. Adherence to a Mediterranean Diet and Survival in a Greek Population. *N. Engl. J. Med.* **2003**, *348*, 2599–2608. [CrossRef] [PubMed]

26. Martínez-González, M.A.; López-Fontana, C.; Varo, J.J.; Sánchez-Villegas, A.; Martinez, J.A. Validation of the Spanish version of the physical activity questionnaire used in the Nurses' Health Study and the Health Professionals' Follow-up Study. *Public Health Nutr.* **2005**, *8*, 920–927. [CrossRef] [PubMed]

27. Ainsworth, B.E.; Haskell, W.L.; Whitt, M.C.; Irwin, M.L.; Swartz, A.M.; Strath, S.J.; O'brien, W.L.; Bassett, D.R.; Schmitz, K.H.; Emplaincourt, P.O. Compendium of physical activities: An update of activity codes and MET intensities. *Med. Sci. Sports Exerc.* **2000**, *32*, S498–S504. [CrossRef] [PubMed]

28. Javier Basterra-Gortari, F.; Bes-Rastrollo, M.; Gea, A.; Núñez-Córdoba, J.; Toledo, E.; Martínez-González, M.Á. Television Viewing, Computer Use, Time Driving and All-Cause Mortality: The SUN Cohort. *J. Am. Heart Assoc.* **2014**, *3*, e000864. [CrossRef] [PubMed]

29. Alonso, Á.; Beunza, J.J.; Delgado-Rodríguez, M.; Martínez-González, M.A. Validation of self reported diagnosis of hypertension in a cohort of university graduates in Spain. *BMC Public Health* **2005**, *5*, 94. [CrossRef] [PubMed]

30. Barrio-Lopez, M.T.; Bes-Rastrollo, M.; Beunza, J.J.; Fernández-Montero, A.; García-López, M.; Martínez-González, M.A. Validation of metabolic syndrome using medical records in the SUN cohort. *BMC Public Health* **2011**, *11*, 867. [CrossRef] [PubMed]

31. Salvayre, R.; Negre-Salvayre, A.; Camaré, C. Oxidative theory of atherosclerosis and antioxidants. *Biochimie* **2016**, *125*, 281–296. [CrossRef] [PubMed]

32. Weber, C.; Erl, W.; Weber, K.; Weber, P.C. Increased Adhesiveness of Isolated Monocytes to Endothelium Is Prevented by Vitamin C Intake in Smokers. *Circulation* **1996**, *93*, 1488–1492. [CrossRef] [PubMed]

33. Siow, R.C.M.; Richards, J.P.; Pedley, K.C.; Leake, D.S.; Mann, G.E. Vitamin C Protects Human Vascular Smooth Muscle Cells Against Apoptosis Induced by Moderately Oxidized LDL Containing High Levels of Lipid Hydroperoxides. *Arterioscler. Thromb. Vasc. Biol.* **1999**, *19*, 2387–2394. [CrossRef] [PubMed]

34. D'Uscio, L.V.; Milstien, S.; Richardson, D.; Smith, L.; Katusic, Z.S. Long-Term Vitamin C Treatment Increases Vascular Tetrahydrobiopterin Levels and Nitric Oxide Synthase Activity. *Circ. Res.* **2003**, *92*, 88–95. [CrossRef] [PubMed]

35. Hu, F.B. Dietary pattern analysis: A new direction in nutritional epidemiology. *Curr. Opin. Lipidol.* **2002**, *13*, 3–9. [CrossRef] [PubMed]

8

Inadequate Vitamin C Status in Prediabetes and Type 2 Diabetes Mellitus: Associations with Glycaemic Control, Obesity and Smoking

Renée Wilson [1], Jinny Willis [2], Richard Gearry [1], Paula Skidmore [3], Elizabeth Fleming [3], Chris Frampton [1] and Anitra Carr [4,*]

[1] Department of Medicine, University of Otago, Christchurch 8011, New Zealand; renee.wilson@postgrad.otago.ac.nz (R.W.); richard.gearry@otago.ac.nz (R.G.); chris.frampton@otago.ac.nz (C.F.)
[2] Lipid and Diabetes Research Group, Canterbury District Health Board, Christchurch 8011, New Zealand; jinny.willis@cdhb.health.nz
[3] Department of Human Nutrition, University of Otago, Dunedin 9016, New Zealand; paula.skidmore@otago.ac.nz (P.S.); liz.fleming@otago.ac.nz (E.F.)
[4] Department of Pathology, University of Otago, Christchurch 8011, New Zealand
* Correspondence: anitra.carr@otago.ac.nz

Abstract: Vitamin C (ascorbate) is an essential micronutrient in humans, being required for a number of important biological functions via acting as an enzymatic cofactor and reducing agent. There is some evidence to suggest that people with type 2 diabetes mellitus (T2DM) have lower plasma vitamin C concentrations compared to those with normal glucose tolerance (NGT). The aim of this study was to investigate plasma vitamin C concentrations across the glycaemic spectrum and to explore correlations with indices of metabolic health. This is a cross-sectional observational pilot study in adults across the glycaemic spectrum from NGT to T2DM. Demographic and anthropometric data along with information on physical activity were collected and participants were asked to complete a four-day weighed food diary. Venous blood samples were collected and glycaemic indices, plasma vitamin C concentrations, hormone tests, lipid profiles, and high-sensitivity C-reactive protein (hs-CRP) were analysed. A total of 89 participants completed the study, including individuals with NGT ($n = 35$), prediabetes ($n = 25$), and T2DM managed by diet alone or on a regimen of Metformin only ($n = 29$). Plasma vitamin C concentrations were significantly lower in individuals with T2DM compared to those with NGT (41.2 µmol/L versus 57.4 µmol/L, $p < 0.05$) and a higher proportion of vitamin C deficiency (i.e. <11.0 µmol/L) was observed in both the prediabetes and T2DM groups. The results showed fasting glucose ($p = 0.001$), BMI ($p = 0.001$), smoking history ($p = 0.003$), and dietary vitamin C intake ($p = 0.032$) to be significant independent predictors of plasma vitamin C concentrations. In conclusion, these results suggest that adults with a history of smoking, prediabetes or T2DM, and/or obesity, have greater vitamin C requirements. Future research is required to investigate whether eating more vitamin C rich foods and/or taking vitamin C supplements may reduce the risk of progression to, and/or complications associated with, T2DM.

Keywords: vitamin C; glycaemic control; metabolic health; prediabetes; type 2 diabetes mellitus

1. Introduction

Type 2 diabetes mellitus (T2DM) is a complex disorder influenced by both genetic and environmental factors. It is characterized by chronic hyperglycemia, altered insulin secretion, and insulin resistance [1]. As in many Western countries, T2DM is associated with increased morbidity and mortality due to microvascular (e.g. retinopathy, nephropathy, and neuropathy) and macrovascular complications (e.g. myocardial infarction, peripheral vascular disease, and stroke) [1]. Diabetes is one of the largest global health emergencies with 415 million people between the ages of 20 and 70 worldwide estimated as having diabetes in 2015 and the prevalence is increasing [2]. T2DM accounts for at least 90% of all cases of diabetes [2]. In 2016, approximately 5% of New Zealanders were living with diabetes compared to an estimated 6.5% of people in the UK [3,4].

Research suggests that chronic low grade inflammation and oxidative stress plays a pivotal role in the development of insulin resistance and T2DM, as well as the related complications [5]. Vitamin C is an essential micronutrient with potent antioxidant properties [6]. Vitamin C can protect important biomolecules from oxidation through participating in oxidation-reduction reactions whereby it is readily oxidized to dehydroascorbic acid, which in turn is rapidly reduced back to ascorbate [7]. Vitamin C is naturally present in fruit and vegetables, is often added as a preservative to foods/beverages, and is also used as a dietary supplement [6]. As a result of being water-soluble, it has a relatively short half-life in the body due to rapid renal clearance and a regular and adequate intake is required to prevent deficiency.

Previous research suggests that people with T2DM have lower plasma vitamin C concentrations than those with normal glucose control [8–10]. There are several proposed mechanisms including: (1) increased ascorbate excretion in those with microalbuminuria, (2) blood glucose may compete with vitamin C for uptake into cells due to its structural similarity to the oxidised form (dehydroascorbic acid), and (3) increased oxidative stress may deplete antioxidant stores [8]. Recent research has indicated that the glucose-dependent inhibition of dehydroascorbic acid uptake into erythrocytes may contribute to enhanced erythrocyte fragility and could potentially contribute to complications such as diabetic microvascular angiopathy [11].

As dietary vitamin C contributes to plasma vitamin C concentrations, potential differences in the intake between those with normal glucose control and T2DM must also be considered. A prospective study of 48,850 men revealed that while the baseline consumption of fruit and vegetables was similar, men who developed T2DM increased their consumption of fruit and vegetables by 1.6 serves/week compared to an increase of 0.7 serves/week in those who remained diabetes free [12]. Therefore, it seems that people with T2DM are altering their diet in an attempt to manage their blood sugar. Indeed, clinical advice to those newly-diagnosed with T2DM focuses on improving the diet. However, the dietary changes appear to be small and, furthermore, those with T2DM appear to have a similar intake of fruit and vegetables to those without T2DM [12].

The lower plasma vitamin C concentrations reported in people with T2DM has led to a growing interest in the role that vitamin C may afford against the development of T2DM and associated complications. A prospective survey of the Dutch and Finnish cohorts within the Seven Countries Study revealed an inverse association between dietary vitamin C intake and glucose intolerance, suggesting that antioxidants such as vitamin C may play a protective role against the development of impaired glucose tolerance and T2DM [13]. Further, the European Prospective Investigation of Cancer (EPIC)-Norfolk Study of some 21,000 individuals ascertained 735 cases of T2DM after a 12 year follow-up, and demonstrated a strong inverse association between plasma vitamin C concentration and T2DM risk [14].

However, studies investigating plasma vitamin C and glycaemic control have often failed to account for factors such as smoking status and dietary vitamin C intake, which are known to impact plasma vitamin C concentrations. When dietary intake is taken into account there are conflicting results, with one study showing a low plasma vitamin C concentration in people with diabetes consuming a similar amount of dietary vitamin C to those without diabetes [15], compared to another study that reported no differences in serum vitamin C concentrations in people grouped by T2DM status after adjustment for dietary vitamin C intake [16]. Therefore, the objective of this study was to determine the association between plasma vitamin C status and glycaemic control accounting for vitamin C intake in adults.

2. Materials and Methods

2.1. Study Participants

This study was approved by the New Zealand Central Health and Disability Ethics Committee (consent no. 14/CEN/34). Written informed consent was obtained from all participants. Individuals aged $\geq$ 18 years meeting the inclusion criteria detailed below were recruited from General Practice, Prediabetes and Diabetes Services, Retinal Screening Services, Pharmacies, and from local advertisements. Fasting glucose cut-off values for normal glucose tolerance (NGT), prediabetes, and T2DM were based on the American Diabetes Association (ADA) criteria [1]. Those taking Metformin were also included in the T2DM group. A total of 101 individuals underwent a screening questionnaire to ascertain the eligibility for the study. Ninety participants were enrolled and 89 participants completed the study. One participant was excluded due to incomplete sample collection.

2.2. Study Design

This was a cross-sectional observational pilot study that was part of a wider study on the gut microbiota and glycaemic control. At their study appointment, participants completed demographic and physical activity questionnaires. Anthropometric data were collected including the body mass index (BMI), waist and hip circumference, and bioelectrical impedance. The completed four-day weighed food diary was reviewed and additional information was added if necessary. A venous blood sample was also collected after an overnight fast and the blood pressure was measured.

2.2.1. Inclusion Criteria

Individuals aged $\geq$18 years with: NGT (fasting glucose $\leq$5.5 mmol/L) (n = 35), prediabetes (fasting glucose $\geq$5.6 mmol/L) (n = 25), T2DM taking no diabetes medication (fasting glucose $\geq$7.0 mmol/L) or on a regimen of Metformin only (n = 29).

2.2.2. Exclusion Criteria

Individuals unable to give informed consent, those who had taken antibiotics in the last month, those with a medical history of significant gastrointestinal disease e.g. inflammatory bowel disease, those who had undergone a previous bowel resection, and individuals taking diabetes medication other than Metformin.

2.3. Demographic Information

Participants recorded their date of birth, sex, ethnicity, qualification, and smoking status. They also recorded information on current medication and supplement use.

2.4. Anthropometric Measures

Weight (kg). Participants were asked to remove their footwear and heavy outer clothing such as jackets and were weighed to the nearest 0.1 kg on calibrated Tanita scales (Model BWB-800A, Tanita Corporation, Tokyo, Japan).

Height (m). Measured once to the nearest mm using calibrated height measures.

BMI (kg/m^2). Widely accepted as an appropriate population-level indicator of excess body fat [17]. BMI is calculated by weight in kilograms divided by height in metres squared.

Waist circumference and the waist-to-hip ratio are alternative anthropometric measures that also indicate whether excess body fat is centrally or peripherally located.

Waist circumference (cm). The World Health Organisation (WHO) STEPwise Approach to Surveillance (STEPS) protocol for measuring the waist circumference was used. The measurement was made at the approximate midpoint between the lower margin of the last palpable rib and the top of the iliac crest [18]. The tightness of the tape was controlled by using a Gulick II Measuring tape

(Model 67020, Country Technology Inc, Gays Mills, Wisconsin, WI, USA). Two to three measures were recorded and if the difference between the measurements exceeded 1.5 cm, a third measure was taken. The measures for each participant were averaged.

Hip circumference (cm). Measured to the nearest mm around the widest portion of the buttocks with the tape parallel to the floor using a Gulick II Measuring tape, as described above.

Waist-to-hip ratio. Calculated by dividing the waist circumference by the hip measurement.

Fat mass (%). Measured using the BIA 450 Bioimpedance Analyser (Biodynamics Corporation, Seattle, Washington, DC, USA). Patient assessments were conducted using a connection between the individual's wrist and ankle and the analyser using standard ECG sensor pad electrodes (CONMED Corporation, Utica, New York, NY, USA).

Blood Pressure. Measured using an automated blood pressure monitor (Bp TRU, BTM-300, Omron Healthcare Co., Ltd, Muko, Kyoto, Japan). The measurement was repeated if the results were outside the normal range. If there was an obvious outlier, this result was removed and the other results were averaged.

2.5. Blood Parameters

Venous blood samples were collected after a 12–hour fast.

Glycated haemoglobin (HbA1c). Determined in EDTA blood by standard methods (Bio-rad Variant HPLC, Bio-Rad, Hercules, California, CA, USA) at an International Accreditation New Zealand (IANZ) laboratory.

Glucose. Fasting glucose was measured in blood collected in fluoride oxalate venoject tubes by standard methods (Glucose Hexokinase Enzymatic Assay, Abbott c series analyser, Abbott Park, Illinois, USA) at an IANZ laboratory.

Lipid parameters. Total cholesterol (TC), HDL-cholesterol (HDL), LDL-cholesterol (LDL), and triglycerides (TG) were determined in lithium heparin blood by standard methods (Abbott c series analyser, Abbott Park, Illinois, IL, USA) at an IANZ laboratory.

High-sensitivity C-reactive protein (hs-CRP). The inflammatory marker hs-CRP was measured using end-point nephelometry at an IANZ laboratory.

Plasma vitamin C and hormones. EDTA blood was collected and centrifuged for 15 min at 1500 g at 4 °C. The plasma was stored −80 °C prior to analysis.

2.5.1. Plasma Vitamin C

Stored plasma was rapidly thawed, and acidified with perchloric acid and a metal chelator (DTPA) to precipitate the protein and stabilise the ascorbate [19]. Following centrifugation, the supernatant was treated with a reducing agent (TCEP) to recover any ascorbate that had become oxidised during the processing and storage of the samples [20]. The vitamin C concentration of the processed samples was determined using high performance liquid chromatography (HPLC) with electrochemical detection in the Department of Pathology, University of Otago Christchurch, as described previously [19].

2.5.2. Plasma Ghrelin, Leptin, and Adiponectin

Plasma hormones were determined by the Christchurch Heart Institute, Department of Medicine, University of Otago, Christchurch.

Plasma ghrelin was measured by an in-house radioimmunoassay (RIA) following extraction from plasma using Sep Pak C_{18} cartridges, as described previously [21]. The assay recognises the total circulating ghrelin (i.e. both octanoyl and non-octanoyl forms). The cross reactivities of other peptides in the assay, including vasointestinal peptide, prolactin, galanin, growth hormone releasing hormone, neuropeptide Y, brain natriuretic peptide, atrial natriuretic peptide, endothelin-1, and angiotensin II were all less than 0.03%. The RIA had a mean detection limit of 10.8 ± 0.8 pmol/L and mean ED_{50} of 136.2 ± 10.0 pmol/L over 23 consecutive assays.

Plasma leptin and adiponectin were measured using commercial enzyme-linked immunosorbent assays (ELISA) from BioVendor (Brno, Czech Republic), Research and Diagnostic products (RD191001100 Human Leptin ELISA and RD191023100 Human Adiponectin ELISA) according to the manufacturer's instructions.

2.5.3. Plasma Insulin

Plasma insulin was measured using the Roche Cobas e411 method in an IANZ laboratory. After storage at −80 °C, thawed plasma was pre-treated using 25% polyethylene glycol to precipitate any unwanted antibodies.

2.6. Dietary Intake of Vitamin C, Macronutrients, and Fibre

Participants completed a four day (non-consecutive) weighed food diary (including one weekend day) prior to their study visit. Participants received training using the Salter digital scales and on how to record the data, either at home or in the clinic, prior to the diary being completed. Once completed, the diary was also reviewed at their second study visit to add any missing information if necessary. The food diaries were entered into the nutrient analysis programme Kai-culator (version 1.08d, Department of Human Nutrition, University of Otago, Dunedin, New Zealand). Kai-culator uses the 2014 version of the New Zealand food composition database "NZ FOODfiles". The methodology for entering the diaries was developed by a dietitian and data entry was undertaken by an experienced dietitian and an experienced nutritionist who cross-checked each other's data and were overseen by an experienced nutritionist and dietitian. A further 16% of the diaries were checked again for accuracy. The Acceptable Macronutrient Distribution Ranges (AMDR) are the recommendations for the balance of protein, fat, and carbohydrate in the diet with respect to the relative contribution to dietary energy [22]. Total daily vitamin C, energy, and fibre were calculated, along with the percent energy values for fat, carbohydrate, and protein. Participants were asked to record the name of dietary supplements taken within the last month, the amount per dose, the frequency, when they started taking the supplement, and when their last dose was.

2.7. Physical Activity

Participants completed the self-administered short form version of the International Physical Activity Questionnaire (IPAQ). The questionnaire asks about physical activity over the previous seven days.

2.8. Statistical Analyses

Standard descriptive statistics including means, standard deviations, frequencies, and percentages as appropriate were used to summarise the demographic, anthropometric, and laboratory results across participants grouped by fasting glucose and T2DM treatment. Four of the laboratory measures (hs-CRP, Ghrelin, Leptin, and Adiponectin) showed a strong positive skew and were therefore $\log_e$ transformed prior to analyses. These variables are described using geometric means and 95% confidence intervals. Associations between the clinical characteristics of the cohorts grouped by fasting glucose (including those treated with Metformin) were tested using one way analysis of variance (ANOVA) and chi-squared tests as appropriate. Where significant associations were identified, these were further explored with pair-wise comparisons amongst the fasting glucose groups. The univariate associations between plasma vitamin C and demographic, anthropometric, and laboratory measures were tested using Pearson's Correlations coefficients and one way ANOVA. Significant predictors identified from these univariate analyses were then combined in a multiple regression analysis to identify significant independent associations with plasma vitamin C. The two-tailed p-value < 0.05 was taken to indicate statistical significance. All statistical analyses were undertaken using SPSS (version 24.0, IBM Corp., Armonk, New York, NY, USA).

3. Results

3.1. Participant Characteristics

The NGT group was slightly younger than the prediabetes and T2DM groups and there were more females in the NGT group and less in the T2DM group. The majority of participants were European and there were a mix of qualifications, as would be expected given the age of the participants (Table 1). There were no significant differences in physical activity between the study groups although those in the NGT and prediabetes groups had reported slightly higher levels of activity than those with T2DM.

Table 1. General characteristics of participants classified as having normal glucose tolerance (NGT) ($n = 35$), prediabetes ($n = 25$), and T2DM ($n = 29$).

Characteristics	NGT	Prediabetes	T2DM	Total
Age * (years)	55 ± 13 [a]	63 ± 9 [b]	61 ± 11 [b]	59 ± 11
Sex *				
Female % (n)	74 (26) [a]	52 (13) [ab]	35 (10) [b]	55% (49)
Male % (n)	26 (9)	48 (12)	66 (19)	45% (40)
Ethnicity				
European % (n)	86 (30)	88 (22)	97 (28)	90% (80)
Maori % (n)	9 (3)	4 (1)	3 (1)	6% (5)
Pacific Island % (n)	0 (0)	4 (1)	0 (0)	1% (1)
Asian % (n)	3 (1)	4 (1)	0 (0)	2% (2)
Other % (n)	3 (1)	0 (0)	0 (0)	1% (1)
Qualification				
No Qualification % (n)	96 (3)	20 (5)	25 (7)	17% (15)
Secondary School % (n)	20 (7)	24 (6)	32 (9)	25% (22)
Post-Secondary Certificate, Diploma or Trade Diploma % (n)	43 (15)	20 (5)	25 (7)	31% (27)
University % (n)	27 (10)	36 (9)	18 (5)	27% (24)
Physical Activity (MET min/week)	1723 ± 1687	2496 ± 3671	1320 ± 1490	1772 ± 2327
Anthropometry				
Weight * (kg)	76 ± 18 [a]	89 ± 19 [b]	96 ± 20 [b]	86 ± 21
BMI * (kg/m^2)	28 ± 6 [a]	30 ± 7 [ab]	33 ± 6 [b]	30 ± 7
Fat Mass (%)	32 ± 8	33 ± 8	35 ± 8	33 ± 8
Waist Circumference * (cm)	89 ± 16 [a]	99 ± 14 [b]	110 ± 15 [c]	99 ± 17
Waist-to-Hip Ratio *	0.9 ± 0.1 [a]	0.9 ± 0.1 [b]	1.0 ± 0.1 [b]	0.9 ± 0.1
Blood Pressure Diastolic (mmHg)	78 ± 9	83 ± 8	79 ± 9	80 ± 9
Blood Pressure Systolic * (mmHg)	125 ± 14 [a]	132 ± 14 [ab]	135 ± 15 [b]	130 ± 15
Smoking Status				
Current Smoker % (n)	7 (2)	5 (1)	3 (1)	5% (4)
Ex-smoker % (n)	28 (8)	439 (9)	38 (11)	35% (28)
Non-smoker % (n)	66 (19)	52 (11)	59 (17)	60% (47)

Values represented as mean $\pm$ SD unless stated otherwise. *All p values from ANOVA tests. Groups sharing a common subscript letter denotes the study groups that do not differ significantly from each other at the 0.05 level based on characteristics from Post Hoc analysis. Note: There was missing data from one participant for qualification (1 × T2DM), 12 participants for physical activity (7 × NGT and 5 × prediabetes), five participants for waist-to-hip ratio (2 × NGT and 3 × prediabetes), nine participants for blood pressure measures (4 × NGT and 5 × prediabetes), and 10 participants did not provide smoking status data (6 × NGT, 4 × prediabetes).

The mean BMI for the NGT and prediabetes groups reflects the international BMI cut-off points for overweight (25.00–29.99 kg/m^2) and the T2DM group were obese ($\geq$30.00 kg/m^2). The waist circumference and waist-to-hip ratio increased across the groups from NGT to T2DM along with fat mass (%), as would be expected given that obesity is a risk factor for T2DM.

3.2. Metabolic and Inflammatory Plasma Biomarkers

Glycaemic measures (fasting glucose and HbA1c), used as the basis for defining prediabetes and T2DM, increased from NGT to T2DM as expected and differed significantly between the study groups ($p < 0.05$, Table 2). Although fasting glucose was used as the basis for classifying participants in the analysis, the mean HbA1c of 35 mmol/mol for the NGT group and 40 mmol/mol for the prediabetes group were consistent with the New Zealand guidelines for the classification of diabetes based on HbA1c [23]. The mean HbA1c of 47 mmol/mol for the T2DM group is lower than the current threshold for the diagnosis of diabetes in New Zealand (50 mmol/mol) using this measure because some of the individuals in this category were treated with the biguanide oral hypoglycaemic drug, Metformin. Fasting and postprandial glucose were likely reduced in these treated individuals. The mean HbA1c for all participants was 41 mmol/mol (Table 2). While hs-CRP was inversely associated with glycaemic control, this was not significant.

Table 2. Laboratory measures of participants classified as having normal glucose tolerance (NGT) (n = 35), prediabetes (n = 25), and T2DM (n = 29).

Laboratory Measures	NGT	Prediabetes	T2DM	Total
Fasting Glucose * (mmol/L)	5.0 ± 0.4 [a]	6.2 ± 0.4 [b]	7.2 ± 1.3 [c]	6.0 ± 1.2
HbA1c * (mmol/mol)	35 ± 4 [a]	40 ± 5 [b]	47 ± 9 [c]	41 ± 8
hs-CRP (mg/L) Mean (95% CI)	1.2 (0.9–1.6)	1.6 (1.0–2.3)	2.1 (1.4–2.8)	1.6 (1.3–1.9)
Total Cholesterol * (mmol/L)	5.3 ± 0.9 [a]	5.9 ± 1.2 [a]	4.3 ± 1.1 [b]	5.0 ± 1.1
Cholesterol HDL * (mmol/L)	1.5 ± 0.4 [a]	1.3 ± 0.3 [b]	1.1 ± 0.2 [b]	1.3 ± 0.3
Cholesterol LDL * (Calc) (mmol/L)	3.4 ± 0.8 [a]	3.3 ± 1.0 [a]	2.5 ± 1.0 [b]	3.1 ± 1.0
Triglycerides * (mmol/L)	1.1 ± 0.4 [a]	1.3 ± 0.7 [ab]	1.4 ± 0.6 [b]	1.3 ± 0.6
Cholesterol (total/HDL) (ratio)	3.8 ± 0.8	4.2 ± 0.8	3.9 ± 1.1	4.0 ± 0.9
Fasting Insulin * (pmol/L)	53 ± 37 [a]	89 ± 53 [b]	95 ± 48 [b]	77 ± 49
Ghrelin * (pmol/L) Mean (95% CI)	171 (142–207) [a]	111 (88–140) [b]	112 (91–139) [b]	132 (117–150)
Leptin (ng/mL) Mean (95% CI)	27 (20–38)	33 (20–54)	33 (23–47)	31 (25–38)
Adiponectin * (μg/mL) Mean (95% CI)	11 (9–13) [a]	9 (7–11) [a]	7 (6–8) [b]	9 (8–10)
Plasma vitamin C * (μmol/L)	57 ± 14 [a]	48 ± 16 [b]	41 ± 18 [b]	49 ± 17

Values represented as mean ± SD unless stated otherwise. *All p values from ANOVA tests. Groups sharing a common subscript letter denotes the study groups that do not differ significantly from each other at the 0.05 level based on characteristics from Post Hoc analysis. Log conversion was carried out for Ghrelin, Leptin, Adiponectin, and hs-CRP. Note: There was missing data from three participants for plasma vitamin C (2 × NGT and 1 × prediabetes).

The average fasting insulin concentrations were consistent with the glycaemic measures and were significantly higher in the T2DM group compared to the NGT group. The increasing BMI across the groups was associated with the increase in leptin concentrations, and the reduction in ghrelin concentrations.

Total, HDL, and LDL cholesterol decreased from the NGT to the T2DM group, which may reflect the use of lipid lowering medications which are routinely used in individuals with T2DM.

There was a slight increase in TG across the groups, with the average for each group remaining below the recommended cut-off in New Zealand (<1.7 mmol/L). There were no significant differences in the total cholesterol/HDL ratio between groups, and each group was below the recommended cut-off in New Zealand of 4.5.

3.3. Dietary Intake of Vitamin C, Macronutrients, and Fibre

There were no significant differences in macronutrient intake and dietary vitamin C intake across the groups (Table 3). The AMDR range for protein is 15–25% of total energy, total fat 20–35% of total energy, and carbohydrate 45–65% of total energy [22]. All study groups had slightly higher average total fat intakes and slightly lower CHO intakes than recommended, but the average protein intake for all groups fell within the recommended range.

The adequate intake (AI) for dietary fibre in New Zealand and Australia is set at the median for dietary fibre intake recorded in the 1995 National Nutrition Survey of Australia (ABS 1998) and the 1997 National Nutrition Survey of New Zealand (MOH 1999) [22]. The AI is 25 g for women and 30 g for men. Although fibre intake is not reported by sex in Table 1, the average daily fibre intake for each group of 24 g, 25 g, and 27 g for the NGT, prediabetes, and T2DM groups, respectively, was similar to recommendations.

Six participants reported taking a high dose vitamin C supplement (≥500 mg vitamin C). The plasma vitamin C concentration of five of these participants ranged from 36–59 μmol/L, which reflects inadequate to adequate plasma vitamin C concentrations and suggests that they didn't take the supplement close to their study appointment. The other participant had a plasma vitamin C concentration of 74 μmol/L, which is a saturating concentration, but they also had an average dietary vitamin C intake of 194 mg/day and so this high plasma concentration could be explained by their dietary intake as 200 mg/day will saturate plasma [19].

Table 3. Dietary intake of participants classified as having normal glucose tolerance (NGT) (*n* = 35), prediabetes (*n* = 25), and T2DM (*n* = 29).

Total Daily Dietary intake	NGT	Prediabetes	T2DM	Total
Energy (KJ)	8192 ± 2336	8430 ± 2260	8033 ± 2416	8204 ± 2321
Fibre (g)	24 ± 9	25 ± 8	27 ± 9	25 ± 9
Protein (% of Energy)	17 ± 3	18 ± 4	17 ± 3	17 ± 3
Fat (% of Energy)	37 ± 6	39 ± 8	36 ± 7	37 ± 7
Carbohydrate (% of Energy)	44 ± 6	40 ± 8	44 ± 8	43 ± 7
Dietary Vitamin C Intake (mg)	103 ± 76	94 ± 58	101 ± 61	100 ± 66

Values represented as mean ± SD unless stated otherwise. Note: There was missing data from one participant for dietary information (1 × prediabetes). There were no significant differences between the study groups for any of the dietary intake measures.

3.4. Plasma Vitamin C Status and Dietary Vitamin C Intakes

A significant decrease in the mean plasma vitamin C concentration was observed between the NGT (57.4 μmol/L) and the prediabetes group (48.2 μmol/L) (*p* = 0.035) and the T2DM (41.2 μmol/L) group (*p* < 0.001) (Table 2). Furthermore, there was a much higher proportion of individuals with prediabetes and T2DM with deficient (4% and 3% respectively), marginal (14% in T2DM group), and inadequate (58% in prediabetes and 52% in T2DM group) plasma vitamin C concentrations, compared with the NGT group (3% marginal and 21% inadequate) (Figure 1).

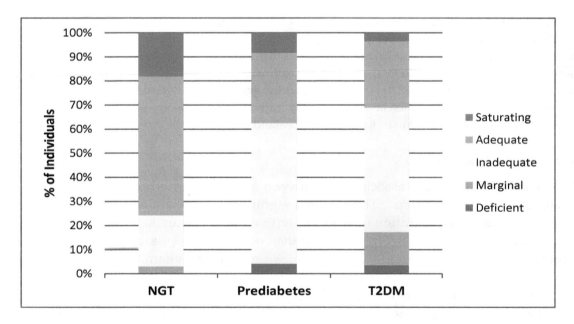

Figure 1. Plasma vitamin C status of individuals within study groups. Percentage of individuals from each study group [normal glucose tolerance (NGT), prediabetes, and type 2 diabetes mellitus (T2DM), including those taking no diabetes medication (fasting glucose ≥ 7.0 mmol/L or on a regimen of Metformin only (T2DM)], classified as having saturating (>70 μmol/L), adequate (51.0–69.9 μmol/L), inadequate (24.0–50.9 μmol/L), marginal (11.0–23.9 μmol/L), and deficient (<11.0 μmol/L) plasma vitamin C concentrations [24].

Although plasma vitamin C decreased from NGT to T2DM, there were no significant differences in dietary vitamin C concentrations between study groups determined from the four day weighed food diaries (Table 3). The majority of participants met the New Zealand recommended dietary intake

(RDI) of 45 mg/day (Figure 2). Furthermore, there were no participants in the T2DM group that had intakes below the New Zealand estimated average requirement (EAR) (30 mg/day). At the group level, it appears that most participants had an adequate fruit and vegetable intake to meet the recommended vitamin C intakes. However, few participants were reaching the New Zealand Ministry of Health's suggested dietary targets (SDT) to reduce chronic disease risk, i.e. 220 mg/day for men and 190 mg/d for women (Figure 2).

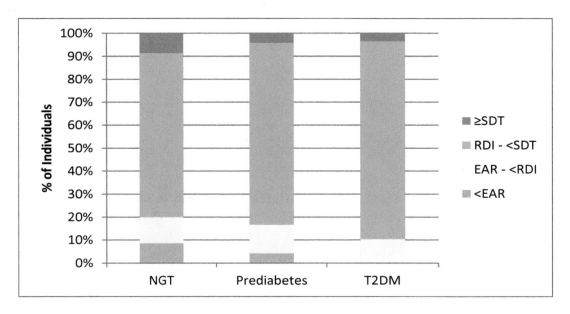

Figure 2. Individuals meeting New Zealand dietary intake recommendations for vitamin C. Percentage of individuals from each study group [normal glucose tolerance (NGT), prediabetes, and type 2 diabetes mellitus (T2DM), including those taking no diabetes medication (fasting glucose ≥7.0 mmol/L or on a regimen of Metformin only (T2DM)], meeting the estimated average requirement (EAR) (30 mg/day), recommended dietary intake (RDI) (45 mg/day), and suggested dietary target (SDT) to reduce chronic disease risk (220 mg/day for men and 190 mg/day for women) for dietary vitamin C intake using the nutrient reference values for Australia and New Zealand [22].

3.5. Plasma Vitamin C Correlations

There were no significant associations between age, gender, ethnicity, education level, and plasma vitamin C concentrations. There was a significant association between smoking history and plasma vitamin C concentration ($p = 0.035$), with current (mean 30.9 μmol/L) and ex-smokers (mean 47.3 μmol/L) having lower concentrations than non-smokers (mean 52.6 μmol/L). There was a significant linear association between vitamin C intake and plasma vitamin C concentration ($r = 0.353$, $p = 0.001$).

The three anthropometric measures (BMI, fat mass, and waist-to-hip ratio) were all significantly negatively associated with plasma vitamin C ($p < 0.05$) when conducting univariate analyses. When these three variables were included in a multiple regression, only BMI was independently negatively associated with plasma vitamin C ($p < 0.001$). Laboratory measurements (HbA1c, fasting glucose, TG, total chol/HDL chol, insulin, and hs-CRP) were negatively associated with plasma vitamin C ($p < 0.05$) and HDL chol and ghrelin were positively associated with plasma vitamin C ($p < 0.05$) in the univariate anlaysis (Table 4). When these variables were included in a multiple regression, only hs-CRP and fasting glucose were independently negatively associated with plasma vitamin C ($p < 0.05$).

A final multiple regression showed fasting glucose ($p = 0.001$), BMI ($p = 0.001$) and smoking history ($p = 0.003$) to be significant independent predictors of plasma vitamin C. Fasting glucose and BMI were negatively associated with plasma vitamin C, and current and ex-smokers had reduced plasma vitamin C concentrations compared to non-smokers. There was a strong positive association between hs-CRP concentrations and BMI ($r = 0.618$, $p < 0.001$). Accordingly, hs-CRP does not feature as an independent predictor of plasma vitamin C. Including dietary vitamin C intake in the above model (Table 5) showed that this was a significant independent predictor ($p = 0.032$) of plasma vitamin C concentrations, and BMI, fasting glucose, and smoking history remained as significant independent predictors ($R^2 = 0.43$).

Table 4. Pearson correlations of plasma vitamin C, glycaemic indices, hormones, lipids, high sensitivity C-reactive protein, and anthropometric measures.

Measure	Pearson Correlation
Fasting Glucose (mmol/L)	−0.411 ***
HbA1c (mmol/mol)	−0.334 ***
Total Cholesterol (mmol/L)	0.093
Triglycerides (mmol/L)	−0.322 **
Cholesterol (HDL)	0.295 **
Cholesterol (total/HDL)	−0.214 *
Cholesterol (LDL) calculated	0.086
Insulin (pmol/L)	−0.353 **
hs-CRP (mg/L)	−0.333 **
Ghrelin (pmol/L)	0.295 **
Leptin (ng/mL)	−0.183
Adiponectin (ng/mL)	0.202
BMI (kg/m2)	−0.446 ***
Waist-to-Hip Ratio	−0.274 *
Fat Mass (%)	−0.295 **

*** correlations significant at 0.001 level (2-tailed); ** correlations significant at the 0.01 level (2-tailed); * correlations significant at the 0.05 level (2-tailed).

Table 5. Multiple regression analysis showing significant associations with plasma vitamin C concentrations.

Measure	B	Lower 95% CI	Upper 95% CI	p Value
BMI	−0.9	−1.4	−0.4	0.001
Current Smoker	−21.9	−35.8	−7.9	0.003
Ex-Smoker	−4.9	−11.2	1.5	0.128
Fasting Glucose	−4.4	−7.1	−1.8	0.001
Dietary vitamin C	0.05	0.01	0.10	0.032

B: coefficient from the multiple linear regression model.

4. Discussion

4.1. Predictors of Plasma Vitamin C

This study showed fasting glucose, BMI, smoking history, and dietary vitamin C intake to be significant independent predictors of plasma vitamin C concentrations. The inverse association between fasting glucose and plasma vitamin C concentration shown in this study is in agreement with earlier studies [8–10]. In addition, the mean plasma vitamin C concentration was significantly lower in the prediabetes group (compared to the NGT group, suggesting that a reduction in plasma vitamin C concentration occurs in parallel with the decline in glucose tolerance during the progression to T2DM. It has been proposed that the uptake of dehydroascorbic acid, the oxidized form of vitamin C, by the glucose transporters (GLUTs), could be competitively inhibited by elevated blood glucose levels [25]. This could contribute to complications such as diabetic microvascular angiopathy due to erythrocyte fragility, as erythrocytes lack the sodium-dependent vitamin C transporters (SVCTs) and are dependent on the GLUTs for the uptake of vitamin C [11]. Our study also found plasma vitamin C concentration to be inversely related to BMI, which concurs with previous research [26]. Individuals with a higher weight are prone to vitamin C inadequacy and are known to require higher intakes of vitamin C in order to reach adequate plasma concentrations [27,28].

Oxidative stress is defined as a significant imbalance between the production of reactive oxygen species (ROS) and antioxidant defenses, and leads to alterations in signalling pathways and to potential tissue damage [29]. ROS activate nuclear factor κB (NFκB), a pro-inflammatory transcription factor, triggering a signalling cascade that leads to the continued synthesis of oxidative species and low-grade chronic inflammation [29]. High-sensitivity CRP, produced by the liver, reflects the presence of inflammation in the body. The concentration of hs-CRP increased with the deterioration of glycaemic control and increase in BMI. This result is consistent with the evidence suggesting that obesity can lead to chronic activation of the innate immune system and low-grade systemic inflammation and oxidative stress, which have been implicated in the development of insulin resistance and T2DM [5,30,31]. Hyperglycaemia, increased plasma concentrations of free fatty acids (FFAs), and hyperinsulinaemia have all been linked to an increased production of ROS [29,31]. Our data showed an inverse relationship between hs-CRP and plasma vitamin C. It is therefore hypothesized that lower plasma vitamin C in those with higher BMI, prediabetes, and T2DM reflects the depletion of the vitamin due to its antioxidant and anti-inflammatory activities.

Consistent with the role of vitamin C as an antioxidant, our data showed a significant inverse relationship between plasma vitamin C concentration and smoking status, with ex- and current-smokers having lower plasma vitamin C concentrations than non-smokers, which is consistent with previous research [32,33]. It has long been recognised that smokers and passive smokers have a lower vitamin C status than non-smokers partly due to poor dietary habits, but also due to the oxidizing properties of tobacco smoke, resulting in an increased turnover of vitamin C [34].

As expected, dietary vitamin C was found to be a predictor for plasma vitamin C concentration. However, when the dietary intake of the vitamin was corrected for by covariate analysis fasting glucose, BMI and smoking status remained as significant independent predictors of plasma vitamin C concentration. That is, the associations observed were not solely explained by differences in dietary intake. This result is at odds with one study that reported no differences in serum vitamin C concentrations in people grouped by diabetes status after adjustment for dietary vitamin C intake [16].

4.2. Metabolic Hormones

The average fasting insulin concentrations were consistent with the glycaemic measures and were significantly higher in the T2DM group compared to the NGT group. A higher fasting insulin concentration indicates insulin resistance, a well-known contributor to impaired glucose tolerance and T2DM. Leptin and ghrelin are two hormones that have a major influence on energy balance [35]. Leptin is a mediator of long-term regulation of energy balance, suppressing food intake and thereby inducing weight loss. Ghrelin, on the other hand, is a fast-acting hormone, seemingly playing a role in meal initiation. In obese patients, the circulating concentration of leptin is increased, whereas surprisingly, ghrelin is decreased [35]. It is now established that obese patients are leptin-resistant [35]. Indeed, in this study, the increasing BMI across the groups was associated with an increase in leptin concentrations and a reduction in ghrelin concentrations. There was an inverse relationship between insulin and leptin and plasma vitamin C, and a positive relationship between ghrelin and plasma vitamin C; however, these hormones were also associated with fasting glucose and were thus not included as independent predictors of plasma vitamin C.

4.3. Clinical Significance

As hyperglycemia is associated with increased oxidative stress, a role for antioxidants such as vitamin C in the prevention of T2DM and/or the reduction of complications is a reasonable proposition. Indeed, a recent meta-analysis of 15 randomized control trials (RCTs) investigating vitamin C supplementation and insulin resistance and biomarkers of glycaemic control (fasting glucose, HbA1c) found that doses of ≥200 mg/day vitamin C significantly reduced glucose concentrations in patients with T2DM, particularly if the intervention was for more than 30 days and in older individuals [36]. Furthermore, a recent 12 month RCT found that treating those with T2DM with both Metformin and vitamin C was more effective at reducing HbA1c and risk factors for diabetes-related long-term complications than treating with Metformin alone [37].

Although T2DM is not traditionally considered a risk factor for vitamin C deficiency, our research indicates that those with prediabetes or T2DM are more likely to have inadequate or deficient plasma vitamin C concentrations. This did not appear to be due to a lower dietary vitamin C intake, so dietary advice needs to emphasise the importance of consuming high vitamin C foods, aiming for an intake of at least 200 mg/day [22]. This is particularly relevant in light of the associated T2DM risk factors of higher BMI and smoking status, both of which impact vitamin C status. Further research into the possibility of a higher RDI for vitamin C for those with prediabetes and T2DM is warranted, in line with what has been recommended in some countries for smokers [38].

4.4. Study Strengths and Limitations

Our study used robust methodology for dietary intake, plasma vitamin C, and statistical analysis, and accounted for other factors that are known to impact plasma vitamin C concentration such as smoking status, dietary vitamin C intake, and supplement use. The participants with T2DM were clinically well defined and were either not treated with diabetes medication or treated with a single oral hypoglycaemic agent only (Metformin). Those taking Metformin were included in the overall analysis. When the Metformin treated cases were excluded, the correlation between fasting glucose and plasma vitamin C concentrations was similar in direction and magnitude ($n = 64$, $r = -0.477$, $p < 0.001$) to the entire cohort ($n = 86$, $r = -0.411$, $p = 0.001$). Further, the current norm is for Metformin treatment to be initiated at diagnosis, rather than after the failure of diet and lifestyle changes to optimize glucose control. As such, it will become increasingly difficult to recruit treatment-naïve individuals with T2DM to studies.

T2DM has been shown to increase the urinary excretion of vitamin C, leading to reduced plasma vitamin C concentrations in a rodent model [39]. Whether this also occurs in humans is unknown. In addition, the duration of T2DM was not reported. Indeed, many individuals have undiagnosed T2DM for a significant period of time prior to formal diagnosis, making it very difficult to interpret data on the duration of the disease. There are always limitations around the self-reporting of dietary data and supplement use, and the study cohort was relatively small with 89 participants. Our study had only one measure of plasma vitamin C per participant and so future research should ideally incorporate repeated samples to account for any temporal fluctuations. There was a limitation around the lack of detail with regards to vitamin C supplement use; however, only six participants reported taking high dose vitamin C supplements and the use was sporadic.

5. Conclusions

Our cross-sectional observational study has identified a moderate inverse relationship between plasma vitamin C and both fasting glucose and BMI in adult subjects across the glycaemic spectrum. The relationship can be explained by the depletion of vitamin C due to oxidative stress and inflammation resulting from dysglycaemia, overweight/obesity, and smoking, rather than lower dietary intakes. Further research is required to determine whether those with an increased dietary intake through fruit and vegetables and/or vitamin C supplementation have a decreased risk of progression to T2DM and/or complications associated with the metabolic syndrome and T2DM.

Acknowledgments: We would like to thank all participants for volunteering their time to take part in the study, Sharon Berry for helping take blood samples, and Angie Anderson and Lizzie Jones for food diary data entry. Rénee Wilson, Jinny Willis, Richard Gearry, and Paula Skidmore are the recipients of a Zespri International Ltd. grant. Anitra Carr is the recipient of a Health Research Council of New Zealand Sir Charles Hercus Health Research Fellowship.

Author Contributions: R.W. conducted participant recruitment and interviews; R.W., P.S., and L.F. completed the dietary analysis, A.C. vitamin C analysis, and C.F. statistical analysis; R.W., A.C., and J.W. undertook the conception and writing of the paper; R.G. and P.S. edited the paper.

References

1.   American Diabetes Association. Diagnosis and classification of diabetes mellitus. *Diabetes Care* **2014**, *37*, S81–S90.
2.   International Diabetes Federation. IDF diabetes atlas 2015. Available online: http://www.diabetesatlas.org. (accessed on 5 June 2017).
3.   Ministry of Health. Virtual diabetes register 2017. Available online: http://www.health.govt.nz/our-work/diseases-and-conditions/diabetes/about-diabetes/virtual-diabetes-register-vdr. (accessed on 11 June 2017).
4.   Primary Care Domain NHS Digital. Quality and outcomes framework-prevalence, achievements and exceptions report 2016. Available online: http://www.content.digital.nhs.uk/catalogue/PUB22266 (accessed on 25 June 2017).
5.   McArdle, M.; Finucane, O.; Connaughton, R.; McMorrow, A.; Roche, H. Mechanisms of obesity-induced inflammation and insulin resistance: insights into the emerging role of nutritional strategies. *Front. Endocrinol. (Lausanne)* **2013**, *4*, 1–23. [CrossRef] [PubMed]
6.   Carr, A.C.; Frei, B. Toward a new recommended dietary allowance for vitamin C based on antioxidant and health effects in humans. *Am. J. Clin. Nutr.* **1999**, *69*, 1086–1107. [PubMed]
7.   Carr, A.; Frei, B. Does vitamin C act as a pro-oxidant under physiological conditions? *FASEB J.* **1999**, *13*, 1007–1024. [PubMed]
8.   Will, J.C.; Byers, T. Does diabetes mellitus increase the requirement for vitamin C? *Nutr. Rev.* **1996**, *54*, 193–202. [CrossRef] [PubMed]
9.   Sargeant, L.; Wareham, N.; Bingham, S.; Day, N. Vitamin C and hyperglycemia in the European prospective investigation into cancer-Norfolk (EPIC-Norfolk) study: A population-based study. *Diabetes Care.* **2000**, *23*, 726–732. [CrossRef] [PubMed]
10.   Kositsawat, J.; Freeman, V.L. Vitamin C and A1c relationship in the National Health and Nutrition Examination Survey (NHANES) 2003–2006. *J. Am. Coll. Nutr.* **2011**, *30*, 477–483. [CrossRef] [PubMed]
11.   Tu, H.; Li, H.; Wang, Y.; Niyyati, M.; Wang, Y.; Leshin, J.; Levine, M. Low red blood cell vitamin C concentrations induce red blood cell fragility: A link to diabetes via glucose, glucose transporters, and dehydroascorbic Acid. *EBioMedicine* **2015**, *2*, 1735–1750. [CrossRef] [PubMed]
12.   Olofsson, C.; Discacciati, A.; Akesson, A.; Orsini, N.; Brismar, K.; Wolk, A. Changes in fruit, vegetable and juice consumption after the diagnosis of type 2 diabetes: A prospective study in men. *Br. J. Nutr.* **2017**, *117*, 712–719. [CrossRef] [PubMed]
13.   Feskens, E.J.M.; Virtanen, S.M.; Räsänen, L.; Tuomilehto, J.; Stengård, J.; Pekkanen, J.; Nissinen, A.; Kromhout, D. Dietary factors determining diabetes and impaired glucose tolerance: A 20-year follow-up of the Finnish and Dutch cohorts of the Seven Countries Study. *Diabetes Care.* **1995**, *18*, 1104–1112. [CrossRef] [PubMed]
14.   Harding, A.H.; Wareham, N.J.; Bingham, S.A.; Khaw, K.; Luben, R.; Welch, A.; Forouhi, N.G. Plasma vitamin C level, fruit and vegetable consumption, and the risk of new-onset type 2 diabetes mellitus: The European prospective investigation of cancer-Norfolk prospective study. *Arch. Intern. Med.* **2008**, *168*, 1493. [CrossRef] [PubMed]
15.   Som, S.; Basu, S.; Mukherjee, D.; Deb, S.; Choudhury, P.R.; Mukherjee, S.; Chatterjee, S.N.; Chatterjee, I.B. Ascorbic acid metabolism in diabetes mellitus. *Metabolism* **1981**, *30*, 572–577. [CrossRef]
16.   Will, J.; Ford, E.; Bowman, B. Serum vitamin C concentrations and diabetes: Findings from the third National Health and Nutrition Examination Survey, 1988–1994. *Am. J. Clin. Nutr.* **1999**, *70*, 49–52. [PubMed]
17.   World Health Organization. Obesity: Preventing and managing the global epidemic. Report of a WHO consultation. 2000. Available online: http://www.who.int/nutrition/publications/obesity/WHO_TRS_894/en/ (accessed on 10 June 2017).
18.   World Health Organization. Section 5: Collecting step 2 data: Physical measurements 2017. Available online: http://www.who.int/chp/steps/Part3_Section5.pdf?ua=1 (accessed on 19 June 2017).

19. Carr, A.C.; Pullar, J.M.; Moran, S.; Vissers, M.C. Bioavailability of vitamin C from kiwifruit in non-smoking males: Determination of 'healthy' and 'optimal' intakes. *J. Nutr. Sci.* **2012**, *1*, e14. [CrossRef] [PubMed]

20. Sato, Y.; Uchiki, T.; Iwama, M.; Kishimoto, Y.; Takahashi, R.; Ishigami, A. Determination of dehydroascorbic acid in mouse tissues and plasma by using tris(2-carboxyethyl)phosphine hydrochloride as reductant in metaphosphoric acid/ethylenediaminetetraacetic acid solution. *Biol. Pharm. Bull.* **2010**, *33*, 364–369. [CrossRef] [PubMed]

21. Bang, A.S.; Soule, S.G.; Yandle, T.G.; Richards, A.M.; Pemberton, C.J. Characterisation of proghrelin peptides in mammalian tissue and plasma. *J. Endocrinol.* **2007**, *192*, 313–323. [CrossRef] [PubMed]

22. National Health and Medical Research Council. Nutrient Reference Values for Australia and New Zealand Including Recommended Dietary Intakes Canberra: ACT: National Health and Medical Research Council. 2006. Available online: https://www.nhmrc.gov.au/_files_nhmrc/file/publications/17122_nhmrc_nrv_update-dietary_intakes-web.pdf (accessed on 12 June 2017).

23. New Zealand Society for the Study of Diabetes. NZSSD position statement on the diagnosis of, and screening for, type 2 diabetes 2011. Available online: http://www.nzssd.org.nz/HbA1c/1.%20NZSSD%20position%20statement%20on%20screening%20for%20type%202%20diabetes%20final%20Sept%202011.pdf (accessed on 20 June 2017).

24. Lykkesfeldt, J.; Poulsen, H.E. Is vitamin C supplementation beneficial? Lessons learned from randomised controlled trials. *Br. J. Nutr.* **2010**, *103*, 1251–1259. [CrossRef] [PubMed]

25. Girgis, C.; Christie-David, D.; Gunton, J. Effects of vitamins C and D in type 2 diabetes mellitus. *Nutr. Diet. Suppl.* **2015**, *7*, 21–28. [CrossRef]

26. Johnston, C.S.; Beezhold, B.L.; Mostow, B.; Swan, P.D. Plasma vitamin C is inversely related to body mass index and waist circumference but not to plasma adiponectin in nonsmoking adults. *J. Nutr.* **2007**, *137*, 1757–1762. [PubMed]

27. Block, G.; Mangels, A.R.; Patterson, B.H.; Levander, O.A.; Norkus, E.P.; Taylor, P.R. Body weight and prior depletion affect plasma ascorbate levels attained on identical Vitamin C intake: A controlled-diet study. *J. Am. Coll. Nutr.* **1999**, *18*, 628–637. [CrossRef] [PubMed]

28. Carr, A.C.; Pullar, J.M.; Bozonet, S.M.; Vissers, M.C. Marginal ascorbate status (hypovitaminosis C) results in an attenuated response to vitamin C supplementation. *Nutrients* **2016**, *8*, 341. [CrossRef] [PubMed]

29. Lamb, R.E.; Goldstein, B.J. Modulating an oxidative-inflammatory cascade: Potential new treatment strategy for improving glucose metabolism, insulin resistance, and vascular function. *Int. J. Clin. Pract.* **2008**, *62*, 1087–1095. [CrossRef] [PubMed]

30. Calle, M.C.; Fernandez, M.L. Inflammation and type 2 diabetes. *Diabetes Metab.* **2012**, *38*, 183–191. [CrossRef] [PubMed]

31. Garcia-Bailo, B.; El-Sohemy, A.; Haddad, P.S.; Arora, P.; Benzaied, F.; Karmali, M.; Badawi, A. Vitamins D, C, and E in the prevention of type 2 diabetes mellitus: Modulation of inflammation and oxidative stress. *Biologics* **2011**, *5*, 7–19. [PubMed]

32. Schectman, G.; Byrd, J.; Gruchow, H. The influence of smoking on vitamin C status in adults. *Am. J. Public Health* **1989**, *79*, 158. [CrossRef] [PubMed]

33. Pfeiffer, C.M.; Sternberg, M.R.; Schleicher, R.L.; Rybak, M.E. Dietary supplement use and smoking are important correlates of biomarkers of water-soluble vitamin status after adjusting for sociodemographic and lifestyle variables in a representative sample of U.S. adults. *J. Nutr.* **2013**, *143*, 957S–965S. [CrossRef] [PubMed]

34. Lykkesfeldt, J.; Michels, A.J.; Frei, B. Vitamin C. *Adv. Nutr.* **2014**, *5*, 16–18. [CrossRef] [PubMed]

35. Klok, M.D.; Jakobsdottir, S.; Drent, M.L. The role of leptin and ghrelin in the regulation of food intake and body weight in humans: A review. *Obes. Rev.* **2007**, *8*, 21–34. [CrossRef] [PubMed]

36. Ashor, A.W.; Werner, A.D.; Lara, J.; Willis, N.D.; Mathers, J.C.; Siervo, M. Effects of vitamin C supplementation on glycaemic control: a systematic review and meta-analysis of randomised controlled trials. *Eur. J. Clin. Nutr.* **2017**. [CrossRef] [PubMed]

37. Gillani, S.W.; Sulaiman, S.A.S.; Abdul, M.I.M.; Baig, M.R. Combined effect of metformin with ascorbic acid versus acetyl salicylic acid on diabetes-related cardiovascular complication a 12-month single blind multicenter randomized control trial. *Cardiovasc. Diabetol.* **2017**, *16*, 103. [CrossRef] [PubMed]

38. Institute of Medicine, Panel on Dietary Antioxidants Related Compounds. *Dietary Reference Intakes for Vitamin C, Vitamin E, Selenium, and Carotenoids: A Report of the Panel on Dietary Antioxidants and Related Compounds, Subcommittees on Upper Reference Levels of Nutrients and of Interpretation and Use of Dietary Reference Intakes, and the Standing Committee on the Scientific Evaluation of Dietary Reference Intakes, Food and Nutrition Board, Institute of Medicine*; National Academy Press: Washington, DC, USA, 2000.

39. Zebrowski, E.J.; Bhatnagar, P.K. Urinary excretion pattern of ascorbic acid in streptozotocin diabetic and insulin treated rats. *Pharmacol. Res. Commun.* **1979**, *11*, 95–103. [CrossRef]

9

Vitamin C and Microvascular Dysfunction in Systemic Inflammation

Karel Tyml [1,2]

[1]   Centre for Critical Illness Research, Lawson Health Research Institute, London, ON N6A 5W9, Canada;
karel.tyml@lhsc.on.ca

[2]   Department of Medical Biophysics, University of Western Ontario, London, ON N6A 5C1, Canada

Abstract: Sepsis, life-threatening organ dysfunction caused by a dysfunctional host response to infection, is associated with high mortality. A promising strategy to improve the outcome is to inject patients intravenously with ascorbate (vitamin C). In animal models of sepsis, this injection improves survival and, among others, the microvascular function. This review examines our recent work addressing ascorbate's ability to inhibit arteriolar dysfunction and capillary plugging in sepsis. Arteriolar dysfunction includes impaired vasoconstriction/dilation (previously reviewed) and impaired conduction of vasoconstriction/dilation along the arteriole. We showed that ascorbate injected into septic mice prevents impaired conducted vasoconstriction by inhibiting neuronal nitric oxide synthase-derived NO, leading to restored inter-endothelial electrical coupling through connexin 37-containing gap junctions. Hypoxia/reoxygenation (confounding factor in sepsis) also impairs electrical coupling by protein kinase A (PKA)-dependent connexin 40 dephosphorylation; ascorbate restores PKA activation required for this coupling. Both effects of ascorbate could explain its ability to protect against hypotension in sepsis. Capillary plugging in sepsis involves P-selectin mediated platelet-endothelial adhesion and microthrombi formation. Early injection of ascorbate prevents capillary plugging by inhibiting platelet-endothelial adhesion and endothelial surface P-selectin expression. Ascorbate also prevents thrombin-induced platelet aggregation and platelet surface P-selectin expression, thus preventing microthrombi formation. Delayed ascorbate injection reverses capillary plugging and platelet-endothelial adhesion; it also attenuates sepsis-induced drop in platelet count in systemic blood. Thrombin-induced release of plasminogen-activator-inhibitor-1 from platelets (anti-fibrinolytic event in sepsis) is inhibited by ascorbate pH-dependently. Thus, under acidotic conditions in sepsis, ascorbate promotes dissolving of microthrombi in capillaries. We propose that protected/restored arteriolar conduction and capillary bed perfusion by ascorbate contributes to reduced organ injury and improved survival in sepsis.

Keywords: sepsis; microvessels; endothelial cells; platelets; electrical coupling; connexins; nitric oxide; P-selectin; coagulation; plasminogen-activator-inhibitor-1

1. Introduction

Local infectious or non-infectious insult can lead to a systemic inflammatory response. Sepsis, life-threatening organ dysfunction caused by a dysfunctional host response to infection [1], can precipitate multiple organ failure and 40% mortality in Intensive Care Units [2]. Sepsis is annually responsible for the loss of more lives than breast, colorectal, pancreatic and prostate cancers combined [3]. The prevalence of septic patients is highest in the elderly (i.e., older than 65 years) where the outcome disproportionately worsens with age [4]. Sepsis involves many pathophysiological processes including increased oxidative stress [5]. The age-aggravated worsening of outcome could be due to increased mitochondrial free radical formation that occurs naturally in aging tissues [6,7].

Among all antioxidants, ascorbate (reduced vitamin C) is considered to be the most effective water-soluble antioxidant [8]. In healthy middle-age humans, plasma ascorbate concentration is 60–80 μM [6,9], but in healthy elderly it drops to ~40 μM [10,11]. Critically, in the septic elderly, plasma ascorbate is clinically considered to be depleted (i.e., ~10 μM) [12–14]. Thus, the major defense by the antioxidant ascorbate against sepsis is nearly absent in the elderly.

A promising strategy to improve the outcome of sepsis is to replete ascorbate in patients quickly after the diagnosis of sepsis [15]. Indeed, a recent clinical study including the septic elderly reported markedly improved survival in patients injected intravenously with vitamin C, hydrocortisone and thiamine [16]. This improved survival is consistent with that observed in septic mice injected with ascorbate [15,17,18].

The sepsis-induced inflammatory response leads to dysfunction of many organ systems, including the cardiovascular system where decreased systemic vascular resistance, hypotension, maldistribution of blood flow in the microcirculation, and impaired oxygen utilization occur [19,20]. Using various animal models of sepsis, our laboratory has examined the dysfunction of the microcirculation, and the possible beneficial effects of intravenous injection of ascorbate against this dysfunction. The models, the dysfunction, and the effects of various doses of ascorbate have been reviewed [5,15,21,22]. However, our recent advances in this area extend our understanding of protection by ascorbate against microvascular dysfunction in sepsis. The objective of the present paper is to review these advances.

2. Arteriolar Dysfunction in Sepsis

Within the systemic vascular system, arterioles represent the key site along the vascular tree responsible for both the control of blood supply to the tissue and the peripheral vascular resistance [23]. The vascular resistance (and flow control) depend on (i) the degree of arteriolar diameter change elicited by local physiological/pharmacological stimuli impinging on the arteriolar wall, and (ii) the degree of conduction (or spread) of the diameter change along the arteriolar length [24]. A local arteriolar dilation without conduction yielded no increase in blood flow in the microvascular network fed by the stimulated arteriole [25].

We have shown that sepsis (cecal ligation and perforation, CLP) in young mice impairs norepinephrine-induced vasoconstriction in 6–10 μm arterioles in skeletal muscle, and that ascorbate intravenous injection protects against this impairment [26]. Similar protection by ascorbate in the vasculature has been shown for other vasoconstrictors as well as for vasodilators [21,27,28]. The mechanism of protection by ascorbate against impaired vasoconstriction has been reviewed [15]. It involves (i) inhibition of nicotinamide adenine dinucleotide phosphate (NADPH) oxidase and inducible nitric oxide synthase (iNOS) in endothelial cells of the vascular wall and (ii) inhibition of the subsequent refractory vasodilation caused by iNOS-derived NO.

2.1. Arteriolar Conducted Response in Vivo

In addition to the arteriolar diameter response, we have also examined the effects of sepsis and ascorbate on arteriolar conduction. The conduction is underpinned by electrical coupling along the arteriolar endothelial layer where connexins (i.e., constituents of inter-cellular gap junctions) are required for this coupling [29]. We used CLP (24 h model of sepsis) and lipopolysaccharide (LPS) in young mice to show that sepsis impairs conducted vasoconstriction in skeletal muscle by tyrosine kinase- and NO-dependent mechanisms [24,30]. We further determined that this impairment is mediated by the neuronal NOS (nNOS)-derived NO production and that the target of NO signaling could be the gap junction protein connexin 37 (Cx37) in the arteriolar wall [31]. Finally, we showed that an intravenous bolus of ascorbate prevented as well as reversed impairment of conducted vasoconstriction at 24 h of sepsis by inhibiting nNOS-derived NO production [32].

These studies indicate that, in addition to iNOS, nNOS is also an important source of vascular NO in our in vivo model of sepsis. Here, nNOS is found in smooth muscle cells and adjacent skeletal muscle cells [33,34]. It is possible that the protective effect of ascorbate against impaired conduction involves the heat shock protein 90 (HSP 90). HSP 90 is up-regulated during sepsis [35] and, when it binds to nNOS, it increases nNOS activity [36]. Because sepsis increases the level of reactive oxygen species (ROS) in skeletal muscle [26], and HSP 90 protein expression increases in response to ROS [37], ascorbate could scavenge ROS, prevent HSP 90 protein up-regulation, inhibit sepsis-induced increased nNOS activity and NO production, and thus prevent the septic impairment of arteriolar conduction [29].

2.2. Inter-Endothelial Electrical Coupling In Vitro

In order to gain further mechanistic insights into the impairment of conduction, we have developed an electrophysiological approach to determine inter-endothelial electrical coupling under conditions that mimic sepsis. We used monolayers of cultured microvascular endothelial cells obtained from the mouse skeletal muscle (i.e., the same tissue studied in vivo). Regarding the role of nNOS-derived NO in the impairment, we mimicked sepsis by applying exogenous NO to the monolayer. NO reduced electrical coupling [38]. Using cells from mice where individual vascular connexins were knocked-out, we determined that NO indeed targets Cx37 to reduce coupling [38]. This reduction could be due to the effect of peroxynitrite (i.e., formed after NO reaction with superoxide), or due to a direct effect of NO. Pretreatment of monolayers with ascorbate or with peroxynitrite scavenger did not affect the reduction in coupling, indicating that NO reduces coupling directly, possibly via Cx37 nitrosylation [38]. Thus, ascorbate appears to protect against impaired arteriolar conduction sepsis by affecting arteriolar function indirectly (i.e., reducing nNOS activity and NO production), rather than by affecting the target molecule Cx37.

In addition to addressing the mechanism of impaired conduction during the advanced stage in sepsis involving NO (i.e., 24 h post-CLP), we also used our electrophysiological approach in endothelial cell monolayers to address the mechanism of impaired conduction caused by LPS (i.e., an initiating factor in sepsis). We discovered that LPS reduces inter-endothelial electrical coupling via tyrosine-, ERK1/2-, PKA-, and PKC-dependent signaling that targets Cx40 [39]. This finding was consistent with the LPS-induced tyrosine-dependent impaired conduction observed in arterioles in vivo [24].

Importantly, impaired arteriolar dilatation/constriction and conduction in sepsis results in impaired microvascular blood flow which, in turn, precipitates episodes of micro-regional ischemia/reperfusion (I/R) in the tissue supplied by the arteriole (i.e., evidenced by intermittent capillary blood flow in septic skeletal muscle, [40]). I/R has been shown to aggravate the sepsis-induced inflammatory response [41,42]. Because ascorbate prevents the development of intermittent capillary blood flow in sepsis in vivo [40], we also sought to determine if ascorbate protects against reduction in inter-endothelial electrical coupling in our endothelial cell monolayer model in vitro. Using a hypoxia/reoxygenation (H/R) protocol to mimic I/R, we discovered that (i) H/R reduces inter-endothelial coupling PKA-dependently, also by targeting Cx40, and (ii) ascorbate pretreatment of the monolayer prevents this reduction by scavenging ROS [43]. This scavenging eliminates PKA inhibition by ROS [43]. Significantly, we were able to corroborate the aggravating effect by I/R on sepsis-induced inflammatory response. Concurrent LPS+H/R application to the monolayer synergistically reduced inter-endothelial electrical coupling, PKA- and PKC-dependently [44]. We demonstrated that LPS+H/R initiates tyrosine kinase- and ERK1/2-sensitive signaling that reduces electrical coupling by dephosphorylating PKA-specific serine residues of Cx40 [44]. Our most recent work pinpointed the residues 345–358 of the Cx40 carboxyl terminal tail as possible sites of this dephosphorylation [45].

Taken together, a complex picture emerges for the impaired arteriolar conduction in sepsis. Initially, LPS and the concurrent H/R may reduce inter-endothelial electrical coupling and arteriolar conduction by targeting Cx40, whereas nNOS-mediated NO overproduction in advanced sepsis reduces coupling and conduction by targeting Cx37 instead. The protection by ascorbate against impaired conduction involves (i) inhibition of the H/R component in the initial stage of sepsis (i.e., ascorbate restores PKA activation required for conduction) and, in the advanced stage, (ii) inhibition of nNOS activation and excess NO production.

Protection by ascorbate against both sepsis-induced impairment in arteriolar vasoconstriction and conduction could explain ascorbate's ability (i) to inhibit hypotension in rat models of sepsis [40,46] and (ii) to markedly reduce duration of vasopressor treatment in septic patients, normally necessitated by falling blood pressure [16].

3. Capillary Plugging in Sepsis

Sepsis-induced inflammation leads to activation of the coagulation pathway [47]. We have used the skeletal muscle in rats and mice as a bioassay to examine this aspect of sepsis in terms of capillary bed plugging, a well-known indicator of sepsis involving pro-coagulant responses [5,15]. Capillary plugging involves P-selectin mediated platelet-endothelial adhesion and fibrin deposition in capillaries [48,49]. This plugging, reported in animal and human organs, leads to inadequate oxygenation of the tissue and organ failure [5,15]. Importantly, we and others have shown that intravenous injection of ascorbate protects against sepsis-induced capillary plugging and organ injury [17,40,48,50]. The experimental details and the mechanism of this protection against capillary plugging have been reviewed [5,15]. A key component of this mechanism is endothelial nitric oxide synthase (eNOS) in endothelial cells of the microvascular wall. Since eNOS-derived NO is anti-coagulatory (i.e., it reduces platelet-endothelial adhesion [51]), and since the protection by ascorbate is absent in eNOS$^{-/-}$ mice [50], ascorbate has been proposed to act indirectly via restoring the eNOS function in the microvasculature in sepsis [50].

Ascorbate intravenous injection early in sepsis prevents capillary plugging, whereas delayed ascorbate injection later in sepsis reverses plugging (i.e., restores blood flow in previously plugged capillaries) [40,46,48]. Recently, we have addressed the mechanisms of both the prevention and reversal of plugging.

3.1. Ascorbate Prevents Capillary Plugging in Sepsis

A key event in the initiation process of sepsis-induced capillary plugging is platelet adhesion to the capillary wall. Pretreatment of mice with platelet-depleting antibody inhibits this plugging [48]. P-selectin is a key platelet-endothelium adhesion molecule [52]. Pretreatment of mice with P-selectin blocking antibody also inhibits plugging [48]. We have carried out a series of experiments designed to tease out whether platelet surface and/or endothelial surface P-selectin expression are involved in the initiation. Using a platelet-endothelial cell adhesion assay in vitro, we determined that activation of endothelial cells by LPS increased platelet adhesion to the endothelial monolayer (mouse skeletal muscle origin) P-selectin-dependently [49]. Further, LPS increased P-selectin protein expression at the surface of endothelial cells, most likely by promoting exocytosis of P-selectin protein already contained in Weibel-Palade granules beneath the endothelial surface [49,53,54]. Significantly, pretreatment of the monolayer with ascorbate inhibited all platelet adhesion to the monolayer, endothelial P-selectin surface expression, and exocytosis [49]. These in vitro studies demonstrated that ascorbate can inhibit platelet-endothelial adhesion in capillaries in vivo directly, rather than indirectly via hemodynamic effects of ascorbate on capillary blood flow.

We have also used a platelet aggregation assay in vitro, to examine the role of P-selectin at the platelet surface. LPS or plasma from septic mice did not alter P-selectin expression at the platelet surface, or platelet aggregation [55]. However, platelet-activating agents known to be released into the bloodstream during sepsis [thrombin, adenosine diphosphate (ADP), thromboxane A2] did increase P-selectin expression and aggregation. Interestingly, ascorbate inhibited these increases independently of platelet-derived NOS [55]. Thus, ascorbate could reduce aggregation directly, independent of its ability to restore eNOS function within the microvasculature. In the context of plugging of septic capillaries, the inhibition of platelet aggregation directly by ascorbate may not be enough to fully prevent plugging. In addition to this direct effect, NO-derived from non-platelet sources (e.g., endothelial eNOS) may be needed for the full in vivo effect of ascorbate.

Our results suggest a complex mechanism in the initiation of capillary plugging and in the protection by ascorbate against this plugging. An early platelet-endothelial adhesion may be followed/paralleled by the generation of platelet-activating stimuli which, in turn, result in platelet aggregation and buildup of other materials (e.g., fibrin deposits, microthrombi) which eventually plug capillaries [48,55]. So far our data indicate that ascorbate can protect against the initial platelet-endothelial adhesion and the subsequent platelet aggregation in the septic capillary. These data are consistent with the reported anti-coagulatory effect of ascorbate in sepsis [17,18].

3.2. Ascorbate Reverses Capillary Plugging

A delayed intravenous injection of ascorbate reverses both the number of plugged capillaries and platelet adhesion/trapping therein (observed in skeletal muscle, in a mouse model of sepsis involving feces injection into peritoneum, FIP) [48]. This reversal is eNOS-dependent [48]. Since platelet trapping in capillaries leads to subsequent reduction in the number of platelets available for detection in systemic blood, the platelet count in systemic blood is a complementary, clinically relevant [56], measure of capillary plugging. To this end, we showed that (i) sepsis at 7 h post-FIP indeed reduces platelet count measured in samples of arterial blood and (ii) ascorbate injection delayed to 6 h post-FIP attenuates this reduction (i.e., previously trapped platelets were released back into the systemic circulation) [48,57].

To address ascorbate's ability to quickly reverse platelet trapping (i.e., over 1 h period) we examined ascorbate's ability to dissolve microthrombi in capillaries. This dissolving will permit restarting of blood flow in these microvessels. To this end, we examined the thrombolytic system. Using our FIP model of sepsis in mice, sepsis increased mRNA of both the pro-fibrinolytic urokinase plasminogen activator (u-PA) and the anti-fibrinolytic plasminogen activator inhibitor 1 (PAI-1) in muscle and liver homogenates [57]. Delayed ascorbate did not affect u-PA mRNA in either tissue; it inhibited PAI-1 mRNA in the muscle (i.e., suggesting enhanced fibrinolysis in this tissue) but not in the liver. Since liver PAI-1 is the dominant source of soluble PAI-1 in systemic blood, we further examined PAI-1 enzymatic activity in this tissue. Ascorbate did not affect sepsis-induced increase in PAI-1 activity in the liver [57]. Consistently, delayed ascorbate also did not affect sepsis-induced increase in PAI-1 protein and activity in systemic blood plasma [57,58]. Thus, based on the PAI-1 protein/enzymatic activity data measured in tissue homogenates and systemic blood, our study did not support the hypothesis that ascorbate reverses capillary plugging in sepsis by promoting fibrinolysis.

Local pro- and anti-fibrinolytic events, which occur at the level of the capillary, may not necessarily be assessed by analyzing tissue homogenates or systemic blood. A clear example of this is the observation that sepsis causes hypocoagulability in systemic blood but hypercoagulability in the microcirculation [15]. To address this issue, we used our in vitro models of cultured microvascular endothelial cells (mouse skeletal muscle origin) and platelets isolated from mice (i.e., both cell types are present in the milieu of capillary microthrombi) [59]. Because both cell types can release PAI-1 into the extracellular space [60,61], we asked whether ascorbate affects PAI-1 release from these cells. We used thrombin or LPS to mimic sepsis. In unstimulated endothelial cells and platelets, PAI-1 was released into the extracellular space and this release was unaffected by ascorbate pretreatment. Thrombin or LPS did not alter PAI-1 release from endothelial cells. However, thrombin, but not LPS, increased PAI-1 release from platelets. Ascorbate inhibited this release pH-dependently [59].

Thus, under acidotic conditions prevalent in sepsis, our in vitro studies suggest that, together with the inhibition by ascorbate of thrombin-induced platelet aggregation discussed above, inhibition by ascorbate of thrombin-induced PAI-1 release from platelets would yield a pro-fibrinolytic effect leading to dissolving of microthrombi in septic capillaries.

3.3. A Multifaceted Mechanism of Capillary Plugging

Our work has focused mainly on the role of endothelial cells and platelets in capillary plugging observed by intravital microscopy in the septic skeletal muscle. Clearly, there are other cell types which could contribute to the formation of microvascular microthrombi. These include red blood cells which become stiff in sepsis and thus may obstruct the capillary lumen [15,62]. Additionally, activated leukocytes, including neutrophils, can adhere to the capillary/venular endothelium and thus increase the hemodynamic resistance to blood flow. The number of adhering leukocytes was negligible in capillaries and venules in the skeletal muscle of septic mice; these cells thus could not account for the capillary plugging, or be involved in the inhibitory effect of ascorbate against plugging in this tissue [48,62]. However, the presence of neutrophils in immunogenic organs such as the lung and liver and their abundance there during sepsis [18,59] would undoubtedly contribute to capillary plugging therein. Recent reports of neutrophil extracellular traps (NETs) contributing to platelet aggregation or leukocyte-platelet aggregation [63], and to microthrombi formation [64], underscore the involvement of neutrophils in capillary plugging. Importantly, ascorbate has been shown to reduce the lung NETs formation in septic mice [65].

Sepsis leads to endothelial barrier dysfunction, involving increased permeability in the microvasculature and increased extravasation of plasma proteins and fluid (reviewed by [15]). This extravasation could form tissue edema, compress the capillary lumen, and thus also contribute to capillary plugging in sepsis. Ascorbate can inhibit this dysfunction by inhibiting NADPH oxidase expression and activity in endothelial cells, by attenuating protein phosphatase 2 (PP2A) activation, and subsequently restoring the phosphorylation and distribution of the tight junction protein occludin in endothelial cells (mechanism reviewed by [15]).

4. Unresolved Issues and Future Directions in Experimental Studies of Systemic Inflammation

Most experimental studies of sepsis have used young animals, but the majority of septic patients are elderly. In septic mice, it has been shown that the levels of plasma inflammatory cytokines, antioxidant defense, and mortality markedly worsen in aged when compared to young mice [66–68]. Thus, studies in young animals may have a limited impact on our understanding and development of therapeutic strategies to treat sepsis in the elderly.

To our knowledge, there are no reports addressing the effect of ascorbate on the outcome of sepsis in aged mice. Relevant to this unresolved issue is a recent study using Gulo$^{-/-}$ mice [69]. These mice are deficient in endogenous vitamin C production and thus require the vitamin supplementation in diet. In Gulo$^{-/-}$ mice without supplementation (i.e., mimicking the nearly-depleted plasma ascorbate status in the septic elderly), sepsis resulted in exacerbated mortality and organ injury when compared to both Gulo$^{-/-}$ mice with ascorbate supplementation and Gulo$^{-/-}$ mice injected with ascorbate after the onset of sepsis [69]. The study suggests that ascorbate repletion would be critical when treating the septic elderly.

Because of the increased incidence of obesity in the present general population, another unresolved issue may be the effect of ascorbate on the outcome of sepsis in obese animals or in animals with other co-morbidities. Similar to the effect of aging, obesity in mice also worsens the inflammatory response to sepsis [70]. However, in a clinical study, sepsis in obese patients [71] did not worsen the outcome as predicted by this animal study, underscoring the complexity of human sepsis. To our knowledge, there are no reports addressing the effect of ascorbate on the outcome of sepsis in obese animals.

The non-infectious insult I/R also leads to a systemic inflammatory response, including lung injury [72], impaired arteriolar conduction [43] and capillary plugging [73]. Ascorbate has been shown to attenuate the I/R-induced injury [72] and H/R-induced impairment of inter-endothelial electrical coupling [43]. A key feature of the H/R-induced coupling impairment is H/R-stimulated increase in ROS production in endothelial cells [43,74]. Intriguingly, the stimulated ROS increase is Cx40-dependent, possibly involving a cross-talk between Cx40 and NADPH oxidase [74]. Thus, Cx40 may not function only as a structural protein in intercellular gap junctions [29,75], but also as a signaling molecule responsible for the H/R-stimulated ROS increase in endothelial cells. Given the reported aggravation by I/R in sepsis-induced inflammatory response [41,42], and the critical roles of NAPDH oxidase in impaired arteriolar vasoconstriction in sepsis and of Cx40 in impaired electrical coupling in endothelial cells exposed to LPS, H/R or LPS+H/R, the possible signaling function of Cx40 warrants further investigation.

5. Conclusions

Despite numerous animal studies and clinical trials, the mortality in sepsis remains unacceptably high. A promising strategy to improve the outcome of sepsis is to intravenously inject patients with ascorbate (vitamin C) to quickly restore its levels in blood plasma and tissues. We have shown that intravenous injection of ascorbate improves the microvascular function in septic rats and mice. These improvements include the arteriolar responsiveness to vasoactive stimuli and capillary bed perfusion.

In particular, our recent work demonstrated that ascorbate inhibits the sepsis-induced impairment of arteriolar conducted vasoconstriction by inhibiting nNOS-derived NO production and ROS production, to restore the inter-endothelial cell electrical coupling and gap junction function. These effects contribute to ascorbate's ability to protect against hypotension in sepsis. Further, we demonstrated that ascorbate inhibits capillary plugging in sepsis by inhibiting platelet-endothelial adhesion and platelet aggregation mediated by P-selectin, and by promoting the dissolution of microthrombi in capillaries. These effects contribute to ascorbate's ability to protect against tissue injury and to improve survival in sepsis.

Acknowledgments: I would like to thank Scott Swarbreck, Dan Secor, Darcy Lidington, Michael Bolon, Feng Wu, Fuyan Li, Rebecca McKinnon, Gail Yu, Mohammad Siddiqui, John Armour, and Nigel Gocan for their lab work and accomplishments summarized in this review, John Wilson, Christopher Ellis, Sean Gill, Yves Ouellette, Gerald Kidder and Dale Laird for stimulating discussions, and the Heart and Stroke Foundation of Ontario and the Canadian Institutes of Health Research for providing financial support. I also acknowledge William Sibbald who, in the 1990s, assembled a group of clinicians and basic scientists to spearhead long-term research into the mechanism of circulatory dysfunction in sepsis, including the microcirculatory dysfunction, at Victoria Hospital Research Institute, London, Ontario.

References

1. Singer, M.; Deutschman, C.S.; Seymour, C.W.; Shankar-Hari, M.; Annane, D.; Bauer, M.; Bellomo, R.; Bernard, G.R.; Chiche, J.D.; Coopersmith, C.M.; et al. The third international consensus definitions for sepsis and septic shock (sepsis-3). *JAMA* **2016**, *315*, 801–810. [CrossRef] [PubMed]

2. Martin, C.M.; Priestap, F.; Fisher, H.; Fowler, R.A.; Heyland, D.K.; Keenan, S.P.; Longo, C.J.; Morrison, T.; Bentley, D.; Antman, N. A prospective, observational registry of patients with severe sepsis: The Canadian Sepsis Treatment and Response Registry. *Crit. Care Med.* **2009**, *37*, 81–88. [CrossRef] [PubMed]

3. Angus, D.C.; Linde-Zwirble, W.T.; Lidicker, J.; Clermont, G.; Carcillo, J.; Pinsky, M.R. Epidemiology of severe sepsis in the United States: Analysis of incidence, outcome, and associated costs of care. *Crit. Care Med.* **2001**, *29*, 1303–1310. [CrossRef] [PubMed]

4. Martin, G.S.; Mannino, D.M.; Moss, M. The effect of age on the development and outcome of adult sepsis. *Crit. Care Med.* **2006**, *34*, 15–21. [CrossRef] [PubMed]

5. Tyml, K. Critical role for oxidative stress, platelets, and coagulation in capillary blood flow impairment in sepsis. *Microcirculation* **2011**, *18*, 152–162. [CrossRef] [PubMed]

6. Bailey, D.M.; McEneny, J.; Mathieu-Costello, O.; Henry, R.R.; James, P.E.; McCord, J.M.; Pietri, S.; Young, I.S.; Richardson, R.S. Sedentary aging increases resting and exercise-induced intramuscular free radical formation. *J. Appl. Physiol.* **2010**, *109*, 449–456. [CrossRef] [PubMed]

7. Miquel, J.; Economos, A.C.; Fleming, J.; Johnson, J.E. Mitochondrial role in cell aging. *Exp. Gerontol.* **1980**, *15*, 575–591. [CrossRef]

8.   Frei, B.; England, L.; Ames, B.N. Ascorbate is an outstanding antioxidant in human blood plasma. *Proc. Natl. Acad. Sci. USA* **1989**, *86*, 6377–6381. [CrossRef] [PubMed]

9.   Levine, M.; Conry-Cantilena, C.; Wang, Y.; Welch, R.W.; Washko, P.W.; Dhariwal, K.R.; Park, J.B.; Lazarev, A.; Graumlich, J.F.; King, J.; et al. Vitamin C pharmacokinetics in healthy volunteers: Evidence for a recommended dietary allowance. *Proc. Natl. Acad. Sci. USA* **1996**, *93*, 3704–3709. [CrossRef] [PubMed]

10.   Heseker, H.; Schneider, R. Requirement and supply of vitamin C, E and beta-carotene for elderly men and women. *Eur. J. Clin. Nutr.* **1994**, *48*, 118–127. [PubMed]

11.   Smith, V.H. Vitamin C deficiency is an under-diagnosed contributor to degenerative disc disease in the elderly. *Med. Hypotheses* **2010**, *74*, 695–697. [CrossRef] [PubMed]

12.   Fain, O.; Pariés, J.; Jacquart, B.T.; Le Moël, G.; Kettaneh, A.; Stirnemann, J.; Héron, C.; Sitbon, M.; Taleb, C.; Letellier, E.; et al. Hypovitaminosis C in hospitalized patients. *Eur. J. Intern. Med.* **2003**, *14*, 419–425. [CrossRef] [PubMed]

13.   Galley, H.F.; Davies, M.J.; Webster, N.R. Ascorbyl radical formation in patients with sepsis: Effect of ascorbate loading. *Free Radic. Biol. Med.* **1996**, *20*, 139–143. [CrossRef]

14.   Paz, H.L.; Martin, A.A. Sepsis in an aging population. *Crit. Care Med.* **2006**, *34*, 234–235. [CrossRef] [PubMed]

15.   Wilson, J.X. Evaluation of vitamin C for adjuvant sepsis therapy. *ARS* **2013**, *19*, 2129–2140. [CrossRef] [PubMed]

16.   Marik, P.E.; Khangoora, V.; Rivera, R.; Hooper, M.H.; Catravas, J. Hydrocortisone, Vitamin C and thiamine for the treatment of severe sepsis and septic shock: A retrospective before–after study. *Chest* **2016**, *151*, 1229–1238. [CrossRef] [PubMed]

17.   Fisher, B.J.; Seropian, I.M.; Kraskauskas, D.; Thakkar, J.N.; Voelkel, N.F.; Fowler, A.A.; Natarajan, R. Ascorbic acid attenuates lipopolysaccharide-induced acute lung injury. *Crit. Care Med.* **2011**, *39*, 1454–1460. [CrossRef] [PubMed]

18.   Fisher, B.J.; Kraskauskas, D.; Martin, E.J.; Farkas, D.; Wegelin, J.A.; Brophy, D.; Ward, K.R.; Voelkel, N.F.; Fowler, A.A.; Natarajan, R. Mechanisms of attenuation of abdominal sepsis induced acute lung injury by ascorbic acid. *Am. J. Physiol. Lung Cell. Mol. Physiol.* **2012**, *303*, 20–32. [CrossRef] [PubMed]

19.   Nguyen, H.B.; Rivers, E.P.; Knoblich, B.P.; Jacobsen, G.; Muzzin, A.; Ressler, J.A.; Tomlanovich, M.C. Early lactate clearance is associated with improved outcome in severe sepsis and septic shock. *Crit. Care Med.* **2004**, *32*, 1637–1642. [CrossRef] [PubMed]

20.   Bone, R.C. Gram-negative sepsis: Background, clinical features, and intervention. *Chest* **1991**, *100*, 802–808. [CrossRef] [PubMed]

21.   Wilson, J.X. Mechanism of action of vitamin C in sepsis: Ascorbate modulates redox signaling in endothelium. *Biofactors* **2009**, *35*, 5–13. [CrossRef] [PubMed]

22.   Wilson, J.X.; Wu, F. Vitamin C in sepsis. *Subcell. Biochem.* **2012**, *56*, 67–83. [PubMed]

23.   Joyner, W.L.; Davis, M.J. Pressure profile along the microvascular network and its control. *Fed. Proc.* **1987**, *46*, 266–269. [PubMed]

24.   Tyml, K.; Wang, X.; Lidington, D.; Ouellette, Y. Lipopolysaccharide reduces intercellular coupling *in vitro* and arteriolar conducted response in vivo. *Am. J. Physiol. Heart Circ. Physiol.* **2001**, *281*, H1397–H1406. [PubMed]

25.   Kurjiaka, D.T.; Segal, S.S. Conducted vasodilation elevates flow in arteriole networks of hamster striated muscle. *Am. J. Physiol.* **1995**, *269*, H1723–H1728. [PubMed]

26.   Wu, F.; Wilson, J.X.; Tyml, K. Ascorbate inhibits iNOS expression and preserves vasoconstrictor responsiveness in skeletal muscle of septic mice. *Am. J. Physiol. Regul. Integr. Comp. Physiol.* **2003**, *285*, R50–R56. [CrossRef] [PubMed]

27.   Wu, F.; Wilson, J.X.; Tyml, K. Ascorbate protects against impaired arteriolar constriction in sepsis by inhibiting inducible nitric oxide synthase expression. *Free Radic. Biol. Med.* **2004**, *37*, 1282–1289. [CrossRef] [PubMed]

28.   Aschauer, S.; Gouya, G.; Klickovic, U.; Storka, A.; Weisshaar, S.; Vollbracht, C.; Krick, B.; Weiss, G.; Wolzt, M. Effect of systemic high dose vitamin C therapy on forearm blood flow reactivity during endotoxemia in healthy human subjects. *Vascul. Pharmacol.* **2014**, *61*, 25–29. [CrossRef] [PubMed]

29.   Tyml, K. Role of connexins in microvascular dysfunction during inflammation. *Can. J. Physiol. Pharmacol.* **2011**, *89*, 1–12. [CrossRef] [PubMed]

30.   Lidington, D.; Ouellette, Y.; Li, F.; Tyml, K. Conducted vasoconstriction is reduced in a mouse model of sepsis. *J. Vasc. Res.* **2003**, *40*, 149–158. [CrossRef] [PubMed]

31. McKinnon, R.L.; Lidington, D.; Bolon, M.; Ouellette, Y.; Kidder, G.M.; Tyml, K. Reduced arteriolar conducted vasoconstriction in septic mouse cremaster muscle is mediated by nNOS-derived NO. *Cardiovasc. Res.* **2006**, *69*, 236–244. [CrossRef] [PubMed]

32. McKinnon, R.L.; Lidington, D.; Tyml, K. Ascorbate inhibits reduced arteriolar conducted vasoconstriction in septic mouse cremaster muscle. *Microcirculation* **2007**, *14*, 697–707. [CrossRef] [PubMed]

33. Gocan, N.C.; Scott, J.A.; Tyml, K. Nitric oxide produced via neuronal NOS may impair vasodilatation in septic rat skeletal muscle. *Am. J. Physiol. Heart Circ. Physiol.* **2000**, *278*, H1480–H1489. [PubMed]

34. Kavdia, M.; Popel, A.S. Contribution of nNOS- and eNOS-derived NO to microvascular smooth muscle NO exposure. *J. Appl. Physiol.* **2004**, *97*, 293–301. [CrossRef] [PubMed]

35. Hashiguchi, N.; Ogura, H.; Tanaka, H.; Koh, T.; Nakamori, Y.; Noborio, M.; Shiozaki, T.; Nishino, M.; Kuwagata, Y.; Shimazu, T.; et al. Enhanced expression of heat shock proteins in activated polymorphonuclear leukocytes in patients with sepsis. *J. Trauma* **2001**, *51*, 1104–1109. [CrossRef] [PubMed]

36. Song, Y.; Zweier, J.L.; Xia, Y. Heat-shock protein 90 augments neuronal nitric oxide synthase activity by enhancing Ca^{2+}/calmodulin binding. *Biochem. J.* **2001**, *355*, 357–360. [CrossRef] [PubMed]

37. Muller, M.; Gauley, J.; Heikkila, J.J. Hydrogen peroxide induces heat shock protein and proto-oncogene mRNA accumulation in Xenopus laevis A6 kidney epithelial cells. *Can. J. Physiol. Pharmacol.* **2004**, *82*, 523–529. [CrossRef] [PubMed]

38. McKinnon, R.L.; Bolon, M.L.; Wang, H.-X.; Swarbreck, S.; Kidder, G.M.; Simon, A.M.; Tyml, K. Reduction of electrical coupling between microvascular endothelial cells by NO depends on connexin37. *Am. J. Physiol. Heart Circ. Physiol.* **2009**, *297*, H93–H101. [CrossRef] [PubMed]

39. Bolon, M.L.; Kidder, G.M.; Simon, A.M.; Tyml, K. Lipopolysaccharide reduces electrical coupling in microvascular endothelial cells by targeting connexin40 in a tyrosine-, ERK1/2-, PKA-, and PKC-dependent manner. *J. Cell. Physiol.* **2007**, *211*, 159–166. [CrossRef] [PubMed]

40. Armour, J.; Tyml, K.; Lidington, D.; Wilson, J.X. Ascorbate prevents microvascular dysfunction in the skeletal muscle of the septic rat. *J. Appl. Physiol.* **2001**, *90*, 795–803. [PubMed]

41. Khadaroo, R.G.; Kapus, A.; Powers, K.A.; Cybulsky, M.I.; Marshall, J.C.; Rotstein, O.D. Oxidative stress reprograms lipopolysaccharide signaling via Src kinase-dependent pathway in RAW 264.7 macrophage cell line. *J. Biol. Chem.* **2003**, *278*, 47834–47841. [CrossRef] [PubMed]

42. Powers, K.A.; Szaszi, K.; Khadaroo, R.G.; Tawadros, P.S.; Marshall, J.C.; Kapus, A.; Rotstein, O.D. Oxidative stress generated by hemorrhagic shock recruits Toll-like receptor 4 to the plasma membrane in macrophages. *JEM* **2006**, *203*, 1951–1961. [CrossRef] [PubMed]

43. Bolon, M.L.; Ouellette, Y.; Li, F.; Tyml, K. Abrupt reoxygenation following hypoxia reduces electrical coupling between endothelial cells of wild-type but not connexin40 null mice in oxidant- and PKA-dependent manner. *FASEB J.* **2005**, *19*, 1725–1727. [CrossRef] [PubMed]

44. Bolon, M.L.; Peng, T.; Kidder, G.M.; Tyml, K. Lipopolysaccharide plus hypoxia and reoxygenation synergistically reduce electrical coupling between microvascular endothelial cells by dephosphorylating connexin40. *J. Cell. Physiol.* **2008**, *217*, 350–359. [CrossRef] [PubMed]

45. Siddiqui, M.; Swarbreck, S.; Shao, Q.; Secor, D.; Peng, T.; Laird, D.W.; Tyml, K. Critical role of Cx40 in reduced endothelial electrical coupling by lipopolysaccharide and hypoxia-reoxygenation. *J. Vasc. Res.* **2015**, *52*, 396–403. [CrossRef] [PubMed]

46. Tyml, K.; Li, F.; Wilson, J.X. Delayed ascorbate bolus protects against maldistribution of microvascular blood flow in septic rat skeletal muscle. *Crit. Care Med.* **2005**, *33*, 1823–1828. [CrossRef] [PubMed]

47. Levi, M.; van der Poll, T.; Büller, H.R. Bidirectional relation between inflammation and coagulation. *Circulation* **2004**, *109*, 2698–2704. [CrossRef] [PubMed]

48. Secor, D.; Li, F.; Ellis, C.G.; Sharpe, M.D.; Gross, P.L.; Wilson, J.X.; Tyml, K. Impaired microvascular perfusion in sepsis requires activated coagulation and P-selectin-mediated platelet adhesion in capillaries. *Intensive Care Med.* **2010**, *36*, 1928–1934. [CrossRef] [PubMed]

49. Secor, D.; Swarbreck, S.; Ellis, C.G.; Sharpe, M.D.; Feng, Q.; Tyml, K. Ascorbate inhibits platelet-endothelial adhesion in an in-vitro model of sepsis via reduced endothelial surface P-selectin expression. *Blood Coagul. Fibrinolysis* **2017**, *28*, 28–33. [CrossRef] [PubMed]

50. Tyml, K.; Li, F.; Wilson, J.X. Septic impairment of capillary blood flow requires nicotinamide adenine dinucleotide phosphate oxidase but not nitric oxide synthase and is rapidly reversed by ascorbate through an endothelial nitric oxide synthase-dependent mechanism. *Crit. Care Med.* **2008**, *36*, 2355–2362. [CrossRef] [PubMed]

51. Cerwinka, W.H.; Cooper, D.; Krieglstein, C.F.; Feelisch, M.; Granger, D.N. Nitric oxide modulates endotoxin-induced platelet-endothelial cell adhesion in intestinal venules. *Am. J. Physiol. Heart Circ. Physiol.* **2002**, *282*, H1111–H1117. [CrossRef] [PubMed]

52. Blann, A.D.; Nadar, S.K.; Lip, G.Y.H. The adhesion molecule P-selectin and cardiovascular disease. *Eur. Heart J.* **2003**, *24*, 2166–2179. [CrossRef] [PubMed]

53. McCarron, R.M.; Doron, D.A.; Sirén, A.L.; Feuerstein, G.; Heldman, E.; Pollard, H.B.; Spatz, M.; Hallenbeck, J.M. Agonist-stimulated release of von willebrand factor and procoagulant factor VIII in rats with and without risk factors for stroke. *Brain Res.* **1994**, *647*, 265–272. [CrossRef]

54. Wang, G.F.; Wu, S.Y.; Rao, J.J.; Lü, L.; Xu, W.; Pang, J.X.; Liu, Z.Q.; Wu, S.G.; Zhang, J.J. Genipin inhibits endothelial exocytosis via nitric oxide in cultured human umbilical vein endothelial cells. *Acta. Pharmacol. Sin.* **2009**, *30*, 589–596. [CrossRef] [PubMed]

55. Secor, D.; Swarbreck, S.; Ellis, C.G.; Sharpe, M.D.; Tyml, K. Ascorbate reduces mouse platelet aggregation and surface P-selectin expression in an ex vivo model of sepsis. *Microcirculation* **2013**, *20*, 502–510. [CrossRef] [PubMed]

56. Moreau, D.; Timsit, J.F.; Vesin, A.; Garrouste-Orgeas, M.; de Lassence, A.; Zahar, J.R.; Adrie, C.; Vincent, F.; Cohen, Y.; Schlemmer, B.; et al. Platelet count decline: an early prognostic marker in critically ill patients with prolonged ICU stays. *Chest* **2007**, *131*, 1735–1741. [CrossRef] [PubMed]

57. Swarbreck, S.; Secor, D.; Li, F.; Gross, P.L.; Ellis, C.G.; Sharpe, M.D.; Wilson, J.X.; Tyml, K. Effect of ascorbate on fibrinolytic factors in septic mouse skeletal muscle. *Blood Coagul. Fibrinolysis* **2014**, *25*, 745–753. [CrossRef] [PubMed]

58. Swarbreck, S.B.; Secor, D.; Ellis, C.G.; Sharpe, M.D.; Wilson, J.X.; Tyml, K. Short-term effect of ascorbate on bacterial content, plasminogen activator inhibitor-1, and myeloperoxidase in septic mice. *J. Surg. Res.* **2014**, *191*, 432–440. [CrossRef] [PubMed]

59. Swarbreck, S.B.; Secor, D.; Ellis, C.G.; Sharpe, M.D.; Wilson, J.X.; Tyml, K. Effect of ascorbate on plasminogen activator inhibitor-1 expression and release from platelets and endothelial cells in an in-vitro model of sepsis. *Blood Coagul. Fibrinolysis* **2015**, *26*, 436–442. [CrossRef] [PubMed]

60. Sagripanti, A.; Morganti, M.; Carpi, A.; Cupisti, A.; Nicolini, A.; Barsotti, M.; Camici, M.; Mittermayer, C.; Barsotti, G. Uremic medium increases cytokine-induced PAI-1 secretion by cultured endothelial cells. *Biomed. Pharmacother.* **1998**, *52*, 298–302. [CrossRef]

61. Nylander, M.; Osman, A.; Ramström, S.; Aklint, E.; Larsson, A.; Lindahl, T.L. The role of thrombin receptors PAR1 and PAR4 for PAI-1 storage, synthesis and secretion by human platelets. *Thromb. Res.* **2012**, *129*, 51–58. [CrossRef] [PubMed]

62. Bateman, R.M.; Jagger, J.E.; Sharpe, M.D.; Ellsworth, M.L.; Mehta, S.; Ellis, C.G. Erythrocyte deformability is a nitric oxide-mediated factor in decreased capillary density during sepsis. *Am. J. Physiol. Heart Circ. Physiol.* **2001**, *280*, H2848–H2856. [PubMed]

63. Tanaka, K.; Koike, Y.; Shimura, T.; Okigami, M.; Ide, S.; Toiyama, Y.; Okugawa, Y.; Inoue, Y.; Araki, T.; Uchida, K.; et al. In vivo characterization of neutrophil extracellular traps in various organs of a murine sepsis model. *PLoS ONE* **2014**. [CrossRef] [PubMed]

64. McDonald, B.; Davis, R.P.; Kim, S.J.; Tse, M.; Esmon, C.T.; Kolaczkowska, E.; Jenne, C.N. Platelets and neutrophil extracellular traps collaborate to promote intravascular coagulation during sepsis in mice. *Blood* **2017**, *129*, 1357–1367. [CrossRef] [PubMed]

65. Mohammed, B.M.; Fisher, B.J.; Kraskauskas, D.; Farkas, D.; Brophy, D.F.; Fowler, A.A.; Natarajan, R. Vitamin C: A novel regulator of neutrophil extracellular trap formation. *Nutrients* **2013**, *5*, 3131–3151. [CrossRef] [PubMed]

66. Starr, M.E.; Ueda, J.; Takahashi, H.; Weiler, H.; Esmon, C.T.; Evers, B.M.; Saito, H. Age-dependent vulnerability to endotoxemia is associated with reduction of anticoagulant factors activated protein C and thrombomodulin. *Blood* **2010**, *115*, 4886–4893. [CrossRef] [PubMed]

67. Starr, M.E.; Ueda, J.; Yamamoto, S.; Evers, B.M.; Saito, H. The effects of aging on pulmonary oxidative damage, protein nitration, and extracellular superoxide dismutase down-regulation during systemic inflammation. *Free Radic. Biol. Med.* **2011**, *50*, 371–380. [CrossRef] [PubMed]

68. Turnbull, I.R.; Clark, A.T.; Stromberg, P.E.; Dixon, D.J.; Woolsey, C.A.; Davis, C.G.; Hotchkiss, R.S.; Buchman, T.G.; Coopersmith, C.M. Effects of aging on the immunopathologic response to sepsis. *Crit. Care Med.* **2009**, *37*, 1018–1023. [CrossRef] [PubMed]

69. Fisher, B.J.; Kraskauskas, D.; Martin, E.J.; Farkas, D.; Puri, P.; Massey, H.D.; Idowu, M.O.; Brophy, D.F.; Voelkel, N.F.; Fowler, A.A.; et al. Attenuation of Sepsis-induced Organ Injury in Mice by Vitamin C. *JPEN* **2013**, *38*, 825–839. [CrossRef] [PubMed]

70. Vachharajani, V.; Russell, J.M.; Scott, K.L.; Conrad, S.; Stokes, K.Y.; Tallam, L.; Hall, J.; Granger, D.N. Obesity exacerbates sepsis-induced inflammation and microvascular dysfunction in mouse brain. *Microcirculation* **2005**, *12*, 183–194. [CrossRef] [PubMed]

71. Arabi, Y.M.; Dara, S.I.; Tamim, H.M.; Rishu, A.H.; Bouchama, A.; Khedr, M.K.; Feinstein, D.; Parrillo, J.E.; Wood, K.E.; Keenan, S.P.; et al. Clinical characteristics, sepsis interventions and outcomes in the obese patients with septic shock: An international multicenter cohort study. *Crit Care.* **2013**, *17*, R72. [CrossRef] [PubMed]

72. Baltalarli, A.; Ozcan, V.; Bir, F.; Ferda, B.; Aybek, H.; Sacar, M.; Onem, G.; Goksin, I.; Demir, S.; Teke, Z.; et al. Ascorbic acid (vitamin C) and iloprost attenuate the lung injury caused by ischemia/reperfusion of the lower extremities of rats. *Ann. Vasc. Surg.* **2006**, *20*, 49–55. [CrossRef] [PubMed]

73. Bihari, A.; Cepinskas, G.; Forbes, T.L.; Potter, R.F.; Lawendy, A.R. Systemic application of carbon monoxide-releasing molecule 3 protects skeletal muscle from ischemia-reperfusion injury. *J. Vasc. Surg.* **2017**. [CrossRef] [PubMed]

74. Yu, G.; Bolon, M.; Laird, D.W.; Tyml, K. Hypoxia and reoxygenation-induced oxidant production increase in microvascular endothelial cells depends on connexin40. *Free Radic. Biol. Med.* **2010**, *49*, 1008–1013. [CrossRef] [PubMed]

75. Guo, R.; Si, R.; Scott, B.T.; Makino, A. Mitochondrial connexin40 regulates mitochondrial calcium uptake in coronary endothelial cells. *Am. J. Physiol. Cell. Physiol.* **2017**, *312*, C398–C406. [CrossRef] [PubMed]

10

Vitamin C and Infections

Harri Hemilä

Department of Public Health, University of Helsinki, Helsinki FI-00014, Finland; harri.hemila@helsinki.fi;

Abstract: In the early literature, vitamin C deficiency was associated with pneumonia. After its identification, a number of studies investigated the effects of vitamin C on diverse infections. A total of 148 animal studies indicated that vitamin C may alleviate or prevent infections caused by bacteria, viruses, and protozoa. The most extensively studied human infection is the common cold. Vitamin C administration does not decrease the average incidence of colds in the general population, yet it halved the number of colds in physically active people. Regularly administered vitamin C has shortened the duration of colds, indicating a biological effect. However, the role of vitamin C in common cold treatment is unclear. Two controlled trials found a statistically significant dose–response, for the duration of common cold symptoms, with up to 6–8 g/day of vitamin C. Thus, the negative findings of some therapeutic common cold studies might be explained by the low doses of 3–4 g/day of vitamin C. Three controlled trials found that vitamin C prevented pneumonia. Two controlled trials found a treatment benefit of vitamin C for pneumonia patients. One controlled trial reported treatment benefits for tetanus patients. The effects of vitamin C against infections should be investigated further.

Keywords: ascorbic acid; bacteria; bacterial toxins; common cold; herpes zoster; pneumonia; protozoa; respiratory tract infections; viruses; tetanus

---

1. Early History on Vitamin C and Infections

Vitamin C was identified in the early twentieth century in the search for a substance, the deficiency of which would cause scurvy [1,2]. Scurvy was associated with pneumonia in the early literature, which implies that the factor that cured scurvy might also have an effect on pneumonia.

Alfred Hess (1920) summarized a series of autopsy findings as follows: "pneumonia, lobular or lobar, is one of the most frequent complications (of scurvy) and causes of death" and "secondary pneumonias, usually broncho-pneumonic in type, are of common occurrence and in many (scurvy) epidemics constitute the prevailing cause of death" [3]. He later commented that in "infantile scurvy ... a lack of the antiscorbutic factor (vitamin C) which leads to scurvy, at the same time predisposes to infections (particularly of the respiratory tract) ... Similar susceptibility to infections goes hand in hand with adult scurvy" [4]. In the early 1900s, Casimir Funk, who coined the word "vitamin", noted that an epidemic of pneumonia in the Sudan disappeared when antiscorbutic (vitamin C-containing) treatment was given to the numerous cases of scurvy that appeared at about the same time [5].

The great majority of mammals synthesize vitamin C in their bodies, but primates and the guinea pig cannot. Therefore, the guinea pig is a useful animal model on which to study vitamin C deficiency. Bacteria were often found in histological sections of scorbutic guinea pigs, so much so that some early authors assumed that scurvy might be an infectious disease. However, Hess (1920) concluded that such results merely showed that the tissues of scorbutic animals frequently harbor bacteria, and "there is no doubt that the invasion of the blood-stream does occur readily in the course of scurvy, but this takes place generally after the disease has developed and must be regarded as a secondary phenomenon and therefore unessential from an etiological standpoint. Indeed one of the striking and important symptoms of scurvy is the marked susceptibility to infection" [3]. When summarizing autopsy findings of experimental scurvy in the guinea pig, Hess also noted that "Pneumonia is met with very frequently and constitutes a common terminal infection".

Vitamin C was considered as an explanation for scurvy, which was regarded as a disease of the connective tissues, since many of the symptoms such as poor wound healing implied crucial effects on the connective tissues. Therefore, the mainstream view in medicine regarded vitamin C as a vitamin that safeguards the integrity of connective tissues [6]. The implications of the earlier research by Hess and others were superseded. This historical background might explain the current lack of interest in the effects of vitamin C on infections, even though firm evidence that vitamin C influences infections has been available for decades.

Early literature on vitamin C and infections was reviewed by Clausen (1934), Robertson (1934), and Perla and Marmorston (1937) [5,7,8]. Those reviews are thorough descriptions of the large number of early studies on the topic of this review. Scanned versions of those reviews and English translations of many non-English papers cited in this review are available at the home page of this author [9]. The book on scurvy by Hess (1920) is available in a digitized format [3].

2. Biology Relevant to the Effects of Vitamin C on Infections

Evidence-based medicine (EBM) emphasizes that in the evaluation of treatments researchers should focus primarily on clinically relevant outcomes, and little weight should be put on biological explanations. Therefore, this review focuses on infections and not on the immune system. Immune system effects are surrogates for clinical effects and there are numerous cases when surrogates had poor correlations with clinically relevant outcomes [10]. Nevertheless, biology provides a useful background when we consider the plausibility of vitamin C to influence infections.

2.1. Dose–Concentration Relationship

The vitamin C level in plasma of people in good health becomes saturated at about 70 μmol/L when the intake is about 0.2 g/day [11]. On the other hand, when vitamin C intake is below 0.1 g/day, there is a steep relationship between plasma vitamin C level and the dose of the vitamin. Clinical scurvy may appear when the plasma concentration falls below 11 μmol/L, which corresponds to an intake of less than 0.01 g/day [12–14]. Thus, when healthy people have a dietary intake of about 0.2 g/day of vitamin C, there is usually no reason to expect a response to vitamin C supplementation. This does not apply universally because certain studies have shown the benefits of supplementation, even though the baseline intake was as high as 0.5 g/day (see below). If the initial vitamin C intake is lower than about 0.1 g/day, effects of vitamin C supplementation may be expected on the basis of the dose–concentration curve. Nevertheless, this argument does not apply to patients with infections since their vitamin C metabolism is altered and they have decreased vitamin C levels (see below).

2.2. Infections Increase Oxidative Stress

Vitamin C is an antioxidant. Therefore, any effects of vitamin C may be most prominent under conditions when oxidative stress is elevated. Many infections lead to the activation of phagocytes, which release oxidizing agents referred to as reactive oxygen species (ROS). These play a role in the processes that lead to the deactivation of viruses and the killing of bacteria [15]. However, many of the ROS appear to be harmful to the host cells, and in some cases they seem to play a role in the pathogenesis of infections [16,17]. Vitamin C is an efficient water-soluble antioxidant and may protect host cells against the actions of ROS released by phagocytes. Phagocytes have a specific transport system by which the oxidized form of vitamin C (dehydroascorbic acid) is imported into the cell where it is converted into the reduced form of vitamin C [18,19].

Influenza A infection in mice resulted in a decrease in vitamin C concentration in bronchoalveolar lavage fluid, which was concomitant with an increase in dehydroascorbic acid, the oxidized form of vitamin C [20], and in vitamin C deficiency influenza led to greater lung pathology [21]. Respiratory syncytial virus decreased the expression of antioxidant enzymes thereby increasing oxidative damage [22]. Bacterial toxins have also led to the loss of vitamin C from many tissues in animal studies [1] (p. 6).

Increased ROS production during the immune response to pathogens can explain the decrease in vitamin C levels seen in several infections. There is evidence that plasma, leukocyte and urinary vitamin C levels decrease in the common cold and in other infections [1,23]. Hume and Weyers (1973) reported that vitamin C levels in leukocytes halved when subjects contracted a cold and returned to the original level one week after recovery [24]. Vitamin C levels are also decreased by pneumonia [25–28].

Decreases in vitamin C levels during various infections imply that vitamin C administration might have a treatment effect on many patients with infections. There is no reason to assume that the saturation of plasma or leukocyte vitamin C levels during infections is reached by the 0.2 g/day intake of vitamin C that applies to healthy people (see above). In particular, Hume and Weyers (1973) showed that supplementation at the level of 0.2 g/day was insufficient to normalize leukocyte vitamin C levels in common cold patients, but when 6 g/day of vitamin C was administered, the decline in leukocyte vitamin C induced by the common cold was essentially abolished [24].

2.3. Vigorous Physical Activity Increases Oxidative Stress

Heavy physical stress leads to the elevation of oxidative stress [29]. Therefore, responses to vitamin C might be observed when people are particularly active physically. Electron spin resonance studies have shown that vitamin C administration decreased the levels of free radicals generated during exercise [30] and vitamin C administration attenuated the increases in oxidative stress markers caused by exercise [31]. Therefore, vitamin C supplementation might have beneficial effects on people who are under physical stress. In such cases there is no reason to assume that 0.2 g/day of vitamin C might lead to maximal effects of the vitamin. Direct evidence of benefits of vitamin C supplementation to physically active people was found in three randomized trials in which 0.5 to 2 g/day of vitamin C prevented exercise-induced bronchoconstriction [32,33].

2.4. Vitamin C May Protect against Stress Caused by Cold and Hot Environments

Studies in animals and humans have indicated that vitamin C may protect against stress caused by cold and hot environments [34–37]. Some common cold studies with positive results investigated physically active participants in cold environments and other studies investigated marathon runners in South Africa (see below). Therefore, the effects of vitamin C in the protection against cold or heat stress might also be relevant when explaining the benefits in those studies.

2.5. Marginally Low Vitamin C Status Might Lead to Benefits of Supplementation

It seems evident that any effects of vitamin C supplementation may be more prominent when the baseline vitamin C level is particularly low. As noted above, a profound vitamin C deficiency was associated with pneumonia in the early literature. It seems plausible that less severe vitamin C deficiency, which may be called "marginal vitamin C deficiency", can also be associated with increased risk and severity of infections, although the effects may be less pronounced than those caused by scurvy.

Low vitamin C levels are not just of historical relevance. Cases of scurvy in hospitals have been described in several recent case reports [38,39]. One survey estimated that about 10% of hospitalized elderly patients had scurvy [40]. Surveys have also shown that plasma vitamin C levels below 11 µmol/L were found for 14% of males and 10% of females in the USA, 19% of males and 13% of females in India, 40% of elderly people living in institutions in the UK, 23% of children and 39% of women in Mexico, and 79%–93% of men in Western Russia. Moreover, 45% of a cohort of pregnant women in rural India had plasma vitamin C levels below 4 µmol/L and the mean plasma vitamin C level fell to 10 µmol/L in a cohort of pregnant or lactating women in Gambian villages in the rainy season [41].

The mean vitamin C intake in adults in the USA has been about 0.10 g/day, but 10% of the population has had intake levels of less than 0.04 g/day [14]. Thus, if low intake levels of vitamin C have adverse effects on the incidence and severity of infections, this may be important also in population groups in western countries, and not just in developing countries.

2.6. Vitamin C Has Effects on the Immune System

Vitamin C levels in white blood cells are tens of times higher than in plasma, which may indicate functional roles of the vitamin in these immune system cells. Vitamin C has been shown to affect the functions of phagocytes, production of interferon, replication of viruses, and maturation of T-lymphocytes, etc. in laboratory studies [1,23,42–44]. Some of the effects of vitamin C on the immune system may be non-specific and in some cases other antioxidants had similar effects.

2.7. The Diverse Biochemical, Physiological, and Psychological Effects of Vitamin C

Biochemistry textbooks usually mention the role of vitamin C in collagen hydroxylation. However, the survival time of vitamin C deficient guinea pigs was extended by carnitine [45] and by glutathione [46], which indicates that scurvy is not solely explained by defects in collagen hydroxylation, and it is not clear whether hydroxylation is important at all in explaining scurvy [6]. Vitamin C participates in the enzymatic synthesis of dopamine, carnitine, a number of neuroendocrine peptides, etc. [6,47–50]. Vitamin C is also a powerful antioxidant, as mentioned above.

Experimentally induced vitamin C deficiency leads to depression and fatigue [11,51]. Recently, vitamin C was reported to improve the mood of acutely hospitalized patients [52,53]. Such effects cannot be explained by collagen metabolism, and vitamin C effects on the immune system are not plausible explanations either. Instead, the effects of vitamin C on the neuroendocrine system or carnitine metabolism might explain such effects. Thus, if vitamin C has beneficial effects on patients with infections, that does not unambiguously indicate that these effects are mediated by the immune system per se.

2.8. The Effects of Antioxidants against Infections May Be Heterogeneous

It is quite a common assumption that the effects of vitamins are uniform. Thus, if there is benefit, it is often assumed that the same benefit applies to all people. However, it seems much more likely that the effects of vitamins, including vitamin C, vary between people depending on biology and their lifestyle. Thus, it is possible that there are benefits (or harms) restricted to special conditions or to particular people. In the case of vitamin E, there is very strong evidence for the heterogeneity in its effects on pneumonia [54,55] and on the common cold [56]. Although the factors modifying the effects of vitamin E cannot be extrapolated to vitamin C, it seems probable that there is comparable heterogeneity in the effects of vitamin C.

3. Infections in Animals

Early research showed that severe deficiency of vitamin C increased the incidence and severity of infections in guinea pigs. Hemilä (2006) carried out a systematic search of animal studies on vitamin C and infections and analyzed their findings [1], which are summarized in Tables 1–3 and discussed below.

3.1. Studies with Diets Containing Vitamin C

Many early studies with guinea pigs did not examine the effect of pure vitamin C. Instead, "vitamin-C-deficient groups" were fed diets that contained only small amounts of vitamin C, whereas the "vitamin C group" was administered oranges or other foods that contained high levels of vitamin C. The findings of studies on guinea pigs with tuberculosis and other bacterial infections are shown in Table 1.

Assuming that vitamin C containing foods do not influence infections, by pure chance only, one positive result at the level of $p < 0.01$ would be expected for a group of 100 studies. However,

20 of the reported 28 studies found significant benefits from feeding diets rich in vitamin C (Table 1). Although these findings are consistent with the notion that low vitamin C intake may increase the susceptibility to and the severity of infections, other substances in fruit and vegetables might also contribute to this effect, thus confounding the differences between the study groups.

As one example of Table 1 studies, McConkey (1936) reported that the administration of tuberculous sputum to 16 guinea pigs that were vitamin C deficient led to intestinal tuberculosis to 15 of them, but none of the five guinea pigs that were administered tomato juice as a source of vitamin C suffered from intestinal tuberculosis [57] (pp. 507–508).

Table 1. Effect of vitamin-C-rich foods on infections in guinea pigs.

Infection	No. of Studies	No. of Studies with Benefit in Any Infectious Disease Outcome with $p \leq 0.01$
All	28	20
Tuberculosis (TB)	11	7
Bacterial infection (non-TB) [a]	15	11
Diphtheria toxin	2	2

One group of guinea pigs was administered a vitamin-C-poor diet, and the other group was administered oranges, cabbage, etc. as supplements to the vitamin-C-poor diet. Based on Appendix 3 in Hemilä (2006) [1] (pp. 119–121). See Supplementary file 1 of this review for the list of the studies. p(1-tail) is used in this table. [a] Bacterial infections included pneumococcus, group C streptococcus, *Staphylococcus*, and *Salmonella typhimurium*.

3.2. Studies with Pure Vitamin C

Table 2 summarizes the animal studies in which pure vitamin C was administered to the "vitamin C" group. Overall, 148 animal studies had been published by 2005.

Out of the 148 studies, over half found a significant benefit, $p < 0.01$, for at least one infectious disease outcome. Furthermore, over a third of the studies found a benefit at the level of $p < 0.001$ [1]. Of the 100 studies with mammals, 58 found a significant benefit, $p < 0.01$, from vitamin C on some infectious disease outcome.

A benefit of vitamin C against infections was found in all animal groups. Although rats and mice synthesize vitamin C in their bodies, half or more of the studies with these species found significant benefits of additional vitamin C. This implies that rats and mice do not necessarily synthesize sufficient amounts of vitamin C to reach optimal levels that prevent or curtail infections. In addition to mammals, vitamin C protected against infections in several studies with birds and fishes.

Vitamin C was found to be beneficial against various groups of infectious agents including bacteria, viruses, *Candida albicans*, and protozoa (Table 2). Over half ($n = 97$) of all the studies evaluated the effect of vitamin C on bacterial infections or bacterial toxins, and 55 out of those studies found significant benefits of vitamin C ($p < 0.01$). Studies in which animals were administered diphtheria toxin, tetanus toxin, or endotoxin are also relevant, because these toxins are essential components in the pathogenesis of the bacterial infections. Over half of the studies on viruses, *Candida albicans* and protozoa also reported significant benefits ($p < 0.01$).

Table 3 shows the distribution of infections in studies that reported decreases in mortality caused by infections ($p < 0.001$). It is apparent that vitamin C reduced mortality in all etiological groups.

As one example of the studies in Tables 2 and 3, Dey (1966) reported that five rats administered twice the minimal lethal dose of tetanus toxin all died, whereas 25 rats administered vitamin C either before or after the same dose of toxin all lived [58].

In addition to the animal studies yielding quantitative data on the effect of vitamin C on infections in Tables 1–3, a few studies reported interesting findings of vitamin C effects against infections in studies without control groups [1] (p. 9). For example, two case-series suggested therapeutic benefit of vitamin C on dogs afflicted by the canine distemper virus. Belfield (1967) described a series of 10 dogs that appeared to benefit from 1–2 g/day of intravenous vitamin C over three days [59]. Leveque (1969) noted that usually only 5%–10% of dogs recovered from canine distemper with signs of central nervous system (CNS) disturbance. He became interested in Belfield's report and in a series of 16 dogs showing CNS disturbance that were treated with vitamin C, the proportion of dogs that recovered was 44% (95% CI: 20%–70%; based on 7/16) [60].

Table 2. Effect of pure vitamin C on infectious disease outcomes in animal studies.

Category	No. of Studies in the Category	No. of Studies with Benefit in Any Infectious Disease Outcome with $p \leq 0.01$
All studies	148	86
Time of publication		
Published in 1935–1949	40	20
Published in 1950–1989	48	32
Published in 1990–2005	60	34
Animal species		
Monkey	13	4
Guinea pig	36	21
Cow, sheep, rabbit	10	8
Cat	1	1
Rat	15	10
Gerbil, hamster	7	5
Mouse	18	9
Mammals [a]	100	58
Birds	13	8
Fish	35	20
Etiological agent		
Tuberculosis (TB)	8	3
Bacteria (non-TB)	70	36
Bacterial toxins	19	16
Virus	22	12
Candida albicans	6	4
Protozoa	23	15

A shorter version of this table was published in Hemilä (2006) [1] (p. 8). This table is based on data collected and analyzed in Appendix 2 of [1] (pp. 105–118). See Supplementary file 1 of this review for the list of the studies and their characteristics. p(1-tail) is used in this table. [a] The mammals category combines all the mammal species from the rows above.

Table 3. Infectious agents in studies in which vitamin C decreased the mortality of mammals by $p \leq 0.025$.

All Studies	29
Tuberculosis (TB)	6
Bacteria (non-TB) [a]	7
Bacterial toxin [b]	6
Virus (rabies)	1
Candida albicans	2
Protozoa [c]	7

Table 3 is restricted to mortality as the outcome, and to studies in which the effect of vitamin C on mortality was statistically significant. See Supplementary file 1 of this review for a list of the studies in which vitamin C decreased mortality by $p \leq 0.025$ (1-tail). In comparison, Table 2 includes studies with all infectious disease outcomes, such as incidence without the animals dying, and various forms of severity of infectious diseases. [a] Bacterial infections included pneumococcus and β-hemolytic streptococci; [b] Bacterial toxins included diphtheria toxin, tetanus toxin, endotoxin, and a set of clostridial toxins; [c] Protozoa infections include *Entamoeba histolytica*, *Leishmania donovani*, *Toxoplasma gondii*, and *Trypanosoma brucei*.

3.3. Implications of the Animal Studies

Many of the studies on vitamin C and infections summarized in Table 2 are old. However, it is unlikely that administering a specified dose of pure vitamin C and evaluating clinical outcomes of infections, such as mortality, will have changed meaningfully since those early days. Furthermore, 60 studies were published in the 1990s or later, and half of these later reports also found significant benefits of vitamin C on at least one infectious disease outcome.

The studies on guinea pigs are most interesting since that species is dependent on dietary vitamin C as are humans. Infections in guinea pigs against which vitamin C was significantly beneficial included *Mycobacterium tuberculosis*, β-hemolytic streptococci, *Fusobacterium necrophorum*, diphtheria toxin, *Entamoeba histolytica*, *Trypanosoma brucei*, and *Candica albicans* [1].

Some of the 148 studies in Table 2 were small and did not have sufficient statistical power to test whether vitamin C and control groups might differ. However, this problem cannot explain the large number of reported significant benefits. In contrast, inclusion of studies with a low statistical power biases the findings towards the opposite direction, leading to false negative findings.

Mortality and severity of infections in animals are definitive outcomes. In this respect, the animal studies with actual infections are much more relevant to humans than studies on laboratory determinations of the human immune system.

Given the universal nature of the effect of vitamin C against infections in diverse animal species as seen in Table 2, it seems obvious that vitamin C also has influences on infections in humans. It seems unlikely that human beings qualitatively differ from all of the animal species that have been used in the experiments listed in Table 2. Nevertheless, it is not clear to what degree the animal studies can be extrapolated to human subjects.

The fundamental question in human beings is not whether vitamin C affects the susceptibility to and severity of infections. Instead, the relevant questions are the following: What are the population groups who might benefit from higher vitamin C intakes? What is the dose-dependency relation between intake and the effects on infections? How does the optimal level of intake differ between healthy people and patients with infections?

4. The Common Cold

The term "the common cold" does not refer to any precisely defined disease, yet the set of symptoms that is called "the common cold" is personally familiar to practically everybody [61]. Typically the symptoms consist of nasal discharge, sore throat, cough, with or without fever. Young children typically have half a dozen colds per year, and the incidence decreases with age so that elderly people have colds about once per year [62]. The common cold is the leading cause of acute morbidity and of visits to a physician in high-income countries, and a major cause of absenteeism from work and school. The economic burden of the common cold is comparable to that of hypertension or stroke [63].

The most relevant definition of the common cold is based on the symptoms; thus the "common cold" does not always entail a viral etiology. Although the majority of common cold episodes are caused by respiratory viruses, similar symptoms are also caused by certain bacterial infections and by some non-infectious causes such as allergic and mechanical irritation. The cough and sore throat after running a marathon does not necessarily imply a viral etiology, although some researchers have assumed so. It is still reasonable to use the term the "common cold" in such a context on the grounds of the symptom-based definition.

4.1. Vitamin C and the Common Cold

Interest in the effects of vitamin C on the common cold originated soon after purified vitamin C became available. The first controlled trials on vitamin C were carried out as early as the 1940s. For example, in the 1950s, a British study examined the clinical effects of vitamin C deprivation, and reported that "the geometric mean duration of colds was 6.4 days in vitamin C-deprived subjects and 3.3 days in non-deprived subjects", and the authors concluded that the absence of vitamin C tended to cause colds to last longer [12].

Figure 1 shows the number of participants in placebo-controlled studies in which ≥1 g/day of vitamin C was administered. It also illustrates the main time points of the history of vitamin C and the common cold.

In 1970, Linus Pauling, a Nobel laureate in chemistry and also a Nobel Peace Prize winner, wrote a book on vitamin C and the common cold [64]. He also published two meta-analyses, which were among the earliest meta-analyses in medicine [65,66]. Pauling identified four placebo-controlled studies from which he calculated that there was strong evidence that vitamin C decreased the "integrated morbidity" of colds ($p = 0.00002$ [65]). By integrated morbidity, Pauling meant the total burden of the common cold: the combination of the incidence and duration of colds. In his analysis, Pauling put the greatest weight on the study by Ritzel (1961), which was a randomized controlled trial (RCT) with double-blinded placebo control and the subjects were schoolchildren in a skiing camp in the Swiss Alps [67]. Ritzel's study was methodologically the best of the four and used the highest dose of vitamin C, 1 g/day, and therefore Pauling concluded that gram doses of vitamin C would be beneficial against colds [64–66].

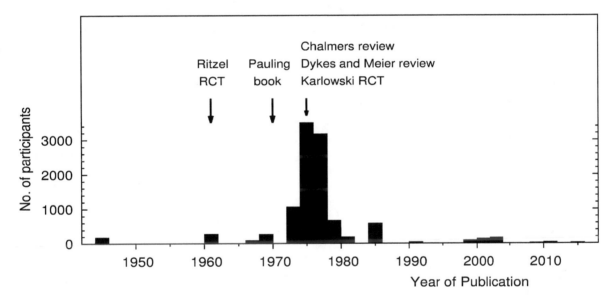

Figure 1. The numbers of participants in the placebo-controlled trials for which ≥1 g/day of vitamin C was administered. The numbers of participants in studies published over two consecutive years are combined and plotted for the first of the two years. This figure is based on data collected by Hemilä and Chalker (2013) [68,69]. See Supplementary file 1 of this review for the list of the studies. RCT, randomized controlled trial.

The activity of Pauling, in turn, led to a great upsurge in interest in vitamin C among lay people and also in academic circles in the early 1970s. From 1972 to 1979, in that eight-year period, 29 placebo-controlled studies were published, which amounted to a total of 8409 participants (Figure 1) [68,69]. Thus, the mean number of participants per study was 290.

In the interval from 1972 to 1975, five placebo-controlled trials were published that used ≥2 g/day of vitamin C. Those five studies were published after Pauling's book and therefore they formally tested Pauling's hypothesis. A meta-analysis by Hemilä (1996) showed that there was very strong evidence from the five studies that colds were shorter or less severe in the vitamin C groups ($p = 10^{-5}$), and therefore those studies corroborated Pauling's hypothesis that vitamin C was indeed effective against colds [70].

After the mid-1970s, however, interest in the topic plummeted so much so that during the 30-year period from 1985 to 2014, only 11 placebo-controlled trials comprising just 538 participants in total were published, with a mean of 49 participants per study (Figure 1). Thus, the number of studies published after 1985 is much lower than during the 1970s. In addition, the few recent studies are much smaller than the trials published in the 1970s. Therefore, the great majority of the data on vitamin C and the common cold that are currently available originated within the decade after the publication of Pauling's book.

This sudden lack of interest after the middle of the 1970s can be explained by three papers published in the same year by Chalmers (1975), Karlowski et al. (1975), and Dykes and Meier (1975) [71–73] (Figure 1). Few trials were started after 1975, which indicates the great impact of these three papers. First, the findings of the placebo controlled studies will be summarized, and then difficulties in the interpretation of common cold studies will be considered, and finally problems in the three papers that were published in 1975 will be discussed.

4.2. Vitamin C Does Not Decrease the Average Incidence of Colds in the General Community

Table 4 summarizes the findings of the studies on vitamin C and the common cold in the Cochrane review by Hemilä and Chalker (2013) [68,69]. Regularly administered vitamin C has not decreased the average number of colds among the general population (Table 4). Another meta-analysis combined the findings of the six largest trials that had used ≥ 1 g/day of vitamin C and calculated that there was no difference in the vitamin and placebo groups with RR = 0.99 (95% CI 0.93, 1.04) [74,75].

Table 4. Effects of regular vitamin C on the incidence and duration of the common cold [a].

Outcome Participants	No. of Studies	No. of Participants	Effect of Vitamin C (95% CI)	p
Incidence of colds [b]				
General population	24	10,708	−3% (−6% to 0%)	
People under heavy short-term physical stress	5	598	−52% (−65% to −36%)	10^{-6}
Duration of colds		No. of colds		
All studies (≥ 0.2 g/day)	31	9745	−9.4% (−13% to −6%)	10^{-7}
Adults (≥ 1 g/day)	13	7095	−8% (−12% to −4%)	10^{-4}
Children (≥ 1 g/day)	10	1532	−18% (−27% to −9%)	10^{-5}
Severity of colds		No. of colds		
All studies	16	7209	−0.12 (−0.17 to −0.07) [c]	10^{-6}

This table summarizes the main findings of the Cochrane review by Hemilä and Chalker (2013) [68,69]. [a] Regular supplementation of vitamin C means that vitamin C was administered each day over the whole study period. Duration and severity of colds indicates the effects on colds that occurred during the study; [b] Incidence indicates here the number of participants who had ≥ 1 cold during the study; [c] The unit in this comparison is the standard deviation. Thus −0.12 means that symptoms were decreased by 0.12 times the SD of the outcome.

Thus, there is no justification for "ordinary people" to take vitamin C regularly in order to prevent colds. However, this conclusion does not mean that regular vitamin C supplementation is ineffective for all people. There is strong evidence that vitamin C decreases the incidence of colds under special conditions and/or among certain population groups.

4.3. Vitamin C May Decrease Common Cold Incidence in Special Conditions

Vitamin C halved the incidence of colds in five RCTs during which the participants were under heavy short-term physical activity (Table 4) [68,76]. Three of the studies used marathon runners in South Africa as subjects, whereas one study used Canadian military personnel on winter exercise, and the fifth study was on schoolchildren in a skiing camp in the Swiss Alps, i.e., the Ritzel (1961) trial [67]. Thus, three studies were conducted under conditions of a hot environment and profound physical stress and the other two were carried out under cold environments and physical stress (see Section 2.4).

Another group in which vitamin C has prevented colds is British men [74,75,77]. Four trials found that vitamin C decreased the incidence of colds by 30%, and in another set of four trials, the proportion of men who had recurrent common cold infections during the study decreased by a mean of 46%. All these studies were carried out in the 1970s or earlier, and according to surveys, the intake of vitamin C in the United Kingdom was low when the studies were carried out, 0.03 to 0.06 g/day, and three of the U.K. trials specifically estimated that the dietary vitamin C intake was between 0.015

to 0.05 g/day [74]. In particular, Baird (1979) administered only 0.08 g/day of vitamin C yet they observed 37% lower incidence of colds in the vitamin C group, indicating that it was the "marginal deficiency" and not a high dose that explained the benefit [77,78].

In addition, the levels of vitamin C are usually lower in men than in women, which may explain the benefit for British males, in comparison to no apparent effect in British females. Evidently, the dietary vitamin C intake in the United Kingdom has increased since the 1970s, and therefore these studies do not indicate that vitamin C supplementation would necessarily influence colds in ordinary British men nowadays. However, if low dietary vitamin C intake increases the risk of respiratory infections, then that may be currently relevant in other contexts, since there are still many population groups that have low intakes of vitamin C. A recent small study in the USA by Johnston (2014) was restricted to 28 males with marginally low vitamin C levels, mean 30 μmol/L, and found a decrease in common cold incidence, RR = 0.55 (95% CI: 0.33–0.94; $p = 0.04$) [79], which may also be explained by the low vitamin C levels.

4.4. Vitamin C Might Protect against the Common Cold in a Restricted Subgroup of the General Community

Although vitamin C has not influenced the average common cold incidence in the general community trials (Table 4), some of them found that there was a subgroup of people who had obtained benefits from vitamin C. In a Canadian trial, Anderson (1972) [80] reported that in the vitamin C group there were 10 percentage points more participants with no "days confined to house" because of colds (57% vs. 47%; $p = 0.01$, [1] (p. 44)). Thus, one in 10 benefited from vitamin C in this outcome. In a trial with Navajo schoolchildren, Coulehan (1974) [81] found that in the vitamin C group there were 16 percentage points more children who were "never ill on active surveillance by a medically trained clerk or the school nurse" (44% vs. 29%; $p < 0.001$; [1] (p. 44)). A more recent study in the UK by van Straten (2002) reported that vitamin C decreased the number of participants who had recurrent colds by 17 percentage points [82] (19% vs. 2%; $p < 0.001$, [1] (p. 47)). Thus, the statistical evidence of benefit for a restricted subgroup in these three trials is strong.

4.5. Vitamin C Shortens and Alleviates the Common Cold

The effect of vitamin C on the duration and severity of the common cold has been studied in regular supplementation trials and in therapeutic trials. Regular supplementation means that vitamin C was administered each day over the whole study period, and the outcome is the duration and severity of colds that occurred during the study. Therapeutic vitamin C trial means that vitamin C administration was started only after the first common cold symptoms had occurred and the duration of colds were then recorded.

In regular supplementation studies, $\geq$0.2 g/day of vitamin C decreased the duration of colds by 9% (Table 4). When the dosage was >1 g/day of vitamin C, the mean duration of colds was shortened by 8% in adults and by 18% in children. Vitamin C also significantly alleviated the severity of the colds.

Therapeutic studies have hitherto not shown consistent benefit from vitamin C. However, therapeutic trials are more complex to conduct and interpret than regular supplementation trials. If the timing of the initiation of supplementation or the duration of supplementation influences the extent of the benefit, false negative findings may result from inappropriate study protocols. For example, four therapeutic studies used only 2–3 days of 2–4 g/day vitamin C supplementation, whereas the mean duration of colds in these studies was about a week. None of these studies detected any benefit from vitamin C [68,83]. On the other hand, Anderson (1974) [84] found that 8 g/day on the first day only reduced the duration of colds significantly (Figure 2). In addition, in a five-day therapeutic trial, Anderson (1975) [85] reported a 25% reduction in "days spent indoors per subject" because of illness ($p = 0.048$) in the vitamin C group (1 to 1.5 g/day) [1] (p. 48). Finally, none of the therapeutic studies investigated children, although the effect of regular vitamin C has been greater in children (Table 4). Thus, although the regular supplementation trials unambiguously show that vitamin C shortens and alleviates the common cold, there is no consistent evidence that therapeutic supplementation is effective.

4.6. Possible Differences in the Effects of Vitamin C between Subgroups

The regular supplementation study by Anderson (1972) is one of the largest that has been carried out [80]. They found that the proportion of participants who were not confined to the house decreased by 10 percentage points in the vitamin C group. In addition, they found that per episode the days confined to the house was 21% shorter in the vitamin C group. Together these combine to a 30% reduction in the days confined to the house per person ($p = 0.001$). Such a large effect gives statistical power for subgroup comparisons.

Anderson (1972) reported that vitamin C decreased total days confined to house by 46% in participants who had contact with young children, but just by 17% in participants who did not have contact with young children (Table 5). Anderson (1972) also reported that vitamin C decreased total days confined to house by 43% in participants who usually had two or more colds per winter, but just by 13% in participants who usually had zero to one cold per winter (Table 5).

In a study with adolescent competitive swimmers, Constantini (2011) found a significant difference between males and females in the effect of vitamin C, whereby the vitamin halved the duration and severity of colds in males but had no effect on females [86]. In a study with British students, Baird (1979) also found a significant difference between males and females, but the outcome was the incidence of colds (Table 5).

Carr (1981) found that vitamin C had a beneficial effect on the duration of colds for twins living separately, but not for twins living together [87]. This subgroup difference might be explained by swapping of tablets by twins living together, which was not possible for twins living separately.

The significant within-trial differences in the effect of vitamin C on the common cold indicate that there is no universal effect of vitamin C valid over the whole population. Instead, the size of the vitamin C effect seems to depend on various characteristics of people (see Section 2.8).

Table 5. Possible differences in the effects of vitamin C on the common cold between subgroups.

Study	Subgroup	Effect of Vitamin C	Outcome	Test of Subgroup Differences (p)
Anderson (1972) [80]	Contact with young children No contact with young children	−46% −17%	total days confined to house	0.036
Anderson (1972) [80]	Usually ≥2 colds per winter Usually 0–1 colds per winter	−43% −13%	total days confined to house	0.033
Constantini (2011) [86]	Male adolescent competitive swimmers Female adolescent competitive swimmers	−47% +16%	duration of colds	0.003
Baird (1979) [78]	Male students in UK Female students in UK	−37% +24%	incidence of colds	0.0001
Carr (1981) [87]	Twins living separately Twins living together	−35% +1%	duration of colds	0.035

Calculation of the subgroup differences for the Anderson (1972) and the Carr (1981) studies is described in Supplementary file 2. The interactions in the Constantini (2011) and Baird (1979) trials were calculated in [77,86]. p(2-tail) is used in this table.

4.7. Dose Dependency of Vitamin C Supplementation Effect

An earlier meta-analysis of dose-dependency calculated that on average 1 g/day of vitamin C shortened the duration of colds in adults on average by 6% and in children by 17%; and ≥2 g/day vitamin C shortened the duration of colds in adults by 21% and in children by 26% [83]. Thus, higher doses were associated with greater effects. In addition, children weigh less than adults and the greater effects in children may be explained by a greater dose per weight. Nevertheless, such a comparison suffers from numerous simultaneous differences between the trials. The most valid examination of dose–response is within a single study so that the virus distribution is similar in each trial arm and the outcome definition is identical.

Coulehan (1974) [81] administered 1 g/day to children and observed a 12% reduction in common cold duration, and in parallel they administered 2 g/day to other children and observed a 29% reduction in cold duration. Although the point estimates suggest a dose–response, the study was small and the 95% CIs overlap widely [68,83].

In a 2 × 2 design, Karlowski (1975) [72] randomized participants to 3 g/day regular vitamin C and to 3 g/day vitamin C treatment for five days when the participant caught a cold. Thus, one study arm was administered placebo, the second was administered regular vitamin C, the third therapeutic, and the fourth arm was administered regular + therapeutic vitamin C (i.e., 6 g/day). The four arms of the Karlowski trial are shown in Figure 2A. The 95% CIs show the comparisons with the placebo group. The test for trend for a linear regression model gives $p = 0.018$.

Anderson (1974) [84] randomized participants to a placebo and two vitamin C treatment arms which were administered vitamin C only on the first day of the cold. One treatment arm (arm #7) was given 4 g/day of, and another (arm #8) was given 8 g/day. These arms are compared with the placebo arm #4 in Figure 2B. The 95% CIs show the comparisons with the placebo group. The test for trend in a linear regression model gives $p = 0.013$.

Finally, some case reports have proposed that vitamin C doses should be over 15 g/day for the best treatment of colds [88,89]. Thus, it is possible that the doses used in most of the therapeutic studies, up to just 6–8 g/day, have not been sufficiently high to properly test the effects of vitamin C that might be achievable.

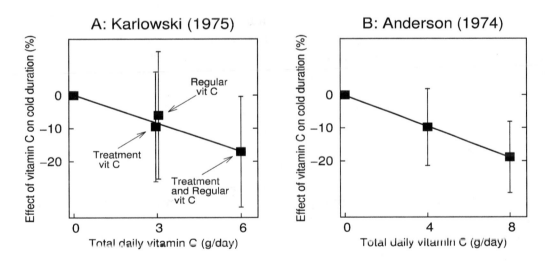

Figure 2. (**A**) Dose–response relationship in the Karlowski (1975) trial. The placebo arm is located at 0 g/day, the 3 g/day regular vitamin C and the 3 g/day treatment vitamin C arms are in the middle and the regular + treatment arm is at 6 g/day [72]. The 95% CIs are shown for the comparison against the placebo arm. With inverse-variance weighing, test for trend in a linear model gives p(2-tail) = 0.018. The addition of the linear vitamin C effect to the statistical model containing a uniform vitamin C effect improved the regression model by $p = 0.002$. Previously, analysis of variance for trend calculated $p = 0.040$ for the linear trend [83]; (**B**) Dose–response relationship in the Anderson (1974) trial. The placebo arm #4 is located at 0 g/day, vitamin C treatment arm #7 at 4 g/day and vitamin C treatment arm #8 at 8 g/day [84]. In the Anderson (1974) trial, vitamin C was administered only on the first day of the common cold. The 95% CIs are shown for the comparison against the placebo arm. With inverse-variance weighing, test for trend in a linear model gives p(2-tail) = 0.013. See Supplementary file 2 for the calculation of the trend for both studies.

4.8. Vitamin C and Complications of the Common Cold

Given the strong evidence that regularly administered vitamin C shortens and alleviates common cold symptoms, it seems plausible that vitamin C might also alleviate complications of the common cold. One frequent complication is the exacerbation of asthma [90].

A systematic review identified three studies that provided information on the potential pulmonary effects of vitamin C in sufferers of common cold–induced asthma [91]. A trial conducted in Nigeria studied asthmatic patients whose asthma exacerbations resulted from respiratory infections. A vitamin C dose of 1 g/day decreased the occurrence of severe and moderate asthma attacks by 89% [92]. Another study on patients who had infection-related asthma reported that 5 g/day vitamin C decreased the prevalence of bronchial hypersensitivity to histamine by 52 percentage points [93]. A third study found that the administration of a single dose of 1 g vitamin C to non-asthmatic common cold patients decreased bronchial sensitivity in a histamine challenge test [94].

It has also been proposed that vitamin C might prevent sinusitis and otitis media [95,96], but to our knowledge there are no data from controlled studies.

A further complication of viral respiratory infections is pneumonia; this is discussed in the section on pneumonia.

5. Problems in the Interpretation: Non-Comparability of the Vitamin C and Common Cold Trials

5.1. Vitamin C Doses in Vitamin C and Control Groups

One great problem in the interpretation of vitamin C trials arises from the fundamental difference between vitamin C and ordinary drugs such as antibiotics. In a trial of an ordinary drug, the control group is not given the drug, which simplifies the interpretation of the findings. In contrast, it is impossible to select control subjects who have zero vitamin C intake and no vitamin C in their system. Thus, all vitamin C trials de facto compare two different vitamin C levels. The lower dose is obtained from the diet, and it has varied considerably among the controlled studies. In addition, the vitamin C supplement doses given to the vitamin C groups have also varied extensively. Finally, the placebo group in some trials was also given extra vitamin C, which further confuses the comparisons. Therefore, the comparison of different vitamin C studies and the generalization of their findings is complicated. As an illustration of these problems, Table 6 shows examples of the variations in vitamin C doses that were used in the common cold trials.

There are 10- to 30-fold differences in the vitamin C intake in the diet of the control groups of the Baird (1979) [78], the Glazebrook (1942) [97], and the Sabiston (1974) [98] trials compared with the Peters (1993) [99] trial, yet all of them are labeled "control groups" of vitamin C trials (Table 6). Evidently, we should not expect similar effects of supplemental vitamin C in such dissimilar studies. Usually the dietary intake of vitamin C is not estimated and therefore cannot be taken into account when comparing studies.

Vitamin C was administered to the placebo group in some studies. For example, Carr (1981) [87] administered 0.07 g/day and some other studies administered 0.01 to 0.05 g/day to the control subjects. This was done to refute the notion that any possible effects of high doses were due to the treatment of marginal deficiencies. Such reasoning does not seem sound, since there are population groups for which ordinary dietary vitamin C intake is particularly low and it would be important to know whether vitamin C supplementation might be beneficial for them. Thus, marginal vitamin C deficiency is also an important issue. The administration of vitamin C to the control group biases the possible effects of vitamin C supplementation downwards.

Finally, there are up to a 240-fold difference between the lowest and highest vitamin C supplementary dose used in the common cold trials, yet the dosage is often ignored. For example, in his influential review (see Figure 1), Chalmers (1975) [71] presented data from the following studies in the same table: Karlowski (1975) study administered up to 6 g/day of vitamin C to their subjects [72], whereas the Cowan (1942) study administered only 0.025 g/day as the lowest dose [100]. Chalmers

(1975) did not list the vitamin C dosages in his table and therefore his readers were unable to consider whether the comparison of such different studies was reasonable or not. Still, Chalmers' review has been widely cited as evidence that vitamin C is not effective against colds [1] (pp. 36–38).

Finally, combinations of the above variations lead to paradoxes. The "vitamin C group" of the Baird (1979) study received about 0.05 g/day of vitamin C from food and 0.08 g/day from supplements, which amounted to 0.13 g/day of total vitamin C [78]. In contrast, the "placebo group" in the study by Peters (1994) received about four times as much, 0.5 g/day, of vitamin C from their usual diet [99]. Furthermore, Baird (1979) administered 0.08 g/day of vitamin C to their vitamin C group [78], whereas Carr (1981) administered 0.07 g/day vitamin C to their placebo group [87]. Thus, the dosages of vitamin C were essentially the same, but the groups were on the opposite sides in the evaluation of vitamin C effects.

High dietary vitamin C intake, and vitamin C supplementation of the placebo group, cannot lead to false positive findings about the efficacy of vitamin C against colds. In contrast, they can lead to false negative findings or estimates biased towards the null effect.

Table 6. Variations in vitamin C dose in the control and vitamin C groups.

Trial Country, Participants	Vitamin C Level (g/Day)		
	Dietary Intake Level in the Control Group	Supplement to the Control Group [a]	Supplement to the Vitamin C Group
Cowan (1942) [100] USA, schoolchildren	?		0.025–0.05
Baird (1979) [78] UK, students	0.05		0.08
Glazebrook (1942) [97] UK, boarding school boys	0.015		0.05–0.3
Peters (1993) [99] South Africa, marathon runners	0.5		0.6
Sabiston (1974) [98] Canada, military recruits	0.04		1
Carr (1981) [87] Australia, twins	?	0.07	1
Karlowski (1975) [72] USA, NIH employees	b		3–6

Modified from Table 12 from Hemilä (2006) [1] (p. 34). [a] In addition to Carr (1981), a few studies administered 0.01 to 0.05 g/day of vitamin C to the placebo group, but they are not listed here; [b] In the 1970s, the average vitamin C intake in the USA was approximately 0.1 g/day. The participants of the Karlowski (1975) study were employees of the National Institutes of Health and therefore their mean dietary intake of vitamin C probably was higher than the national average, but intake of vitamin C was not estimated.

5.2. Non-Compliance of Participants

Carr (1981) studied twins, some of whom lived together, whereas others lived apart [87]. Vitamin C had a significant effect on the duration and severity of colds in twins living apart, but no effect in twins living together (Table 5). Furthermore, the duration of colds among twins living together (5.4 days in vitamin C and placebo groups) was in the middle of the duration of colds among the vitamin C group (4.9 days) and placebo group (7.5 days) of twins living apart. An evident explanation for such a difference between twins living together and twins living apart, is that twins who lived together exchanged their tablets to some extent, whereas the twins who lived apart could not do so. Two studies on children found an increase in vitamin C levels in the plasma of boys and in the urine of boys of the placebo (sic) groups [81,101], which indicates tablet swapping among the children on vitamin C and placebo. Thus, non-compliance may have confounded the results and the true effects of vitamin C might be greater than those reported.

5.3. Implications of the Common Cold Studies

Given the great variations in the vitamin C dosage levels in the vitamin C and control groups, and the apparent problem of non-compliance in some studies, it is obvious that the comparison of different "vitamin C trials" can be complicated. The generalization of the findings of any particular trial is limited irrespective of its methodological quality and statistical power. However, the large variations in vitamin C levels in the vitamin C and control groups, and the non-compliance in some studies, both predispose against a false positive differences between the study groups. In contrast, they make it more difficult to detect true differences, and therefore the findings on common cold duration and severity shown in Table 4 may be biased downwards and might camouflage even stronger true effects.

6. Evaporation of Interest in Vitamin C and the Common Cold after 1975

Given the strong evidence from studies published before 1970 that vitamin C has beneficial effects against the common cold [65], and from the ≥ 2 g/day vitamin C studies published between 1972 and 1975 [70], it is puzzling that the interest in vitamin C and the common cold collapsed after 1975 so that few small trials on vitamin C and the common cold have been conducted thereafter (Figure 1).

This sudden loss of interest can be explained by the publication of the three highly important papers in 1975 (Figure 1). These papers are particularly influential because of their authors and the publication forums. Two of the papers were published in *JAMA* [72,73], and the third paper was published in the *American Journal of Medicine* [71]. Both of these journals are highly influential medical journals with extensive circulations. Two of the papers were authored by Thomas Chalmers [71,72], who was a highly respected and influential pioneer of RCTs [1,102,103], and the third paper was authored by Paul Meier [73], who was a highly influential statistician, e.g., one of the authors of the widely used Kaplan–Meier method [1,104,105].

Karlowski, Chalmers, et al. (1975) [72] published the results of a RCT in *JAMA*, in which 6 g/day of vitamin C significantly shortened the duration of colds (Figure 2A). However, these authors claimed that the observed benefit was not caused by the physiological effects of vitamin C, but by the placebo effect. However, the "placebo-effect explanation" was shown afterwards to be erroneous. For example, Karlowski et al. had excluded 42% of common cold episodes from the subgroup analysis that was the basis for their conclusion, without giving any explanation of why so many participants were excluded. The numerous problems of the placebo explanation are detailed in a critique by Hemilä [1,106,107]. Chalmers wrote a response [108], but did not answer the specific issues raised [109].

In the same year (1975), Chalmers published a review of the vitamin C and common cold studies. He pooled the results of seven studies and calculated that vitamin C would shorten colds only by 0.11 (SE 0.24) days [71]. Such a small difference has no clinical importance and the SE indicates that it is simply explained by random variation. However, there were errors in the extraction of data, studies that used very low doses of vitamin C (down to 0.025 g/day) were included, and there were errors in the calculations [1,110]. Pauling had proposed that vitamin C doses should be ≥ 1 g/day. When Hemilä and Herman (1995) included only those studies that had used ≥ 1 g/day of vitamin C and extracted data correctly, they calculated that colds were 0.93 (SE 0.22) days shorter, which is over eight times that calculated by Chalmers, and highly significant ($p = 0.01$) [110].

The third paper was a review published in *JAMA* by Michael Dykes and Paul Meier (1975). They analyzed selected studies and concluded that there was no convincing evidence that vitamin C has effects on colds [73]. However, they did not calculate the estimates of the effect nor any *p*-values, and many comments in their analysis were misleading. Pauling wrote a manuscript in which he commented upon the review by Dykes and Meier and submitted it to *JAMA*. Pauling stated afterwards that his paper was rejected even after he twice made revisions to meet the suggestions of the referees and the manuscript was finally published in a minor journal [111,112]. The rejection of Pauling's papers was strange since the readers of *JAMA* were effectively prevented from seeing the other side of an important controversy. There were also other problems that were not pointed out by Pauling; see [1,70].

Although the three papers have serious biases, they have been used singly or in the combinations of two as references in nutritional recommendations, in medical textbooks, in texts on infectious diseases and on nutrition, when the authors claimed that vitamin C had been shown to be ineffective for colds [1] (pp. 21–23, 36–38, 42–45). The American Medical Association, for example, officially stated that "One of the most widely misused vitamins is ascorbic acid. There is no reliable evidence that large doses of ascorbic acid prevent colds or shorten their duration" [113], a statement that was based entirely on Chalmers's 1975 review.

These three papers are the most manifest explanation for the collapse in the interest in vitamin C and the common cold after 1975, despite the strong evidence that had emerged by that time that ≥2 g/day vitamin C shortens and alleviates colds [70].

7. Pneumonia

Pneumonia is the most common severe infection, which is usually caused by bacteria and viruses.

As recounted at the beginning of this review, the association between frank vitamin C deficiency and pneumonia was noted by Alfred Hess and other early authors, when the chemical identity of vitamin C was not yet known. Vitamin C was purified in the early 1930s and soon thereafter a few German and U.S. physicians proposed that vitamin C might be beneficial in the treatment of pneumonia. For example, Gander and Niederberger (1936) concluded from a series of 15 cases that "the general condition is always favorably influenced (by vitamin C) to a noticeable extent, as is the convalescence, which proceeds better and more quickly than in cases of pneumonia, which are not treated with vitamin C" [114] and other German physicians also claimed benefits of vitamin C [115,116]. Translations of these papers are available [9]. Case reports from the USA also suggested that vitamin C was beneficial against pneumonia [117–119].

A Cochrane review on vitamin C and pneumonia identified three controlled trials that reported the number of pneumonia cases in participants who were administered vitamin C and two therapeutic trials in which pneumonia patients were given vitamin C [27,28].

7.1. Vitamin C and the Incidence of Pneumonia

Table 7 shows the findings of the three vitamin C and pneumonia trials. Each of them found a ≥80% lower incidence of pneumonia for their vitamin C group [27,28,120].

Glazebrook (1942) studied male students (15–20 years) in a boarding school in Scotland during World War II [97]. No formal placebo was used; however, 0.05 to 0.3 g/day of vitamin C was added to the morning cocoa and to an evening glass of milk in the kitchen. Thus, the placebo effect does not seem to be a relevant concern in the dining hall. The ordinary diet of the schoolboys contained only 0.015 g/day vitamin C so that their intake was particularly low.

Kimbarowski (1967) studied the effect of 0.3 g/day of vitamin C on military recruits who had been hospitalized because of influenza type-A in the former Soviet Union [121]. Thus, these pneumonia cases were complications of the viral respiratory infection. Vitamin C also shortened the mean stay in hospital for pneumonia treatment (9 vs. 12 days).

The latest of the three pneumonia prevention trials was carried out during a two-month recruit training period with U.S. Marine recruits by Pitt (1979) [122]. The dose of vitamin C was 2 g/day. This was a randomized double-blind placebo-controlled trial, whereas the two earlier studies were not.

The findings of the three studies are consistent with the notion that the level of vitamin C intake may influence the risk of pneumonia. However, all the three studies were carried out using special participants under particular conditions, and their findings cannot be generalized to the ordinary current Western population. Dietary vitamin C intake was particularly low in the oldest study, and may also have been low in the second study. Thus, the benefit of vitamin C supplementation may be explained by the correction of marginal deficiency in these two older studies. However, in the study by Pitt (1979), the baseline plasma level of vitamin C, 57 μmol/L, corresponds to the dietary vitamin C intake of about 0.1 g/day [11]. Furthermore, although the dose of 2 g/day was high, the plasma level of vitamin C increased only by 36% for the vitamin C group. This also indicates that the basal dietary intake vitamin C was high. Thus, treating marginal vitamin C deficiency is not a reasonable explanation for that latest study.

It is also worth noting that two of these trials used military recruits, and the third used young males who were accommodated in a boarding school [123]. Therefore, the exposure to viruses and bacteria causing pneumonia may have been much higher compared to children and young adults living at home. In each of the three trials, the incidence of pneumonia in the control group was very high when compared with the incidence in the ordinary population [124,125]. A high incidence of pneumonia has been reported in military recruits [126], but the incidence of pneumonia has been even higher in some child populations of the developing countries [127] (Table 7).

It seems reasonable to consider that these three studies observed a true effect of vitamin C against pneumonia in their specific circumstances. However, these findings should not be extrapolated to different circumstances. It would seem worthwhile to examine the effect of vitamin C in population groups that have a high incidence of pneumonia concomitantly with a low intake of vitamin C [27,41].

Table 7. Effect of vitamin C on the incidence of pneumonia.

Study	Pneumonia Cases/Total		p [a]	Incidence of Pneumonia in the Control Group (1/1000 Person-Years)
	Vitamin C	Control		
Glazebrook (1942) [97]	0/335	17/1100	0.006	30
Kimbarowski (1967) [121]	2/114	10/112	0.022	9% [b]
Pitt (1979) [122]	1/331	7/343	0.009	120
	Incidence of pneumonia in selected populations:			
Merchant (2004) [124]	Middle-aged males in the USA			3
Hemilä (2004) [125]	Middle-aged males in Finland			5
Pazzaglia (1983) [126]	Military recruits in the USA			60
Paynter (2010) [127]	Children in developing countries, up to			400

Modified from Hemilä (2006) [1] (p. 51). [a] Mid-p (1-tail); combined test for all three sets of data: $p = 0.00002$ [120]; [b] 9% of the hospitalized influenza A patients contracted pneumonia.

7.2. Vitamin C in the Treatment of Pneumonia

Two studies have reported on the therapeutic effect of vitamin C for pneumonia patients [27,28].

Hunt (1994) carried out a randomized, double-blind placebo controlled trial with elderly people in the UK (mean age 81 years), who were hospitalized because of acute bronchitis or pneumonia [26]. The mean plasma vitamin C level at baseline was 23 μmol/L and one third of the patients had a vitamin C level of just ≤11 μmol/L. There was a significant difference in the effect of 0.2 g/day of vitamin C between patients who were more ill and those who were less ill when admitted to the hospital. Vitamin C reduced the respiratory symptom score in the more ill patients but not in their less ill counterparts. There were also six deaths during the study, all among the more ill participants: five in the placebo group, but only one in the vitamin C group.

Mochalkin (1970) examined the effect of vitamin C on pneumonia patients in the former Soviet Union [25]. Although a placebo was not administered to the control group, two different doses of vitamin C were used and the observed difference between the low and high dosage cannot be explained by the placebo effect. The high-dose regime administered on average twice the quantity of vitamin C of the low dose, but both of them were related to the dosage of antibiotics so that the low dose vitamin C ranged from 0.25 to 0.8 g/day, and the high dose ranged from 0.5 to 1.6 g/day. The duration of hospital stay in the control group (no vitamin C supplementation) was 23.7 days. In the low dose vitamin C group the hospital stay was 19% shorter and in the high dose vitamin C group it was 36% shorter. A benefit was also reported on the normalization of chest X-ray, temperature, and erythrocyte sedimentation rate.

Although both of these therapeutic studies give support to the old case reports stating that vitamin C is beneficial for pneumonia patients, the findings cannot be directly generalized to typical pneumonia patients of Western countries.

8. Tetanus

Tetanus is a disease caused by the toxin of *Clostridium tetani*, which may contaminate wounds. An early case report claimed that vitamin C was beneficial against tetanus in an unvaccinated six-year-old boy in the USA [128]. A Cochrane review identified one controlled trial in which the effect of vitamin C on tetanus patients was examined [129,130].

Jahan (1984) studied the effect of 1 g/day of intravenous vitamin C on tetanus patients in Bangladesh [131]. In children aged one to 12 years, there were no deaths in the vitamin C group, whereas there were 23 deaths in the control group ($p = 10^{-9}$) [1] (p. 17). In tetanus patients aged 13 to 30 years, there were 10 deaths in the vitamin C group compared with 19 deaths in the control group ($p = 0.03$). The significant difference between the above-described age groups may be caused by the difference in the body weights of the patients. In the young children the same dose of vitamin C corresponds to a substantially higher dose per unit of weight. Although there were methodological weaknesses in the trial, they are unlikely explanations for the dramatic difference in the younger participants [129].

9. Other Infections

The effect of vitamin C supplementation on the common cold has been most extensively studied. One important reason for extensive research on vitamin C and the common cold seems to be the wide publicity given to it by Pauling [1,132]. Probably some researchers wanted to show that Pauling was either right or wrong, whereas others just wanted to study a topic about which a Nobel Prize winner had put his credibility on the line. Another reason for the large number of studies on the common cold is that it is a non-severe ubiquitous infection, and it is very easy to find common cold patients in schools and work places. It is much more difficult to study more serious infections.

The three infections discussed above, the common cold, pneumonia, and tetanus, were selected on the basis that the effects of vitamin C have been evaluated in Cochrane reviews, which entails a thorough literature search and a careful analysis of the identified trials. However, the selection of these three infections does not imply that the effects of vitamin C are limited to them.

Table 2 indicates that vitamin C may have effects on various infections caused by viruses, bacteria, *Candida albicans* and protozoa. Vitamin C might have similar effects in humans. However, it also seems evident that the role of additional vitamin C depends on various factors such as the initial dietary intake level, other nutritional status, the exposure level to pathogens, the level of exercise and temperature stress, etc.

Three extensive searches of the older literature on vitamin C and infections have been published, and they give an extensive list of references, but none of these publications gave a balanced discussion of the findings [133–135]. A few studies on the possible effects of vitamin C on other infections are outlined below, but this selection is not systematic.

Terezhalmy (1978) [136] used a double-blind placebo-controlled RCT and found that the duration of pain caused by herpes labialis was shortened by 51%, from 3.5 to 1.3 days ($p = 10^{-8}$), when patients were administered 1 g/day of vitamin C together with bioflavonoids [1] (pp. 15–17). Furthermore, when vitamin C treatment was initiated within 24 hours of the onset of the symptoms, only six out of 26 patients (23%) developed herpes vesicles, whereas with later initiation of vitamin C, eight out of 12 patients (67%) developed vesicles ($p = 0.003$ in the test of interaction). Vitamin C was administered with bioflavonoids, so the study was not specific to vitamin C, but there is no compelling evidence to indicate that bioflavonoids affect infections.

Herpes zoster (reactivation of varicella zoster virus) can cause long lasting post-herpetic neuralgia (PHN). Chen (2009) found that patients with PHN had significantly lower plasma vitamin C plasma than healthy volunteers, and their RCT showed that vitamin C administration significantly decreased the pain level of PHN [137]. A number of other reports have also suggested that vitamin C may be effective against the pain caused by herpes zoster [138–142].

Patrone (1982) and Levy (1996) reported that vitamin C administration was beneficial to patients who had recurrent infections, mainly of the skin [143,144]. Many of the patients had impaired neutrophil functions and therefore the findings cannot be generalized to the ordinary population.

Galley (1997) reported that vitamin C increased the cardiac index in patients with septic shock [145]. Pleiner (2002) reported that intravenous vitamin C administration preserved vascular reactivity to acetylcholine in study participants who had been experimentally administered *Escherichia coli* endotoxin [146].

It seems unlikely that the effects of vitamin C on herpetic pain, cardiac index and the vascular system are mediated through effects on the immune system. Such effects are probably caused by other mechanisms instead. The question of the possible benefits of vitamin C against infections is therefore not just a question about the immune system effects of the vitamin, as was discussed earlier in this review (see Section 2.7).

Some physicians used vitamin C for a large set of infectious disease patients and described their experiences in case reports that are worth reading [89,147].

10. Observational Studies on Vitamin C and Infections

Cohort studies on vitamins are often unreliable because diet is strongly associated with numerous lifestyle factors that cannot be fully adjusted for in statistical models. Therefore, there may always remain an unknown level of residual confounding [148]. The main source of vitamin C in the diet is fruit, and high dietary vitamin C intake essentially always means a high fruit intake [149]. Thus, any substantial correlations between vitamin C intake and infections could also reflect some other substances in fruit. Only two observational studies are commented upon in this section.

Merchant (2004) studied men whose ages ranged from 40 to 75 years in the USA and found no association between their vitamin C intake and community-acquired pneumonia [124]. These males were U.S. health professionals; thus they were of a population that has a great interest in factors that affect health. The incidence of pneumonia was only three cases per 1000 person-years (Table 7). The median vitamin C intake of the lowest quintile was 0.095 g/day and of the highest quintile it was 1.1 g/day. In contrast, the overall median of the adult U.S. population is about 0.1 g/day, and 10% of the U.S. population has an intake level of less than 0.04 g/day [14]. Thus, Merchant and colleagues' cohort study indicates that increasing the vitamin C intake upwards from the median level in the USA will not lead to any further decline in the already low pneumonia incidence among male health professionals. However, the study is uninformative about whether decreasing vitamin C level downwards from 0.1 g/day might increase pneumonia risk, or about whether vitamin C might have effects in populations that have particularly high incidences of pneumonia (Table 7). Even though we must be cautious about interpreting observational studies, it seems that biological differences, rather than methodological differences, are most reasonable explanations for the divergence between the findings in the Merchant et al. cohort study and the three controlled trials shown in Table 7.

A cohort analysis of Finnish male smokers that is part of the Alpha-Tocopherol Beta-Carotene Cancer prevention (ATBC) Study found a significant inverse association between dietary vitamin C intake and tuberculosis risk in participants who were not administered vitamin E supplements [150,151]. The highest quartile had the median dietary vitamin C intake level of 0.15 g/day, whereas the lowest quartile had an intake level of only 0.052 g/day. The adjusted risk of tuberculosis in the lowest vitamin C intake quartile was 150% higher than that of the highest intake quartile. This is consistent with the animal studies that found that low vitamin C intake increases the susceptibility to, and severity of, tuberculosis (Tables 1–3).

11. Potentially Harmful Interactions between Vitamins C and E

Vitamin C and vitamin E are both antioxidants and they protect against ROS. Therefore, these substances are of parallel interest as water-soluble vitamin C regenerates the lipid-soluble vitamin E in vitro [152]. Dietary vitamin C intake modified the effect of vitamin E on mortality in the ATBC Study, which indicates that these substances may also have clinically important interactions [153]. However, the major sources of the vitamin C in this subgroup were fruit, vegetables and berries and other substances in these foods might also have explained the modification of the vitamin E effect. Such a possibility was refuted by calculating the residual intake of fruit, vegetables and berries, and showing that the residual did not modify the effect of vitamin E. Vitamin C was thus indicated as the specific modifying factor. A similar approach was used to show that vitamin C specifically modified the effect of vitamin E on pneumonia [154].

Two subgroups of the ATBC Study were identified in which the combination of high dietary vitamin C intake and vitamin E supplementation increased the risk of pneumonia by 248% and 1350% when compared with high vitamin C intake without vitamin E (Table 8). In the former subgroup, one extra case of pneumonia was caused for every 13 participants and in the latter subgroup, for every 28 participants. In both subgroups, the residual intake of fruit, vegetables and berries did not modify the effect of vitamin E, indicating specificity of vitamin C. The total number of participants in the ATBC Study was 29,133 and in that respect the identified subgroups were relatively small and at 1081 individuals only amounted to 4% of all the ATBC participants. However, in these two subgroups the harm arising from the combination of vitamins C and E was substantial [154].

Another subgroup analysis of the ATBC Study found that the combination of high vitamin C intake together with vitamin E supplementation increased the risk of tuberculosis in heavy smokers by 125% compared with high vitamin C alone subgroup (Table 8). Thus, one extra case of tuberculosis arose in every 240 participants who had high intakes of vitamins C and E [150,151].

ROS have been implicated in the pathogenesis of diverse diseases, including infections. Antioxidants have been assumed to be beneficial since they react with ROS. However, given the suggestions that people should take vitamins C and E to improve their immune system, the subgroup findings in Table 8 are somewhat alarming. Nevertheless, the harm in the three subgroups is limited to the combination of vitamins C and E. This author does not know of any findings that indicate that similar doses of vitamin C alone might cause harm.

Table 8. Increase in pneumonia and tuberculosis risk with the combination of vitamins C and E.

Infection, ATBC Study Subgroup	No. of Participants	Effect of Vitamin E RR (95% CI)	Test of Interaction p	NNH
Pneumonia Body weight < 60 kg who started smoking at ≤20 years Dietary vitamin C				
<median	467	0.98 (0.48 to 2.0)	0.026	
≥median (75 mg/day)	468	3.48 (1.61 to 7.5)		13
Pneumonia Body weight ≥ 100 kg who started smoking at ≤20 years Dietary vitamin C				
<median	613	1.37 (0.46 to 4.0)	0.019	
≥median (95 mg/day)	613	14.5 (1.84 to 114)		28
Tuberculosis Smoking ≥ 20 cigarettes/day Dietary vitamin C				
<median	9073	0.82 (0.50 to 1.33)	0.011 [a]	
≥median (90 mg/day)	8172	2.25 (1.19 to 4.23)		240

Subgroups of the ATBC Study in which vitamin C increased the risk of pneumonia and tuberculosis [150,151,154]. ATBC Study, Alpha-Tocopherol Beta-Carotene Cancer prevention Study. NNH, number needed to harm: how many people in the particular subgroup need to be exposed to the treatment to cause harm to one person. RR, relative risk. [a] Interaction test was calculated for this review.

12. Misconceptions and Prejudices about Vitamin C and Infections

In the first half of the 20th century, a large number of papers were published in the medical literature on vitamin C and infections and several physicians were enthusiastic about vitamin C. The topic was not dismissed because of large-scale controlled trials showing that vitamin C was ineffective. Instead, many rather large trials found benefits of vitamin C. There seem to be four particular reasons why the interest in vitamin C and infections disappeared.

First, antibiotics were introduced in the mid-20th century. They have specific and sometimes very dramatic effects on bacterial infections and therefore are much more rational first line drugs for patients with serious infections than vitamin C. Secondly, vitamin C was identified as the explanation for scurvy, which was considered a disease of the connective tissues. Evidently it seemed irrational to consider that a substance that "only" participates in collagen metabolism might also have effects on infections. However, the biochemistry and actions of vitamin C are complex and not limited to collagen metabolism. Thirdly, the three papers published in 1975 appeared to herald the loss of interest in vitamin C and the common cold (Figure 1) and it seems likely that they increased the negative attitude towards vitamin C for other infections as well. Fourthly, "if a treatment bypasses the medical establishment and is sold directly to the public ... the temptation in the medical community is to accept uncritically the first bad news that comes along" [155].

The belief that vitamin C is "ineffective" has been widely spread. For example, a survey of general practitioners in the Netherlands revealed that 47% of respondents considered that homeopathy is efficacious for the treatment of the common cold, whereas only 20% of those respondents considered that vitamin C was [156]. Prejudices against vitamin C are not limited to the common cold. Richards compared the attitudes and arguments of physicians to three putative cancer medicines, 5-fluorouracil, interferon and vitamin C, and documented unambiguous bias against vitamin C [157–159]. Goodwin and Tangum gave several examples to support the conclusion that there has been a systematic bias against the concept that vitamins may yield benefits in levels higher than the minimum needed to avoid the classic deficiency diseases [160].

The use of vitamin C for preventing and treating colds falls into the category of alternative medicine under the classifications used by the National Institutes of Health in the USA and of the Cochrane collaboration. However, such categorization does not reflect the level of evidence for vitamin C, but reflects the low level of acceptance amongst the medical community, and may further amplify the inertia and prejudices against vitamin C [161].

13. Conclusions

From a large series of animal studies we may conclude that vitamin C plays a role in preventing, shortening, and alleviating diverse infections. It seems evident that vitamin C has similar effects in humans. Controlled studies have shown that vitamin C shortens and alleviates the common cold and prevents colds under specific conditions and in restricted population subgroups. Five controlled trials found significant effects of vitamin C against pneumonia. There is some evidence that vitamin C may also have effects on other infections, but there is a paucity of such data. The practical importance and optimally efficacious doses of vitamin C for preventing and treating infections are unknown. Vitamin C is safe and costs only pennies per gram, and therefore even modest effects may be worth exploiting.

Acknowledgments: No external funding. Parts of this review were published as earlier versions in the dissertation by Hemilä (2006) [1]. Links to translations of the non-English papers cited in this review and many other references are available at [9].

References

1. Hemilä, H. Do vitamins C and E affect Respiratory Infections? Ph.D. Thesis, University of Helsinki, Helsinki, Finland, 2006. Available online: https://hdl.handle.net/10138/20335 (accessed on 17 March 2017).
2. Carpenter, K.J. *The History of Scurvy and Vitamin C*; Cambridge University Press: Cambridge, UK, 1986.
3. Hess, A.F. *Scurvy: Past and Present*; Lippincott: Philadelphia, PA, USA, 1920. Available online: http://chla.library.cornell.edu (accessed on 17 March 2017).
4. Hess, A.F. Diet, nutrition and infection. *N. Engl. J. Med.* **1932**, *207*, 637–648. [CrossRef]
5. Robertson, E.C. The vitamins and resistance to infection: Vitamin C. *Medicine* **1934**, *13*, 190–206. [CrossRef]
6. Englard, S.; Seifter, S. The biochemical functions of ascorbic acid. *Annu. Rev. Nutr.* **1986**, *6*, 365–406. [PubMed]
7. Clausen, S.W. The influence of nutrition upon resistance to infection. *Physiol. Rev.* **1934**, *14*, 309–350.
8. Perla, D.; Marmorston, J. Role of vitamin C in resistance. Parts I and II. *Arch. Pathol.* **1937**, *23*, 543–575, 683–712.
9. Hemilä, H. Vitamin C and Infections. Available online: http://www.mv.helsinki.fi/home/hemila/N2017 (accessed on 17 March 2017).
10. De Gruttola, V.; Fleming, T.; Lin, D.Y.; Coombs, R. Validating surrogate markers—Are we being naive? *J. Infect. Dis.* **1997**, *175*, 237–246. [CrossRef] [PubMed]
11. Levine, M.; Conry-Cantilena, C.; Wang, Y.; Welch, R.W.; Washko, P.W.; Dhariwal, K.R.; Park, J.B.; Lazarev, A.; Graumlich, J.F.; King, J.; et al. Vitamin C pharmacokinetics in healthy volunteers: Evidence for a recommended dietary allowance. *Proc. Natl. Acad. Sci. USA* **1996**, *93*, 3704–3709. [CrossRef] [PubMed]
12. Bartley, W.; Krebs, H.A.; O'Brien, J.R.P. *Vitamin C Requirement of Human Adults*; A Report by the Vitamin C Subcommittee of the Accessory Food Factors Committee; Her Majesty's Stationery Office (HMSO): London, UK, 1953.
13. Hodges, R.E.; Hood, J.; Canham, J.E.; Sauberlich, H.E.; Baker, E.M. Clinical manifestations of ascorbic acid deficiency in man. *Am. J. Clin. Nutr.* **1971**, *24*, 432–443. [PubMed]
14. Food and Nutrition Board. *Food and Nutrition Board, Institute of Medicine: Dietary Reference Intakes for Vitamin C, Vitamin E, Selenium and Carotenoids*; National Academy Press: Washington, DC, USA, 2000; pp. 95–185.
15. Segal, A.W. How neutrophils kill microbes. *Annu. Rev. Immunol.* **2005**, *23*, 197–223. [CrossRef] [PubMed]
16. Akaike, T. Role of free radicals in viral pathogenesis and mutation. *Rev. Med. Virol.* **2001**, *11*, 87–101. [CrossRef] [PubMed]
17. Peterhans, E. Oxidants and antioxidants in viral diseases. *J. Nutr.* **1997**, *127*, 962S–965S. [PubMed]
18. Wang, Y.; Russo, T.A.; Kwon, O.; Chanock, S.; Rumsey, S.C.; Levine, M. Ascorbate recycling in human neutrophils: Induction by bacteria. *Proc. Natl. Acad. Sci. USA* **1997**, *94*, 13816–13819. [CrossRef] [PubMed]
19. Nualart, F.J.; Rivas, C.I.; Montecinos, V.P.; Godoy, A.S.; Guaiquil, V.H.; Golde, D.W.; Vera, J.C. Recycling of vitamin C by a bystander effect. *J. Biol. Chem.* **2003**, *278*, 10128–10133. [CrossRef] [PubMed]
20. Buffinton, G.D.; Christen, S.; Peterhans, E.; Stocker, R. Oxidative stress in lungs of mice infected with influenza A virus. *Free Radic. Res. Commun.* **1992**, *16*, 99–110. [CrossRef] [PubMed]
21. Li, W.; Maeda, N.; Beck, A. Vitamin C deficiency increases the lung pathology of influenza virus-infected gulo−/− mice. *J. Nutr.* **2006**, *136*, 2611–2616. [PubMed]
22. Hosakote, Y.M.; Jantzi, P.D.; Esham, D.L.; Spratt, H.; Kurosky, A.; Casola, A.; Garofalo, R.P. Viral-mediated inhibition of antioxidant enzymes contributes to the pathogenesis of severe respiratory syncytial virus bronchiolitis. *Am. J. Respir. Crit. Care Med.* **2011**, *183*, 1550–1560. [CrossRef] [PubMed]
23. Hemilä, H. Vitamin C and the common cold. *Br. J. Nutr.* **1992**, *67*, 3–16. [CrossRef] [PubMed]
24. Hume, R.; Weyers, E. Changes in leucocyte ascorbic acid during the common cold. *Scott. Med. J.* **1973**, *18*, 3–7. [CrossRef] [PubMed]
25. Mochalkin, N.I. Ascorbic acid in the complex therapy of acute pneumonia. *Voenno-Meditsinskii Zhurnal* **1970**, *9*, 17–21. (In Russian). [PubMed]
26. Hunt, C.; Chakravorty, N.K.; Annan, G.; Habibzadeh, N.; Schorah, C.J. The clinical effects of vitamin C supplementation in elderly hospitalised patients with acute respiratory infections. *Int. J. Vitam. Nutr. Res.* **1994**, *64*, 212–219. [PubMed]
27. Hemilä, H.; Louhiala, P. Vitamin C for preventing and treating pneumonia. *Cochrane Database Syst. Rev.* **2013**, *8*, CD005532.

28. Hemilä, H.; Louhiala, P. Vitamin C for Preventing and Treating Pneumonia. Available online: http://www. mv.helsinki.fi/home/hemila/CP (accessed on 17 March 2017).

29. Powers, S.K.; Jackson, M.J. Exercise-induced oxidative stress: Cellular mechanisms and impact on muscle force production. *Physiol. Rev.* **2008**, *88*, 1243–1276. [CrossRef] [PubMed]

30. Ashton, T.; Young, I.S.; Peters, J.R.; Jones, E.; Jackson, S.K.; Davies, B.; Rowlands, C.C. Electron spin resonance spectroscopy, exercise, and oxidative stress: An ascorbic acid intervention study. *J. Appl. Physiol.* **1999**, *87*, 2032–2036. [PubMed]

31. Mullins, A.L.; van Rosendal, S.P.; Briskey, D.R.; Fassett, R.G.; Wilson, G.R.; Coombes, J.S. Variability in oxidative stress biomarkers following a maximal exercise test. *Biomarkers* **2013**, *18*, 446–454. [CrossRef] [PubMed]

32. Hemilä, H. Vitamin C may alleviate exercise-induced bronchoconstriction: A meta-analysis. *BMJ Open* **2013**, *3*, e002416. [CrossRef] [PubMed]

33. Hemilä, H. The effect of vitamin C on bronchoconstriction and respiratory symptoms caused by exercise: A review and statistical analysis. *Allergy Asthma Clin. Immunol.* **2014**, *10*, 58. [CrossRef] [PubMed]

34. LeBlanc, J.; Stewart, M.; Marier, G.; Whillans, M.G. Studies on acclimatization and on the effect of ascorbic acid in men exposed to cold. *Can. J. Biochem. Physiol.* **1954**, *32*, 407–427. [CrossRef] [PubMed]

35. Dugal, L.P. Vitamin C in relation to cold temperature tolerance. *Ann. N. Y. Acad. Sci.* **1961**, *92*, 307–317. [CrossRef] [PubMed]

36. Strydom, N.B.; Kotze, H.F.; van der Walt, W.H.; Rogers, G.G. Effect of ascorbic acid on rate of heat acclimatization. *J. Appl. Physiol.* **1976**, *41*, 202–205. [PubMed]

37. Chang, C.Y.; Chen, J.Y.; Chen, S.H.; Cheng, T.J.; Lin, M.T.; Hu, M.L. Therapeutic treatment with ascorbate rescues mice from heat stroke-induced death by attenuating systemic inflammatory response and hypothalamic neuronal damage. *Free Radic. Biol. Med.* **2016**, *93*, 84–93. [CrossRef] [PubMed]

38. Holley, A.D.; Osland, E.; Barnes, J.; Krishnan, A.; Fraser, J.F. Scurvy: Historically a plague of the sailor that remains a consideration in the modern intensive care unit. *Intern. Med. J.* **2011**, *41*, 283–285. [CrossRef] [PubMed]

39. Smith, A.; Di Primio, G.; Humphrey-Murto, S. Scurvy in the developed world. *Can. Med. Assoc. J.* **2011**, *183*, E752–E752. [CrossRef] [PubMed]

40. Raynaud-Simon, A.; Cohen-Bittan, J.; Gouronnec, A.; Pautas, E.; Senet, P.; Verny, M.; Boddaert, J. Scurvy in hospitalized elderly patients. *J. Nutr. Health Aging* **2010**, *14*, 407–410. [PubMed]

41. Hemilä, H.; Louhiala, P. Vitamin C may affect lung infections. *J. R. Soc. Med.* **2007**, *100*, 495–498. [CrossRef] [PubMed]

42. Beisel, W.R. Single nutrients and immunity: Vitamin C. *Am. J. Clin. Nutr.* **1982**, *35*, 423–428, 460–461.

43. Webb, A.L.; Villamor, E. Update: Effects of antioxidant and non-antioxidant vitamin supplementation on immune function. *Nutr. Rev.* **2007**, *65*, 181–217. [CrossRef] [PubMed]

44. Manning, J.; Mitchell, B.; Appadurai, D.A.; Shakya, A.; Pierce, L.J.; Wang, H.; Nganga, V.; Swanson, P.C.; May, J.M.; Tantin, D.; et al. Vitamin C promotes maturation of T-cells. *Antioxid. Redox Signal.* **2013**, *19*, 2054–2067. [PubMed]

45. Jones, E.; Hughes, R.E. Influence of oral carnitine on the body weight and survival time of avitaminotic-C guinea pigs. *Nutr. Rep. Int.* **1982**, *25*, 201–204.

46. Mårtensson, J.; Han, J.; Griffith, O.W.; Meister, A. Glutathione ester delays the onset of scurvy in ascorbate-deficient guinea pigs. *Proc. Natl. Acad. Sci. USA* **1993**, *90*, 317–321. [CrossRef] [PubMed]

47. Padh, H. Cellular functions of ascorbic acid. *Biochem. Cell Biol.* **1990**, *68*, 1166–1173. [CrossRef] [PubMed]

48. Rebouche, C.J. Ascorbic acid and carnitine biosynthesis. *Am. J. Clin. Nutr.* **1991**, *54*, 1147S–1152S. [PubMed]

49. Rice, M.E. Ascorbate regulation and its neuroprotective role in the brain. *Trends Neurol. Sci.* **2000**, *23*, 209–216.

50. May, J.M.; Harrison, F.E. Role of vitamin C in the function of the vascular endothelium. *Antioxid. Redox Signal.* **2013**, *19*, 2068–2083. [CrossRef] [PubMed]

51. Kinsman, R.A.; Hood, J. Some behavioral effects of ascorbic acid deficiency. *Am. J. Clin. Nutr.* **1971**, *24*, 455–464. [PubMed]

52. Zhang, M.; Robitaille, L.; Eintracht, S.; Hoffer, L.J. Vitamin C provision improves mood in acutely hospitalized patients. *Nutrition* **2011**, *27*, 530–533. [CrossRef] [PubMed]

53. Wang, Y.; Liu, X.J.; Robitaille, L.; Eintracht, S.; MacNamara, E.; Hoffer, L.J. Effects of vitamin C and vitamin D administration on mood and distress in acutely hospitalized patients. *Am. J. Clin. Nutr.* **2013**, *98*, 705–711. [CrossRef] [PubMed]

54. Hemilä, H.; Kaprio, J. Subgroup analysis of large trials can guide further research: A case study of vitamin E and pneumonia. *Clin. Epidemiol.* **2011**, *3*, 51–59. [CrossRef] [PubMed]

55. Hemilä, H. Vitamin E and the risk of pneumonia: Using the I^2-statistic to quantify heterogeneity within a controlled trial. *Br. J. Nutr.* **2016**, *116*, 1530–1536. [CrossRef] [PubMed]

56. Hemilä, H.; Virtamo, J.; Albanes, D.; Kaprio, J. The effect of vitamin E on common cold incidence is modified by age, smoking and residential neighborhood. *J. Am. Coll. Nutr.* **2006**, *25*, 332–339. [CrossRef] [PubMed]

57. McConkey, M.; Smith, D.T. The relation of vitamin C deficiency to intestinal tuberculosis in the guinea pig. *J. Exp. Med.* **1933**, *58*, 503–517. [CrossRef] [PubMed]

58. Dey, P.K. Efficacy of vitamin C in counteracting tetanus toxin toxicity. *Naturwissenschaften* **1966**, *53*, 310. [CrossRef] [PubMed]

59. Belfield, W.O. Vitamin C in treatment of canine and feline distemper complex. *Vet. Med. Small Anim. Clin.* **1967**, *62*, 345–348. [PubMed]

60. Leveque, J.I. Ascorbic acid in treatment of the canine distemper complex. *Vet. Med. Small Anim. Clin.* **1969**, *64*, 997–1001. [PubMed]

61. Eccles, R. Is the common cold a clinical entity or a cultural concept? *Rhinology* **2013**, *51*, 3–8. [PubMed]

62. Monto, A.S.; Ullman, B.M. Acute respiratory illness in an American community: The Tecumseh Study. *JAMA* **1974**, *227*, 164–169. [PubMed]

63. Fendrick, A.M.; Monto, A.S.; Nightengale, B.; Sarnes, M. The economic burden of non-influenza-related viral respiratory tract infection in the United States. *Arch. Int. Med.* **2003**, *163*, 487–494. [CrossRef]

64. Pauling, L. *Vitamin C and the Common Cold*; Freeman: San Francisco, CA, USA, 1970.

65. Pauling, L. The significance of the evidence about ascorbic acid and the common cold. *Proc. Natl. Acad. Sci. USA* **1971**, *68*, 2678–2681. [CrossRef] [PubMed]

66. Pauling, L. Ascorbic acid and the common cold. *Am. J. Clin. Nutr.* **1971**, *24*, 1294–1299. [CrossRef] [PubMed]

67. Ritzel, G. Critical analysis of the role of vitamin C in the treatment of the common cold. *Helv. Med. Acta* **1961**, *28*, 63–68. (In German). [PubMed]

68. Hemilä, H.; Chalker, E. Vitamin C for preventing and treating the common cold. *Cochrane Database Syst. Rev.* **2013**, *1*, CD000980.

69. Hemilä, H.; Chalker, E. Vitamin C for Preventing and Treating the Common Cold. Available online: http://www.mv.helsinki.fi/home/hemila/CC (accessed on 17 March 2017).

70. Hemilä, H. Vitamin C supplementation and common cold symptoms: Problems with inaccurate reviews. *Nutrition* **1996**, *12*, 804–809. [CrossRef]

71. Chalmers, T.C. Effects of ascorbic acid on the common cold: An evaluation of the evidence. *Am. J. Med.* **1975**, *58*, 532–536. [CrossRef]

72. Karlowski, T.R.; Chalmers, T.C.; Frenkel, L.D.; Kapikian, A.Z.; Lewis, T.L.; Lynch, J.M. Ascorbic acid for the common cold: A prophylactic and therapeutic trial. *JAMA* **1975**, *231*, 1038–1042. [PubMed]

73. Dykes, M.H.M.; Meier, P. Ascorbic acid and the common cold: Evaluation of its efficacy and toxicity. *JAMA* **1975**, *231*, 1073–1079. [CrossRef] [PubMed]

74. Hemilä, H. Vitamin C intake and susceptibility to the common cold. *Br. J. Nutr.* **1997**, *77*, 59–72. [CrossRef] [PubMed]

75. Bates, C.J.; Schorah, C.J.; Hemilä, H. Vitamin C intake and susceptibility to the common cold: Invited comments and Reply. *Br. J. Nutr.* **1997**, *78*, 857–866. [PubMed]

76. Hemilä, H. Vitamin C and common cold incidence: A review of studies with subjects under heavy physical stress. *Int. J. Sports Med.* **1996**, *17*, 379–383. [CrossRef] [PubMed]

77. Hemilä, H. Vitamin C and sex differences in respiratory tract infections. *Respir. Med.* **2008**, *102*, 625–626. [CrossRef] [PubMed]

78. Baird, I.M.; Hughes, R.E.; Wilson, H.K.; Davies, J.E.; Howard, A.N. The effects of ascorbic acid and flavonoids on the occurrence of symptoms normally associated with the common cold. *Am. J. Clin. Nutr.* **1979**, *32*, 1686–1690. [PubMed]

79. Johnston, C.S.; Barkyoumb, G.M.; Schumacher, S.S. Vitamin C supplementation slightly improves physical activity levels and reduces cold incidence in men with marginal vitamin C status: A randomized controlled trial. *Nutrients* **2014**, *6*, 2572–2583. [CrossRef] [PubMed]

80. Anderson, T.W.; Reid, D.B.W.; Beaton, G.H. Vitamin C and the common cold: A double-blind trial. *Can. Med. Assoc. J.* **1972**, *107*, 503–508. [PubMed]

81. Coulehan, J.L.; Reisinger, K.S.; Rogers, K.D.; Bradley, D.W. Vitamin C prophylaxis in a boarding school. *N. Engl. J. Med.* **1974**, *290*, 6–10. [CrossRef] [PubMed]

82. Van Straten, M.; Josling, P. Preventing the common cold with a vitamin C supplement: A double-blind, placebo-controlled survey. *Adv. Ther.* **2002**, *19*, 151–159. [CrossRef] [PubMed]

83. Hemilä, H. Vitamin C supplementation and common cold symptoms: Factors affecting the magnitude of the benefit. *Med. Hypotheses* **1999**, *52*, 171–178. [PubMed]

84. Anderson, T.W.; Suranyi, G.; Beaton, G.H. The effect on winter illness of large doses of vitamin C. *Can. Med. Assoc. J.* **1974**, *111*, 31–36. [PubMed]

85. Anderson, T.W.; Beaton, G.H.; Corey, P.N.; Spero, L. Winter illness and vitamin C: The effect of relatively low doses. *Can. Med. Assoc. J.* **1975**, *112*, 823–826. [PubMed]

86. Constantini, N.W.; Dubnov-Raz, G.; Eyal, B.B.; Berry, E.M.; Cohen, A.H.; Hemilä, H. The effect of vitamin C on upper respiratory infections in adolescent swimmers: A randomized trial. *Eur. J. Pediatr.* **2011**, *170*, 59–63. [CrossRef] [PubMed]

87. Carr, A.B.; Einstein, R.; Lai, Y.C.; Martin, N.G.; Starmer, G.A. Vitamin C and the common cold: A second MZ co-twin control study. *Acta Genet. Med. Gemellol.* **1981**, *30*, 249–255. [CrossRef] [PubMed]

88. Bee, D.M. The vitamin C controversy. *Postgrad. Med.* **1980**, *67*, 64. [CrossRef] [PubMed]

89. Cathcart, R.F. Vitamin, C.; titrating to bowel tolerance, anascorbemia, and acute induced scurvy. *Med. Hypotheses* **1981**, *7*, 1359–1376. [CrossRef]

90. Gern, J.E. The ABCs of rhinoviruses, wheezing, and asthma. *J. Virol.* **2010**, *84*, 7418–7426. [CrossRef] [PubMed]

91. Hemilä, H. Vitamin C and common cold-induced asthma: A systematic review and statistical analysis. *Allergy Asthma Clin. Immunol.* **2013**, *9*, 46. [CrossRef] [PubMed]

92. Anah, C.O.; Jarike, L.N.; Baig, H.A. High dose ascorbic acid in Nigerian asthmatics. *Trop. Geogr. Med.* **1980**, *32*, 132–137. [PubMed]

93. Schertling, M.; Winsel, K.; Müller, S.; Henning, R.; Meiske, W.; Slapke, J. Action of ascorbic acid on clinical course of infection related bronchial asthma and on reactive oxygen metabolites by BAL cells. *Z. Klin. Med.* **1990**, *45*, 1770–1774. (In German).

94. Bucca, C.; Rolla, G.; Arossa, W.; Caria, E.; Elia, C.; Nebiolo, F.; Baldi, S. Effect of ascorbic acid on increased bronchial responsiveness during upper airway infection. *Respiration* **1989**, *55*, 214–219. [CrossRef] [PubMed]

95. Miegl, H. Acute upper respiratory tract infection and its treatment with vitamin C. *Wien. Med. Wochenschr.* **1957**, *107*, 989–992. (In German). [PubMed]

96. Miegl, H. About the use of vitamin C in otorhinolaryngology. *Wien. Med. Wochenschr.* **1958**, *108*, 859–864. (In German) [PubMed]

97. Glazebrook, A.J.; Thomson, S. The administration of vitamin C in a large institution and its effect on general health and resistance to infection. *J. Hyg.* **1942**, *42*, 1–19. [CrossRef] [PubMed]

98. Sabiston, B.H.; Radomski, M.W. *Health Problems and Vitamin C in Canadian Northern Military Operations*; DCIEM Report No. 74-R-1012; Defence and Civil Institute of Environmental Medicine: Downsview, ON, Canada, 1974.

99. Peters, E.M.; Goetzsche, J.M.; Grobbelaar, B.; Noakes, T.D. Vitamin C supplementation reduces the incidence of postrace symptoms of upper-respiratory-tract infection in ultramarathon runners. *Am. J. Clin. Nutr.* **1993**, *57*, 170–174. [PubMed]

100. Cowan, D.W.; Diehl, H.S.; Baker, A.B. Vitamins for the prevention of colds. *JAMA* **1942**, *120*, 1268–1271. [CrossRef]

101. Miller, J.Z.; Nance, W.E.; Norton, J.A.; Wolen, R.L.; Griffith, R.S.; Rose, R.J. Therapeutic effect of vitamin C: A co-twin control study. *JAMA* **1977**, *237*, 248–251. [CrossRef] [PubMed]

102. Liberati, A. Thomas C Chalmers. *Lancet* **1996**, *347*, 188. [CrossRef]

103. Dickersin, K. Thomas Clark Chalmers. *JAMA* **1996**, *276*, 656–657. [CrossRef]

104. Pincock, S. Paul Meier. *Lancet* **2011**, *378*, 978. [CrossRef]

105. Betts, K. Paul Meier: A man behind the method. *Am. J. Public Health* **2012**, *102*, 2026–2029. [CrossRef] [PubMed]

106. Hemilä, H. Vitamin, C.; the placebo effect, and the common cold: A case study of how preconceptions influence the analysis of results. *J. Clin. Epidemiol.* **1996**, *49*, 1079–1084.

107. Hemilä, H. Analysis of clinical data with breached blindness. *Stat. Med.* **2006**, *25*, 1434–1437. [CrossRef] [PubMed]

108. Chalmers, T.C. Dissent to the preceding article by H. Hemilä. *J. Clin. Epidemiol.* **1996**, *49*, 1085. [CrossRef]

109. Hemilä, H. To the dissent by Thomas Chalmers. *J. Clin. Epidemiol.* **1996**, *49*, 1087. [CrossRef]

110. Hemilä, H.; Herman, Z.S. Vitamin C and the common cold: A retrospective analysis of Chalmers' review. *J. Am. Coll. Nutr.* **1995**, *14*, 116–123. [CrossRef] [PubMed]

111. Pauling, L. Ascorbic acid and the common cold: Evaluation of its efficacy and toxicity. Part I. *Med. Tribune* **1976**, *17*, 18–19. [CrossRef] [PubMed]

112. Pauling, L. Ascorbic acid and the common cold. Part II. *Med. Tribune* **1976**, *17*, 37–38.

113. Council of Scientific Affairs, American Medical Association. Vitamin preparations as dietary supplements and as therapeutic agents. *JAMA* **1987**, *257*, 1929–1936.

114. Gander, J.; Niederberger, W. Vitamin C in the treatment of pneumonia. *Münch. Med. Wochenschr.* **1936**, *83*, 2074–2077. (In German).

115. Bohnholtzer, E. Contribution to the question of pneumonia treatment with vitamin C. *Dtsch. Med. Wochenschr.* **1937**, *63*, 1001–1003. (In German). [CrossRef]

116. Hochwald, A. Vitamin C in the treatment of croupous pneumonia. *Dtsch. Med. Wochenschr.* **1937**, *63*, 182–184. (In German). [CrossRef]

117. Klenner, F.R. Virus pneumonia and its treatment with vitamin C. *South. Med. Surg.* **1948**, *110*, 36–38. [PubMed]

118. Klenner, F.R. Massive doses of vitamin C and the virus diseases. *South. Med. Surg.* **1951**, *113*, 101–107. [PubMed]

119. Dalton, W.L. Massive doses of vitamin C in the treatment of viral diseases. *J. Indiana State Med. Assoc.* **1962**, *55*, 1151–1154. [PubMed]

120. Hemilä, H. Vitamin C intake and susceptibility to pneumonia. *Pediatr. Infect. Dis. J.* **1997**, *16*, 836–837. [CrossRef] [PubMed]

121. Kimbarowski, J.A.; Mokrow, N.J. Colored precipitation reaction of the urine according to Kimbarowski as an index of the effect of ascorbic acid during treatment of viral influenza. *Dtsch. Gesundheitsw.* **1967**, *22*, 2413–2418. (In German). [PubMed]

122. Pitt, H.A.; Costrini, A.M. Vitamin C prophylaxis in marine recruits. *JAMA* **1979**, *241*, 908–911. [PubMed]

123. Hemilä, H. Vitamin C supplementation and respiratory infections: A systematic review. *Mil. Med.* **2004**, *169*, 920–925. [CrossRef] [PubMed]

124. Merchant, A.T.; Curhan, G.; Bendich, A.; Singh, V.N.; Willett, W.C.; Fawzi, W.W. Vitamin intake is not associated with community-acquired pneumonia in US men. *J. Nutr.* **2004**, *134*, 439–444. [PubMed]

125. Hemilä, H.; Virtamo, J.; Albanes, D.; Kaprio, J. Vitamin E and beta carotene supplementation and hospital-treated pneumonia incidence in male smokers. *Chest* **2004**, *125*, 557–565. [CrossRef] [PubMed]

126. Pazzaglia, G.; Pasternack, M. Recent trends of pneumonia morbidity in US Naval personnel. *Mil. Med.* **1983**, *148*, 647–651. [PubMed]

127. Paynter, S.; Ware, R.S.; Weinstein, P.; Williams, G.; Sly, P.D. Childhood pneumonia: A neglected, climate-sensitive disease? *Lancet* **2010**, *376*, 1804–1805. [CrossRef]

128. Klenner, F.R. Recent discoveries in the treatment of lockjaw with vitamin C and tolserol. *Tri State Med. J.* **1954**, *2*, 7–11.

129. Hemilä, H.; Koivula, T. Vitamin C for preventing and treating tetanus. *Cochrane Database Syst. Rev.* **2013**, *11*, CD006665.

130. Hemilä, H.; Koivula, T. Vitamin C for Preventing and Treating Tetanus. Available online: http://www.mv.helsinki.fi/home/hemila/CT (accessed on 17 March 2017).

131. Jahan, K.; Ahmad, K.; Ali, M.A. Effect of ascorbic acid in the treatment of tetanus. *Bangladesh Med. Res. Counc. Bull.* **1984**, *10*, 24–28. [PubMed]

132. Hemilä, H. Vitamin C supplementation and the common cold—Was Linus Pauling right or wrong? *Int. J. Vitamin Nutr. Res.* **1997**, *67*, 329–335.

133. Stone, I. *The Healing Factor: Vitamin C against Disease*; Grosset Dunlap: New York, NY, USA, 1972.

134. Briggs, M. Vitamin C and infectious disease: A review of the literature and the results of a randomized, double-blind, prospective study over 8 years. In *Recent Vitamin Research*; Briggs, M.H., Ed.; CRC Press: Boca Raton, FL, USA, 1984; pp. 39–82.

135. Levy, T.E. *Vitamin C, Infectious Diseases, and Toxins*; Xlibris: Philadelphia, PA, USA, 2002.

136. Terezhalmy, G.T.; Bottomley, W.K.; Pelleu, G.B. The use of water-soluble bioflavonoid-ascorbic acid complex in the treatment of recurrent herpes labialis. *Oral Surg. Oral Med. Oral Pathol.* **1978**, *45*, 56–62. [CrossRef]

137. Chen, J.Y.; Chang, C.Y.; Feng, P.H.; Chu, C.C.; So, E.C.; Hu, M.L. Plasma vitamin C is lower in postherpetic neuralgia patients and administration of vitamin C reduces spontaneous pain but not brush-evoked pain. *Clin. J. Pain* **2009**, *25*, 562–569. [CrossRef] [PubMed]

138. Orient, J.M. Treating herpes zoster with vitamin C: Two case reports. *J. Am. Phys. Surg.* **2006**, *11*, 26–27.

139. Byun, S.H.; Jeon, Y. Administration of vitamin C in a patient with herpes zoster—A case report. *Korean J. Pain* **2011**, *24*, 108–111. [CrossRef] [PubMed]

140. Schencking, M.; Sandholzer, H.; Frese, T. Intravenous administration of vitamin C in the treatment of herpetic neuralgia: Two case reports. *Med. Sci. Monit.* **2010**, *16*, CS58–CS61. [PubMed]

141. Schencking, M.; Vollbracht, C.; Weiss, G.; Lebert, J.; Biller, A.; Goyvaerts, B.; Kraft, K. Intravenous vitamin C in the treatment of shingles: Results of a multicenter prospective cohort study. *Med. Sci. Monit.* **2012**, *18*, CR215–CR224. [PubMed]

142. Kim, M.S.; Kim, D.J.; Na, C.H.; Shin, B.S. A Study of Intravenous Administration of Vitamin C in the Treatment of Acute Herpetic Pain and Postherpetic Neuralgia. *Ann. Dermatol.* **2016**, *28*, 677–683. [CrossRef] [PubMed]

143. Patrone, F.; Dallegri, F.; Bonvini, E.; Minervini, F.; Sacchetti, C. Disorders of neutrophil function in children with recurrent pyogenic infections. *Med. Microbiol. Immunol.* **1982**, *171*, 113–122. [CrossRef] [PubMed]

144. Levy, R.; Shriker, O.; Porath, A.; Riesenberg, K.; Schlaeffer, F. Vitamin C for the treatment of recurrent furunculosis in patients with impaired neutrophil functions. *J. Infect. Dis.* **1996**, *173*, 1502–1505. [CrossRef] [PubMed]

145. Galley, H.F.; Howdle, P.D.; Walker, B.E.; Webster, N.R. The effects of intravenous antioxidants in patients with septic shock. *Free Radic. Biol. Med.* **1997**, *23*, 768–774. [CrossRef]

146. Pleiner, J.; Mittermayer, F.; Schaller, G.; MacAllister, R.J.; Wolzt, M. High doses of vitamin C reverse Escherichia coli endotoxin-induced hyporeactivity to acetylcholine in the human forearm. *Circulation* **2002**, *106*, 1460–1464. [CrossRef] [PubMed]

147. Klenner, F.R. Observations on the dose and administration of ascorbic acid when employed beyond the range of a vitamin in human pathology. *J. Appl. Nutr.* **1971**, *23*, 61–88.

148. Smith, G.D.; Lawlor, D.A.; Harbord, R.; Timpson, N.; Day, I.; Ebrahim, S. Clustered environments and randomized genes: A fundamental distinction between conventional and genetic epidemiology. *PLoS Med.* **2007**, *4*, e352. [CrossRef] [PubMed]

149. Block, G.; Norkus, E.; Hudes, M.; Mandel, S.; Helzlsouer, K. Which plasma antioxidants are most related to fruit and vegetable consumption? *Am. J. Epidemiol.* **2001**, *154*, 1113–1118. [CrossRef] [PubMed]

150. Hemilä, H.; Kaprio, J. Vitamin E supplementation may transiently increase tuberculosis risk in males who smoke heavily and have high dietary vitamin C intake. *Br. J. Nutr.* **2008**, *100*, 896–902. [CrossRef] [PubMed]

151. Hemilä, H.; Kaprio, J. Vitamin E supplementation may transiently increase tuberculosis risk in males who smoke heavily and have high dietary vitamin C intake—Reply by Hemilä & Kaprio. *Br. J. Nutr.* **2009**, *101*, 145–147.

152. Packer, J.E.; Slater, T.F.; Wilson, R.L. Direct observation of a free radical interaction between vitamin E and vitamin C. *Nature* **1979**, *278*, 737–738. [CrossRef] [PubMed]

153. Hemilä, H.; Kaprio, J. Modification of the effect of vitamin E supplementation on the mortality of male smokers by age and dietary vitamin C. *Am. J. Epidemiol.* **2009**, *169*, 946–953. [CrossRef] [PubMed]

154. Hemilä, H.; Kaprio, J. Vitamin E supplementation and pneumonia risk in males who initiated smoking at an early age: Effect modification by body weight and vitamin C. *Nutr. J.* **2008**, *7*, 33. [CrossRef] [PubMed]

155. Goodwin, J.S.; Goodwin, J.M. The tomato effect: Rejection of highly efficacious therapies. *JAMA* **1984**, *251*, 2387–2390. [CrossRef] [PubMed]

156. Knipschild, P.; Kleijnen, J.; Riet, G. Belief in the efficacy of alternative medicine among general practitioners in the Netherlands. *Soc. Sci. Med.* **1990**, *31*, 625–626. [CrossRef]

157. Richards, E. The politics of therapeutic evaluation: The vitamin C and cancer controversy. *Soc. Stud. Sci.* **1988**, *18*, 653–701. [CrossRef]

158. Richards, E. *Vitamin C and Cancer: Medicine or Politics?* St. Martins Press: New York, NY, USA, 1991.

159. Segerstråle, U. Vitamin C and cancer—Medicine or politics. *Science* **1992**, *255*, 613–615. [PubMed]

160. Goodwin, J.S.; Tangum, M.R. Battling quackery: Attitudes about micronutrient supplements in American Academic medicine. *Arch. Intern. Med.* **1998**, *158*, 2187–2191. [CrossRef] [PubMed]

161. Louhiala, P.; Hemilä, H. Can CAM treatments be evidence-based? *Focus Altern. Complement. Ther.* **2014**, *19*, 84–89. [CrossRef]

11

The Use of Intravenous Vitamin C as a Supportive Therapy for a Patient with Glioblastoma Multiforme

Nicola Baillie [1,*], Anitra C. Carr [2] and Selene Peng [3]

[1] Integrated Health Options Ltd., Auckland 1050, New Zealand

[2] Department of Pathology & Biomedical Science, University of Otago, Christchurch 8140, New Zealand; anitra.carr@otago.ac.nz

[3] Feedback Research Ltd., Auckland 1050, New Zealand; selene@feedbackresearch.co.nz

* Correspondence: nicky@integratedhealthoptions.co.nz

Abstract: Glioblastoma multiforme is a high grade malignant brain tumour with a poor prognosis. Here we report the case of a woman with glioblastoma who lived for over four years from diagnosis (median survival 12 months and 2% survival for three years), experiencing good quality of life for most of that time. She underwent initial debulking craniotomy, radiotherapy and chemotherapy, as well as having intravenous vitamin C infusions 2–3 times weekly over the four years from diagnosis. Her progress was monitored by blood tests, regular computerised tomography (CT) and magnetic resonance imaging (MRI) scans, clinical reviews and European Organization for the Research and Treatment of Cancer quality of life questionnaires (EORTC QLQ C30). Our case report highlights the benefits of intravenous vitamin C as a supportive therapy for patients with glioblastoma.

Keywords: vitamin C; intravenous vitamin C; ascorbic acid; glioblastoma; neoplasms; quality of life

1. Introduction

Glioblastoma multiforme is a high grade malignant brain tumour with a poor prognosis; median survival 12 months and 2% survive for three years [1,2]. We describe the case of a 55-year-old woman who responded much better than expected, with good quality of life for almost four years from diagnosis. She chose to combine conventional treatments with intravenous (IV) vitamin C therapy. Although there are limited clinical trials on the use of IV vitamin C for people with cancer, the available evidence indicates it is safe and generally well tolerated when combined with standard cancer therapies [3–5]. A small trial of IV vitamin C in combination with standard therapy in glioblastoma patients indicated a trend towards enhanced median survival [6]. In our case, the IV vitamin C was well tolerated, quality of life improved markedly in the first year, and then stabilised, and the patient had improved or stable blood tests throughout, including normal renal function.

2. Case Report

The enduring power of attorney provided consent for the presentation of the patient's case. The 55 years old woman was diagnosed in November 2010 with glioblastoma multiforme following a 10 days history of headaches and constipation. Concurrently, she was diagnosed with extranodal marginal zone lymphoma, affecting the left parotid gland and bladder. She was previously fit and healthy, with no significant past medical history, and no history of renal stones. She did not drink alcohol and was a nonsmoker. Her sister died of a brain tumour age 40, and her father of prostate and bladder cancer age 84. She underwent craniotomy and debulking surgery in December 2010, followed by a course of radiotherapy and temozolomide. She had no specific conventional treatment for the lymphoma.

Overall, the patient received 25 radiation treatments March to April 2011, and a further 10 treatments April 2014, and temozolomide for six cycles from March to June 2011, and a further six cycles from April 2014. She had no conventional cancer treatments for almost three years, from July 2011 until April 2014.

2.1. IV Vitamin C Treatment

When the patient first presented to our clinic mid-January 2011 she had fatigue, lethargy and an early chest infection. She was diagnosed with pneumonia the following day, which was treated with IV antibiotics in hospital, at which time she also had a blood transfusion for anaemia. The patient commenced regular IV vitamin C infusions a few days later, approximately three weeks following her brain surgery for glioblastoma multiforme. Baseline blood tests showed normal renal function and normal glucose-6-phosphate dehydrogenase (G6PD) status. If G6PD deficiency is present we do not recommend more than 25 grams IV vitamin C as there is an increased risk of haemolysis. Her non-fasting baseline plasma vitamin C level was 1.2 mg/dL (68 μmol/L); she had consumed a 1 g vitamin C supplement prior to coming to the clinic. The patient received IV vitamin C working up to 85 g/infusion, three times/week for the first six months to June 2011, then twice/week for over three years, stopping October 2014. Post-infusion plasma vitamin C levels were monitored for the first four months after she commenced IV vitamin C infusion to ensure that the proposed ascorbic acid therapeutic level was achieved. The average post-infusion plasma vitamin C level was 393 mg/dL (22 mmol/L), with a dose of 85 g (1.1 g/kg). The patient's renal function tests were normal throughout IV vitamin C treatments with creatinine ranging from 51–67 μmol/L and eGFR mostly >90 mL/min/1.73 m^2. The IV vitamin C was well tolerated.

2.2. Outcome and Follow-Up

CT scans or MRI scans with contrast were carried out every 3–6 months over the four years from diagnosis. These indicated stable disease until March 2014 (Table 1). In July 2011, her extranodal marginal zone lymphoma, eight months after diagnosis with no specific lymphoma treatments, showed stable disease on CT scan of the left parotid gland, with a possible decrease in the size of bladder mass. Six monthly follow-ups reported stable disease until March 2014 when a MRI scan noted lymphoma increase in both orbits, but the comment was made that 'overall lymphoma was reasonably stable'.

Table 1. Computerised tomography (CT) and magnetic resonance imaging (MRI) scans of brain.

Date	CT Scan of Brain	MRI Scan of Brain
July 2011	Residual tumour	
January 2012		Stable
May 2012		Stable
September 2012	Reduced tumour size	
August 2013	Stable	
October 2013		Stable
March 2014		Progression of brain tumour with new and increasing foci
June 2014		Likely disease progression
September 2014		Increase size of brain tumour over 1 year, 4 discrete lesions

Following the initiation of IV vitamin C treatments (January 2011), the patient reported clinical improvements that were maintained for almost four years following diagnosis. She noticed improved energy and walking distance four weeks after initially commencing IV vitamin C, prior to starting her first course of radiation therapy. She chose to continue IV vitamin C throughout her two courses of chemotherapy and radiotherapy, despite being advised that we do not recommend IV vitamin C concurrently with these treatments as there is limited research into benefits or interactions in this area. She felt it helped her symptoms and reported tolerating the radiotherapy 'pretty well'.

The patient's health-related quality of life (QoL) was monitored using the EORTC QLQ C30 for the first 12 months, and subsequently through clinical reviews. Compared to the patient's QoL data prior to commencing IV vitamin C treatment, dramatic improvement was reported in the three months survey following initiation of IV vitamin C treatment (at that time the patient had just completed radiotherapy and started chemotherapy) and the improvement was maintained for the first 12 months (Table 2). Clinical symptoms such as fatigue, dyspnoea, insomnia, appetite loss and diarrhoea resolved and the patient's physical and role functioning increased significantly, as well as 'global health status', which improved from 'very poor' to 'excellent'.

Table 2. Health-related quality of life following intravenous vitamin C (IVC) treatments.

Scales	Before IVC	3 Months after IVC	12 Months after IVC
Symptoms scales			
Fatigue	100	0	0
Nausea	0	0	0
Pain	0	0	0
Dyspnoea	100	0	0
Insomnia	100	0	0
Appetite loss	100	0	0
Constipation	0	0	0
Diarrhoea	67	0	0
Functional scales			
Physical functioning	27	100	100
Role functioning	0	100	100
Emotional functioning	100	100	100
Cognitive functioning	100	100	100
Social Functioning	100	100	100
Global health status	0	100	83

Formal QoL monitoring was not collected after the first 12 months, but from clinical reviews the patient maintained a good QoL, feeling 'very well' until April 2014 when she developed seizures. These were well controlled with medication and she continued working full-time until October 2014. Early November she deteriorated with reduced alertness, right sided weakness, and expressive dysphasia. She ceased IV vitamin C at this time. She continued to deteriorate until 26 February 2015 when she passed away at home, four years and three months from the initial diagnosis.

3. Discussion

The use of pharmacological ascorbate as an adjuvant cancer therapy was proposed as early as 1976 [7]. More recent studies have consistently shown selective toxicity to cancer cells compared to normal cells in vitro and in vivo [6,8–11]. The mechanism of action for selective cancer cell toxicity is not fully understood, although several research studies have suggested that the cytotoxic effect is mediated through ascorbate-mediated reduction of catalytic metal ions and subsequent generation of hydrogen peroxide, which can induce oxidative damage to macromolecules (i.e., DNA, proteins and lipids), deplete cellular adenosine triphosphate (ATP), and thereby cause cell death [12–14]. Another plausible mechanism of action has been recently proposed, as high dose ascorbate administration has been shown to slow tumour growth and decrease hypoxia through suppressing the activity of hypoxia-inducible factor (HIF-1), which is known to contribute to tumour progression [11,15,16]. Clinical trials in the use of IV vitamin C in critically ill patients [17–19] and patients with cancer [3–5,20,21] have demonstrated lack of toxicity, good safety and tolerability [22].

Our case report outlines the unexpected increase in progression free and overall survival in a woman with glioblastoma who had IV vitamin C from shortly after diagnosis, for almost four years, stopping three months before she died. She chose to continue IV vitamin C throughout her two courses of chemotherapy and radiotherapy and her increased survival time supports the findings of a small

Phase 1 clinical trial in the concurrent use of IV vitamin C in patients with glioblastoma receiving chemotherapy and radiotherapy [6]. Although the IV vitamin C was the only additional treatment she was undertaking we cannot conclude that it was the primary factor in her increased progression free survival. However, it is interesting to note that epigenetic dysregulation of the vitamin C-dependent DNA hydroxylase ten-eleven translocation-2 (TET2) is observed in human glioblastoma and decreased hydroxymethylcytosine is associated with shorter malignant glioma survival [23,24], suggesting a possible mechanism by which vitamin C could aid in glioblastoma therapy. Nevertheless, it is likely that the IV vitamin C contributed to the patient's improved quality of life, as has been observed in numerous other studies [25].

4. Conclusions

Our case report indicates that IV vitamin C may be a useful supportive therapy in the management of people with glioblastoma multiforme. IV vitamin C even at doses of over 1 g/kg body weight was very well tolerated. There were no renal stones or impairment of renal function throughout four years of treatment with IV vitamin C in this case. Overall, IV vitamin C given concurrently with chemotherapy and radiotherapy had no apparent adverse reactions and contributed to an improved quality of life and potentially an increase in progression free and overall survival. Further trials on the use of IV vitamin C as an adjuvant therapy in people with glioblastoma are warranted. Currently there is a Phase II trial underway investigating pharmacological vitamin C combined with radiation and temozolomide in glioblastoma multiforme (NCT02344355).

Author Contributions: Conceptualization, N.B.; Investigation, N.B. and S.P.; Writing–Original Draft Preparation, N.B., A.C. and S.P.

Acknowledgments: A.C. is supported by a Health Research Council of New Zealand Sir Charles Hercus Health Research Fellowship.

References

1. Yersal, O. Clinical outcome of patients with glioblastoma multiforme: Single center experience. *J. Oncol. Sci.* **2017**, *3*, 123–126. [CrossRef]
2. Adeberg, S.; Bostel, T.; König, L.; Welzel, T.; Debus, J.; Combs, S.E. A comparison of long-term survivors and short-term survivors with glioblastoma, subventricular zone involvement: A predictive factor for survival? *Radiat. Oncol.* **2014**, *9*, 1–6. [CrossRef] [PubMed]
3. Monti, D.A.; Mitchell, E.; Bazzan, A.J.; Littman, S.; Zabrecky, G.; Yeo, C.J.; Pillai, M.V.; Newberg, A.B.; Deshmukh, S.; Levine, M. Phase I evaluation of intravenous ascorbic acid in combination with gemcitabine and erlotinib in patients with metastatic pancreatic cancer. *PLoS ONE* **2012**, *7*, e29794. [CrossRef] [PubMed]
4. Welsh, J.L.; Wagner, B.A.; van't Erve, T.J.; Zehr, P.S.; Berg, D.J.; Halfdanarson, T.R.; Yee, N.S.; Bodeker, K.L.; Du, J.; Roberts, L.J., 2nd; et al. Pharmacological ascorbate with gemcitabine for the control of metastatic and node-positive pancreatic cancer (PACMAN): Results from a phase I clinical trial. *Cancer Chemother. Pharmacol.* **2013**, *71*, 765–775. [CrossRef] [PubMed]
5. Hoffer, L.J.; Robitaille, L.; Zakarian, R.; Melnychuk, D.; Kavan, P.; Agulnik, J.; Cohen, V.; Small, D.; Miller, W.H., Jr. High-dose intravenous vitamin C combined with cytotoxic chemotherapy in patients with advanced cancer: A Phase I-II clinical trial. *PLoS ONE* **2015**, *10*, e0120228. [CrossRef] [PubMed]
6. Schoenfeld, J.D.; Sibenaller, Z.A.; Mapuskar, K.A.; Wagner, B.A.; Cramer-Morales, K.L.; Furqan, M.; Sandhu, S.; Carlisle, T.L.; Smith, M.C.; Abu Hejleh, T.; et al. O_2- and H_2O_2-Mediated Disruption of Fe Metabolism Causes the Differential Susceptibility of NSCLC and GBM Cancer Cells to Pharmacological Ascorbate. *Cancer Cell* **2017**, *31*, 487–500.e8. [CrossRef] [PubMed]
7. Cameron, E.; Pauling, L. Supplemental ascorbate in the supportive treatment of cancer: Prolongation of survival times in terminal human cancer. *Proc. Natl. Acad. Sci. USA* **1976**, *73*, 3685–3689. [CrossRef] [PubMed]

8. Du, J.; Martin, S.M.; Levine, M.; Wagner, B.A.; Buettner, G.R.; Wang, S.H.; Taghiyev, A.F.; Du, C.; Knudson, C.M.; Cullen, J.J. Mechanisms of ascorbate-induced cytotoxicity in pancreatic cancer. *Clin. Cancer Res.* **2010**, *16*, 509–520. [CrossRef] [PubMed]

9. Ma, Y.; Chapman, J.; Levine, M.; Polireddy, K.; Drisko, J.; Chen, Q. High-dose parenteral ascorbate enhanced chemosensitivity of ovarian cancer and reduced toxicity of chemotherapy. *Sci. Transl. Med.* **2014**, *6*, 222ra18. [CrossRef] [PubMed]

10. Yun, J.; Mullarky, E.; Lu, C.; Bosch, K.N.; Kavalier, A.; Rivera, K.; Roper, J.; Chio, I.I.; Giannopoulou, E.G.; Rago, C.; et al. Vitamin C selectively kills KRAS and BRAF mutant colorectal cancer cells by targeting GAPDH. *Science* **2015**, *350*, 1391–1396. [CrossRef] [PubMed]

11. Campbell, E.J.; Vissers, M.C.; Wohlrab, C.; Hicks, K.O.; Strother, R.M.; Bozonet, S.M.; Robinson, B.A.; Dachs, G.U. Pharmacokinetic and anti-cancer properties of high dose ascorbate in solid tumours of ascorbate-dependent mice. *Free Radic. Biol. Med.* **2016**, *99*, 451–462. [CrossRef] [PubMed]

12. Chen, Q.; Espey, M.G.; Krishna, M.C.; Mitchell, J.B.; Corpe, C.P.; Buettner, G.R.; Shacter, E.; Levine, M. Pharmacologic ascorbic acid concentrations selectively kill cancer cells: Action as a pro-drug to deliver hydrogen peroxide to tissues. *Proc. Natl. Acad. Sci. USA* **2005**, *102*, 13604–13609. [CrossRef] [PubMed]

13. Chen, Q.; Espey, M.G.; Sun, A.Y.; Lee, J.H.; Krishna, M.C.; Shacter, E.; Choyke, P.L.; Pooput, C.; Kirk, K.L.; Buettner, G.R.; et al. Ascorbate in pharmacologic concentrations selectively generates ascorbate radical and hydrogen peroxide in extracellular fluid in vivo. *Proc. Natl. Acad. Sci. USA* **2007**, *104*, 8749–8754. [CrossRef] [PubMed]

14. Olney, K.E.; Du, J.; van't Erve, T.J.; Witmer, J.R.; Sibenaller, Z.A.; Wagner, B.A.; Buettner, G.R.; Cullen, J.J. Inhibitors of hydroperoxide metabolism enhance ascorbate-induced cytotoxicity. *Free Radic. Res.* **2013**, *47*, 154–163. [CrossRef] [PubMed]

15. Fischer, A.P.; Miles, S.L. Ascorbic acid, but not dehydroascorbic acid increases intracellular vitamin C content to decrease Hypoxia Inducible Factor -1 alpha activity and reduce malignant potential in human melanoma. *Biomed. Pharmacother.* **2017**, *86*, 502–513. [CrossRef] [PubMed]

16. Wilkes, J.G.; O'Leary, B.R.; Du, J.; Klinger, A.R.; Sibenaller, Z.A.; Doskey, C.M.; Gibson-Corley, K.N.; Alexander, M.S.; Tsai, S.; Buettner, G.R.; et al. Pharmacologic ascorbate (P-AscH(-)) suppresses hypoxia-inducible Factor-1alpha (HIF-1alpha) in pancreatic adenocarcinoma. *Clin. Exp. Metastasis* **2018**. [CrossRef] [PubMed]

17. Fowler, A.A.; Syed, A.A.; Knowlson, S.; Sculthorpe, R.; Farthing, D.; DeWilde, C.; Farthing, C.A.; Larus, T.L.; Martin, E.; Brophy, D.F.; et al. Phase I safety trial of intravenous ascorbic acid in patients with severe sepsis. *J. Transl. Med.* **2014**, *12*, 32. [CrossRef] [PubMed]

18. Zabet, M.H.; Mohammadi, M.; Ramezani, M.; Khalili, H. Effect of high-dose Ascorbic acid on vasopressor's requirement in septic shock. *J. Res. Pharm. Pract.* **2016**, *5*, 94–100. [PubMed]

19. Tanaka, H.; Matsuda, T.; Miyagantani, Y.; Yukioka, T.; Matsuda, H.; Shimazaki, S. Reduction of resuscitation fluid volumes in severely burned patients using ascorbic acid administration: A randomized, prospective study. *Arch. Surg.* **2000**, *135*, 326–331. [CrossRef] [PubMed]

20. Polireddy, K.; Dong, R.; Reed, G.; Yu, J.; Chen, P.; Williamson, S.; Violet, P.C.; Pessetto, Z.; Godwin, A.K.; Fan, F.; et al. High dose parenteral ascorbate inhibited pancreatic cancer growth and metastasis: Mechanisms and a Phase I/IIa study. *Sci. Rep.* **2017**, *7*, 17188. [CrossRef] [PubMed]

21. Stephenson, C.M.; Levin, R.D.; Spector, T.; Lis, C.G. Phase I clinical trial to evaluate the safety, tolerability, and pharmacokinetics of high-dose intravenous ascorbic acid in patients with advanced cancer. *Cancer Chemother. Pharmacol.* **2013**, *72*, 139–146. [CrossRef] [PubMed]

22. Nauman, G.; Gray, J.C.; Parkinson, R.; Levine, M.; Paller, C.J. Systematic review of intravenous ascorbate in cancer clinical trials. *Antioxidants* **2018**, *7*, 89. [CrossRef] [PubMed]

23. Garcia, M.G.; Carella, A.; Urdinguio, R.G.; Bayon, G.F.; Lopez, V.; Tejedor, J.R.; Sierra, M.I.; Garcia-Torano, E.; Santamarina, P.; Perez, R.F.; et al. Epigenetic dysregulation of TET2 in human glioblastoma. *Oncotarget* **2018**, *9*, 25922–25934. [CrossRef] [PubMed]

24. Orr, B.A.; Haffner, M.C.; Nelson, W.G.; Yegnasubramanian, S.; Eberhart, C.G. Decreased 5-hydroxymethylcytosine is associated with neural progenitor phenotype in normal brain and shorter survival in malignant glioma. *PLoS ONE* **2012**, *7*, e41036. [CrossRef] [PubMed]
25. Carr, A.C.; Vissers, M.C.M.; Cook, J.S. The effect of intravenous vitamin C on cancer- and chemotherapy-related fatigue and quality of life. *Front. Oncol.* **2014**, *4*, 1–7. [CrossRef] [PubMed]

12

Vitamin C and Immune Function

Anitra C. Carr [1,*] **and Silvia Maggini** [2]

[1]   Department of Pathology, University of Otago, Christchurch, P.O. Box 4345, Christchurch 8140, New Zealand
[2]   Bayer Consumer Care Ltd., Peter-Merian-Strasse 84, 4002 Basel, Switzerland; silvia.maggini@bayer.com

Abstract: Vitamin C is an essential micronutrient for humans, with pleiotropic functions related to its ability to donate electrons. It is a potent antioxidant and a cofactor for a family of biosynthetic and gene regulatory enzymes. Vitamin C contributes to immune defense by supporting various cellular functions of both the innate and adaptive immune system. Vitamin C supports epithelial barrier function against pathogens and promotes the oxidant scavenging activity of the skin, thereby potentially protecting against environmental oxidative stress. Vitamin C accumulates in phagocytic cells, such as neutrophils, and can enhance chemotaxis, phagocytosis, generation of reactive oxygen species, and ultimately microbial killing. It is also needed for apoptosis and clearance of the spent neutrophils from sites of infection by macrophages, thereby decreasing necrosis/NETosis and potential tissue damage. The role of vitamin C in lymphocytes is less clear, but it has been shown to enhance differentiation and proliferation of B- and T-cells, likely due to its gene regulating effects. Vitamin C deficiency results in impaired immunity and higher susceptibility to infections. In turn, infections significantly impact on vitamin C levels due to enhanced inflammation and metabolic requirements. Furthermore, supplementation with vitamin C appears to be able to both prevent and treat respiratory and systemic infections. Prophylactic prevention of infection requires dietary vitamin C intakes that provide at least adequate, if not saturating plasma levels (i.e., 100–200 mg/day), which optimize cell and tissue levels. In contrast, treatment of established infections requires significantly higher (gram) doses of the vitamin to compensate for the increased inflammatory response and metabolic demand.

Keywords: ascorbate; ascorbic acid; immunity; immune system; neutrophil function; microbial killing; lymphocytes; infection; vitamin C

---

1. Introduction

The immune system is a multifaceted and sophisticated network of specialized organs, tissues, cells, proteins, and chemicals, which has evolved in order to protect the host from a range of pathogens, such as bacteria, viruses, fungi, and parasites, as well as cancer cells [1]. It can be divided into epithelial barriers, and cellular and humoral constituents of either innate (non-specific) and acquired (specific) immunity [1]. These constituents interact in multiple and highly complex ways. More than half a century of research has shown vitamin C to be a crucial player in various aspects of the immune system, particularly immune cell function [2,3].

Vitamin C is an essential nutrient which cannot be synthesized by humans due to loss of a key enzyme in the biosynthetic pathway [4,5]. Severe vitamin C deficiency results in the potentially fatal disease scurvy [6]. Scurvy is characterized by weakening of collagenous structures, resulting in poor wound healing, and impaired immunity. Individuals with scurvy are highly susceptible to potentially fatal infections such as pneumonia [7]. In turn, infections can significantly impact on vitamin C levels due to enhanced inflammation and metabolic requirements. Early on, it was noted that scurvy often followed infectious epidemics in populations [7], and cases of scurvy have been reported following respiratory infection [8]. This is particularly apparent for individuals who are already malnourished.

Although the amount of vitamin C required to prevent scurvy is relatively low (i.e., ~10 mg/day) [9], the recommended dietary intakes for vitamin C are up to one hundred-fold higher than that for many other vitamins [10]. A diet that supplies 100–200 mg/day of vitamin C provides adequate to saturating plasma concentrations in healthy individuals and should cover general requirements for the reduction of chronic disease risk [11,12]. Due to the low storage capacity of the body for the water-soluble vitamin, a regular and adequate intake is required to prevent hypovitaminosis C. Epidemiological studies have indicated that hypovitaminosis C (plasma vitamin C < 23 μmol/L) is relatively common in Western populations, and vitamin C deficiency (<11 μmol/L) is the fourth leading nutrient deficiency in the United States [13,14]. There are several reasons why vitamin C dietary recommendations are not met, even in countries where food availability and supply would be expected to be sufficient. These include poor dietary habits, life-stages and/or lifestyles either limiting intakes or increasing micronutrient requirements (e.g., smoking and alcohol or drug abuse), various diseases, exposure to pollutants and smoke (both active and passive), and economic reasons (poor socioeconomic status and limited access to nutritious food) [15,16]. Even otherwise 'healthy' individuals in industrialized countries can be at risk due to lifestyle-related factors, such as those on a diet or eating an unbalanced diet, and people facing periods of excessive physical or psychological stress [15,16].

Vitamin C has a number of activities that could conceivably contribute to its immune-modulating effects. It is a highly effective antioxidant, due to its ability to readily donate electrons, thus protecting important biomolecules (proteins, lipids, carbohydrates, and nucleic acids) from damage by oxidants generated during normal cell metabolism and through exposure to toxins and pollutants (e.g., cigarette smoke) [17]. Vitamin C is also a cofactor for a family of biosynthetic and gene regulatory monooxygenase and dioxygenase enzymes [18,19]. The vitamin has long been known as a cofactor for the lysyl and prolyl hydroxylases required for stabilization of the tertiary structure of collagen, and is a cofactor for the two hydroxylases involved in carnitine biosynthesis, a molecule required for transport of fatty acids into mitochondria for generation of metabolic energy (Figure 1) [19].

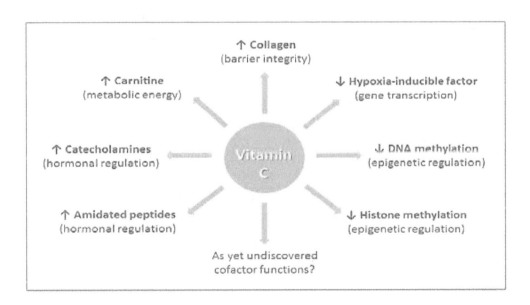

Figure 1. The enzyme cofactor activities of vitamin C. Vitamin C is a cofactor of a family of biosynthetic and gene regulatory monooxygenase and dioxygenase enzymes. These enzymes are involved in the synthesis of collagen, carnitine, catecholamine hormones, e.g., norepinephrine, and amidated peptide hormones, e.g., vasopressin. These enzymes also hydroxylate transcription factors, e.g., hypoxia-inducible factor 1α, and methylated DNA and histones, thus playing a role in gene transcription and epigenetic regulation. ↑ indicates an increase and ↓ indicates a decrease.

Vitamin C is also a cofactor for the hydroxylase enzymes involved in the synthesis of catecholamine hormones, e.g., norepinephrine, and amidated peptide hormones e.g., vasopressin, which are central to the cardiovascular response to severe infection [20]. Furthermore, research over the past 15 years or so has uncovered new roles for vitamin C in the regulation of gene transcription and cell signaling pathways through regulation of transcription factor activity and epigenetic marks (Figure 1) [21,22]. For example, the asparagyl and prolyl hydroylases required for the downregulation of the pleiotropic transcription factor hypoxia-inducible factor-1α (HIF-1α) utilize vitamin C as a cofactor [21]. Recent research has also indicated an important role for vitamin C in regulation of DNA and histone methylation by acting as a cofactor for enzymes which hydoxylate these epigenetic marks [22].

Our review explores the various roles of vitamin C in the immune system, including barrier integrity and leukocyte function, and discusses potential mechanisms of action. We discuss the relevance of the immune-modulating effects of vitamin C in the context of infections and conditions leading to vitamin C insufficiency.

2. Barrier Integrity and Wound Healing

The skin has numerous essential functions, the primary of which is to act as a barrier against external insults, including pathogens. The epidermal layer is highly cellular, comprising primarily keratinocytes, whilst the dermal layer comprises fibroblasts which secrete collagen fibers, the major component of the dermis [23]. Skin contains millimolar concentrations of vitamin C, with higher levels found in the epidermis than the dermis [24–26]. Vitamin C is actively accumulated into the epidermal and dermal cells via the two sodium-dependent vitamin C transporter (SVCT) isoforms 1 and 2 [27], suggesting that the vitamin has crucial functions within the skin. Clues to the role of vitamin C in the skin come from the symptoms of the vitamin C deficiency disease scurvy, which is characterized by bleeding gums, bruising, and impaired wound healing [28,29]. These symptoms are thought to be a result of the role of vitamin C as a co-factor for the prolyl and lysyl hydroxylase enzymes that stabilize the tertiary structure of collagen (Table 1) [30]. Further research has shown that vitamin C can also increase collagen gene expression in fibroblasts [31–35].

Table 1. Role of vitamin C in immune defense.

Immune System	Function of Vitamin C	Refs.
Epithelial barriers	Enhances collagen synthesis and stabilization	[30–35]
	Protects against ROS-induced damage [1]	[36–40]
	Enhances keratinocyte differentiation and lipid synthesis	[41–45]
	Enhances fibroblast proliferation and migration	[46,47]
	Shortens time to wound healing in patients	[48,49]
Phagocytes (neutrophils, macrophages)	Acts as an antioxidant/electron donor	[50–53]
	Enhances motility/chemotaxis	[54–63]
	Enhances phagocytosis and ROS generation	[64–71]
	Enhances microbial killing	[54,55,57,58,70,72]
	Facilitates apoptosis and clearance	[71,73,74]
	Decreases necrosis/NETosis	[73,75]
B- and T-lymphocytes	Enhances differentiation and proliferation	[62,63,76–82]
	Enhances antibody levels	[78,83–85]
Inflammatory mediators	Modulates cytokine production	[75,77,86–94]
	Decreases histamine levels	[56,61,95–101]

[1] ROS, reactive oxygen species; NET, neutrophil extracellular trap. Note that many of these studies comprised marginal or deficient vitamin C status at baseline. Supplementation in situations of adequate vitamin C status may not have comparable effects.

Vitamin C intervention studies in humans (using both dietary and gram doses of vitamin C) have shown enhanced vitamin C uptake into skin cells [26,36] and enhanced oxidant scavenging activity of the skin [36,37]. The elevated antioxidant status of the skin following vitamin C supplementation could potentially protect against oxidative stress induced by environmental pollutants [38,39]. The antioxidant effects of vitamin C are likely to be enhanced in combination with vitamin E [40,102].

Cell culture and preclinical studies have indicated that vitamin C can enhance epithelial barrier functions via a number of different mechanisms. Vitamin C supplementation of keratinocytes in culture enhances differentiation and barrier function via modulating signaling and biosynthetic pathways, with resultant elevations in barrier lipid synthesis [41–45]. Dysfunctional epithelial barrier function in the lungs of animals with serious infection can be restored by administration of vitamin C [74]. This was attributed to enhanced expression of tight junction proteins and prevention of cytoskeletal rearrangements.

Animal studies using the vitamin C-dependent Gulo knockout mouse indicated that deficiency did not affect the formation of collagen in the skin of unchallenged mice [103]; however, following full thickness excisional wounding there was significantly decreased collagen formation in vitamin C-deficient mice [46]. This finding is in agreement with an earlier study carried out with scorbutic guinea pigs [104]. Thus, vitamin C appears to be particularly essential during wound healing, also decreasing the expression of pro-inflammatory mediators and enhancing the expression of various wound healing mediators [46]. Fibroblast cell culture experiments have also indicated that vitamin C can alter gene expression profiles within dermal fibroblasts, promoting fibroblast proliferation and migration which is essential for tissue remodeling and wound healing [46,47]. Following surgery, patients require relatively high intakes of vitamin C in order to normalize their plasma vitamin C status (e.g., $\geq$500 mg/day) [105], and administration of antioxidant micronutrients, including vitamin C, to patients with disorders in wound healing can shorten the time to wound closure [48,49,106,107].

Leukocytes, particularly neutrophils and monocyte-derived macrophages, are major players in wound healing [108]. During the initial inflammatory stage, neutrophils migrate to the wound site in order to sterilize it via the release of reactive oxygen species (ROS) and antimicrobial proteins [109]. The neutrophils eventually undergo apoptosis and are cleared by macrophages, resulting in resolution of the inflammatory response. However, in chronic, non-healing wounds, such as those observed in diabetics, the neutrophils persist and instead undergo necrotic cell death which can perpetuate the inflammatory response and hinder wound healing [109,110]. Vitamin C is thought to influence several important aspects of neutrophil function: migration in response to inflammatory mediators (chemotaxis), phagocytosis and killing of microbes, and apoptosis and clearance by macrophages (see below).

3. Vitamin C and Leukocyte Function

Leukocytes, such as neutrophils and monocytes, actively accumulate vitamin C against a concentration gradient, resulting in values that are 50- to 100-fold higher than plasma concentrations [111–113]. These cells accumulate maximal vitamin C concentrations at dietary intakes of ~100 mg/day [114,115], although other body tissues likely require higher intakes for saturation [116,117]. Neutrophils accumulate vitamin C via SVCT2 and typically contain intracellular levels of at least 1 mM [111,118]. Following stimulation of their oxidative burst neutrophils can further increase their intracellular concentration of vitamin C through the non-specific uptake of the oxidized form, dehydroascorbate (DHA), via glucose transporters (GLUT) [118,119]. DHA is then rapidly reduced to ascorbate intracellularly, to give levels of about 10 mM [119]. It is believed that the accumulation of such high vitamin C concentrations indicates important functions within these cells.

Accumulation of millimolar concentrations of vitamin C into neutrophils, particularly following activation of their oxidative burst, is thought to protect these cells from oxidative damage [119]. Vitamin C is a potent water-soluble antioxidant that can scavenge numerous reactive oxidants and can also regenerate the important cellular and membrane antioxidants glutathione and vitamin E [120]. Upon phagocytosis or activation with soluble stimulants, vitamin C is depleted from neutrophils in an oxidant-dependent manner [50–53]. An alteration in the balance between oxidant generation and antioxidant defenses can lead to alterations in multiple signaling pathways, with the pro-inflammatory transcription factor nuclear factor κB (NFκB) playing a central role [121]. Oxidants can activate NFκB, which triggers a signaling cascade leading to continued synthesis of oxidative species and other inflammatory mediators [122,123]. Vitamin C has been shown to attenuate both oxidant generation and NFκB activation in dendritic cells in vitro, and NFκB activation in neutrophils isolated from septic Gulo knockout mice [75,124]. Thiol-containing proteins can be particularly sensitive to redox alterations within cells and are often central to the regulation of redox-related cell signaling pathways [125]. Vitamin C-dependent modulation of thiol-dependent cell signaling and gene expression pathways has been reported in T-cells [126,127].

Thus, vitamin C could modulate immune function through modulation of redox-sensitive cell signaling pathways or by directly protecting important cell structural components. For example, exposure of neutrophils to oxidants can inhibit motility of the cells, which is thought to be due to oxidation of membrane lipids and resultant effects on cell membrane fluidity [63]. Neutrophils contain high levels of polyunsaturated fatty acids in their plasma membranes, and thus improvements in neutrophil motility observed following vitamin C administration (see below) could conceivably be attributed to oxidant scavenging as well as regeneration of vitamin E [120].

3.1. Neutrophil Chemotaxis

Neutrophil infiltration into infected tissues is an early step in innate immunity. In response to pathogen- or host-derived inflammatory signals (e.g., N-formylmethionyl-leucyl-phenylalanine (fMLP), interleukin (IL)-8, leukotriene B4, and complement component C5a), marginated neutrophils literally swarm to the site of infection [128]. Migration of neutrophils in response to chemical stimuli is termed chemotaxis, while random migration is termed chemokinesis (Figure 2). Neutrophils express more than 30 different chemokine and chemoattractant receptors in order to sense and rapidly respond to tissue damage signals [128]. Early studies carried out in scorbutic guinea pigs indicated impaired leukocyte chemotactic response compared with leukocytes isolated from guinea pigs supplemented with adequate vitamin C in their diet (Table 1) [54–56,64]. These findings suggest that vitamin C deficiency may impact on the ability of phagocytes to migrate to sites of infection.

Patients with severe infection exhibit compromised neutrophil chemotactic ability [129–132]. This neutrophil 'paralysis' is believed to be partly due to enhanced levels of anti-inflammatory and immune-suppressive mediators (e.g., IL-4 and IL-10) during the compensatory anti-inflammatory response observed following initial hyper-stimulation of the immune system [133]. However, it is also possible that vitamin C depletion, which is prevalent during severe infection [20], may contribute. Studies in the 1980s and 1990s indicated that patients with recurrent infections had impaired leukocyte chemotaxis, which could be restored in response to supplementation with gram doses of vitamin C [57–60,65–67]. Furthermore, supplementation of neonates with suspected sepsis with 400 mg/day vitamin C dramatically improved neutrophil chemotaxis [134].

Recurrent infections can also result from genetic disorders of neutrophil function, such as chronic granulomatous disease (CGD), an immunodeficiency disease resulting in defective leukocyte generation of ROS [135], and Chediak-Higashi syndrome (CHS), a rare autosomal recessive disorder affecting vesicle trafficking [136]. Although vitamin C administration would not be expected to affect the underlying defects of these genetic disorders, it may support the function of redundant antimicrobial mechanisms in these cells. For example, patients with CGD showed improved leukocyte chemotaxis following supplementation with gram doses of vitamin C administered either enterally or parenterally [137–139]. This was associated with decreased infections and clinical improvement [137,138]. A mouse model of CHS showed improved neutrophil chemotaxis following vitamin C supplementation [140], and neutrophils isolated from two children with CHS showed improved chemotaxis following supplementation with 200–500 mg/day vitamin C [141,142], although this effect has not been observed in all cases [140,143]. The vitamin C-dependent enhancement of chemotaxis was thought to be mediated in part via effects on microtubule assembly [144,145], and more recent research has indicated that intracellular vitamin C can stabilize microtubules [146].

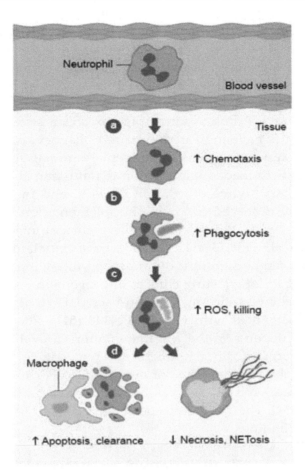

Figure 2. Role of vitamin C in phagocyte function. Vitamin C has been shown to: (**a**) enhance neutrophil migration in response to chemoattractants (chemotaxis), (**b**) enhance engulfment (phagocytosis) of microbes, and (**c**) stimulate reactive oxygen species (ROS) generation and killing of microbes. (**d**) Vitamin C supports caspase-dependent apoptosis, enhancing uptake and clearance by macrophages, and inhibits necrosis, including NETosis, thus supporting resolution of the inflammatory response and attenuating tissue damage.

Supplementation of healthy volunteers with dietary or gram doses of vitamin C has also been shown to enhance neutrophil chemotactic ability [61–63,147]. Johnston et al., proposed that the antihistamine effect of vitamin C correlated with enhanced chemotaxis [61]. In participants who had inadequate vitamin C status (i.e., <50 μM), supplementation with a dietary source of vitamin C (providing ~250 mg/day) resulted in a 20% increase in neutrophil chemotaxis [147]. Furthermore, supplementation of elderly women with 1 g/day vitamin C, in combination with vitamin E, enhanced neutrophil functions, including chemotaxis [148]. Thus, members of the general population may benefit from improved immune cell function through enhanced vitamin C intake, particularly if they have inadequate vitamin C status, which can be more prevalent in the elderly. However, it should be noted that it is not yet certain to what extent improved ex vivo leukocyte chemotaxis translates into improved in vivo immune function.

3.2. Phagocytosis and Microbial Killing

Once neutrophils have migrated to the site of infection, they proceed to engulf the invading pathogens (Figure 2). Various intracellular granules are mobilized and fuse with the phagosome, emptying their arsenal of antimicrobial peptides and proteins into the phagosome [149]. Components of the nicotinamide adenine dinucleotide phosphate (NADPH) oxidase assemble in the phagosomal membrane and generate superoxide, the first in a long line of ROS generated by neutrophils to kill pathogens. The enzyme superoxide dismutase converts superoxide to hydrogen peroxide, which can then be utilized to form the oxidant hypochlorous acid via the azurophilic granule enzyme myeloperoxidase [149]. Hypochlorous acid can further react with amines to form secondary oxidants known as chloramines. These various neutrophil-derived oxidants have different reactivities and specificities for biological targets, with protein thiol groups being particularly susceptible.

Neutrophils isolated from scorbutic guinea pigs exhibit a severely impaired ability to kill microbes [54,55,70], and studies have indicated impaired phagocytosis and/or ROS generation in neutrophils from scorbutic compared with ascorbate replete animals [68–70]. Generation of ROS by neutrophils from volunteers with inadequate vitamin C status can be enhanced by 20% following supplementation with a dietary source of vitamin C [147], and increases in both phagocytosis and oxidant generation were observed following supplementation of elderly participants with a combination of vitamins C and E [148]. Patients with recurrent infections [57,58,66,67,72], or the genetic conditions CGD or CHS [138,139,141,143,150], have impaired neutrophil bacterial killing and/or phagocytosis, which can be significantly improved following supplementation with gram doses of vitamin C, resulting in long lasting clinical improvement. A couple of studies, however, showed no improvement of ex vivo anti-fungal or anti-bacterial activity in neutrophils isolated from CGD or CHS patients supplemented with vitamin C [140,151]. The reason for these differences is not clear, although it may depend on the baseline vitamin C level of the patients, which is not assessed in most cases. Furthermore, different microbes have variable susceptibility to the oxidative and non-oxidative anti-microbial mechanisms of neutrophils. For example, *Staphylococcus aureus* is susceptible to oxidative mechanisms, whereas other microorganisms are more susceptible to non-oxidative mechanisms [152]. Therefore, the type of microbe used to assess the ex vivo neutrophil functions could influence the findings.

Patients with severe infection (sepsis) exhibit a decreased ability to phagocytose microbes and a diminished ability to generate ROS [153]. Decreased neutrophil phagocytosis was associated with enhanced patient mortality [154]. Interestingly, Stephan et al. [155] observed impaired neutrophil killing activity in critically ill patients prior to acquiring nosocomial infections, suggesting that critical illness itself, without prior infection, can also impair neutrophil function. This resulted in subsequent susceptibility to hospital-acquired infections. Impaired phagocytic and oxidant-generating capacity of leukocytes in patients with severe infection has been attributed to the compensatory anti-inflammatory response, resulting in enhanced levels of immunosuppressive mediators such as IL-10 [133], as well as to the hypoxic conditions of inflammatory sites, which diminishes substrate for ROS generation [156]. Another explanation is the larger numbers of immature neutrophils released from the bone marrow due to increased demands during severe infection. These immature 'band' cells have decreased functionality compared with differentiated neutrophils [157]. Thus, conflicting findings in severe infection could be due to variability in the total numbers of underactive immature neutrophils compared with activated fully-differentiated neutrophils [158,159]. Despite displaying an activated basal state, the mature neutrophils from patients with severe infection do not generate ROS to the same extent as healthy neutrophils following ex vivo stimulation [160]. The effect of vitamin C supplementation on phagocytosis, oxidant generation, and microbial killing by leukocytes from septic patients has not yet been explored.

3.3. Neutrophil Apoptosis and Clearance

Following microbial phagocytosis and killing, neutrophils undergo a process of programmed cell death called apoptosis [161]. This process facilitates subsequent phagocytosis and clearance of the spent neutrophils from sites of inflammation by macrophages, thus supporting resolution of inflammation and preventing excessive tissue damage (Figure 2). Caspases are key effector enzymes in the apoptotic process, culminating in phosphatidyl serine exposure, thus marking the cells for uptake and clearance by macrophages [162]. Interestingly, caspases are thiol-dependent enzymes, making them very sensitive to inactivation by ROS generated by activated neutrophils [163,164]. Thus, vitamin C may be expected to protect the oxidant-sensitive caspase-dependent apoptotic process following activation of neutrophils. In support of this premise, in vitro studies have shown that loading human neutrophils with vitamin C can enhance *Escherichia coli*-mediated apoptosis of the neutrophils (Table 1) [71]. Peritoneal neutrophils isolated from vitamin C-deficient Gulo mice exhibited attenuated apoptosis [75], and instead underwent necrotic cell death [73]. These vitamin C-deficient neutrophils were not phagocytosed by macrophages in vitro, and persisted at inflammatory loci in vivo [73]. Furthermore, administration of vitamin C to septic animals decreased the numbers of neutrophils in the lungs of these animals [74].

Numerous studies have reported attenuated neutrophil apoptosis in patients with severe infection compared with control participants [165–172]. The delayed apoptosis appears to be related to disease severity and is thought to be associated with enhanced tissue damage observed in patients with sepsis [173,174]. Immature 'band' neutrophils released during severe infection were also found to be resistant to apoptosis and had longer life spans [157]. Plasma from septic patients has been found to suppress apoptosis in healthy neutrophils, suggesting that pro-inflammatory cytokines were responsible for the increased in vivo survival of neutrophils during inflammatory conditions [165,174–176]. Interestingly, high-dose vitamin C administration has been shown to modulate cytokine levels in patients with cancer [177] and, although this has not yet been assessed in patients with severe infection, could conceivably be another mechanism by which vitamin C may modulate neutrophil function in these patients. To date, only one study has investigated the effect of vitamin C supplementation on neutrophil apoptosis in septic patients [178]. Intravenous supplementation of septic abdominal surgery patients with 450 mg/day vitamin C was found to decrease caspase-3 protein levels and, thus was presumed to have an anti-apoptotic effect on peripheral blood neutrophils. However, caspase activity and apoptosis of the neutrophils following activation was not assessed. Furthermore, circulating neutrophils may not reflect the activation status of neutrophils at inflammatory tissue loci. Clearly, more studies need to be undertaken to tease out the role of vitamin C in neutrophil apoptosis and clearance from inflammatory loci.

3.4. Neutrophil Necrosis and NETosis

Neutrophils that fail to undergo apoptosis instead undergo necrotic cell death (Figure 2). The subsequent release of toxic intracellular components, such as proteases, can cause extensive tissue damage [179,180]. One recently discovered form of neutrophil death has been termed NETosis. This results from the release of 'neutrophil extracellular traps' (NETs) comprising neutrophil DNA, histones, and enzymes [181]. Although NETs have been proposed to comprise a unique method of microbial killing [182,183], they have also been implicated in tissue damage and organ failure [184,185]. NET-associated histones can act as damage-associated molecular pattern proteins, activating the immune system and causing further damage [186]. Patients with sepsis, or who go on to develop sepsis, have significantly elevated levels of circulating cell-free DNA, which is thought to indicate NET formation [184,187].

Pre-clinical studies in vitamin C-deficient Gulo knockout mice indicated enhanced NETosis in the lungs of septic animals and increased circulating cell-free DNA [75]. The levels of these markers were attenuated in vitamin C sufficient animals or in deficient animals that were administered vitamin C (Table 1). The same investigators showed that in vitro supplementation of human neutrophils with vitamin C attenuated phorbol ester-induced NETosis [75]. Administration of gram doses of vitamin C to septic patients over four days, however, did not appear to decrease circulating cell-free DNA levels [188], although the duration of treatment may have been too short to see a sustained effect. It should be noted that cell-free DNA is not specific for neutrophil-derived DNA, as it may also derive from necrotic tissue; however, the association of neutrophil-specific proteins or enzymes, such as myeloperoxidase, with the DNA can potentially provide an indication of its source [184].

The transcription factor HIF-1α facilitates neutrophil survival at hypoxic loci through delaying apoptosis [189]. Interestingly, vitamin C is a cofactor for the iron-containing dioxygenase enzymes that regulate the levels and activity of HIF-1α [190]. These hydroxylase enzymes downregulate HIF-1α activity by facilitating degradation of constitutively expressed HIF-1α and decreasing binding of transcription coactivators. In vitamin C-deficient Gulo knockout mice, up-regulation of HIF-1α was observed under normoxic conditions, along with attenuated neutrophil apoptosis and clearance by macrophages [73]. HIF-1α has also been proposed as a regulator of NET generation by neutrophils [191], hence providing a potential mechanism by which vitamin C could downregulate NET generation by these cells [75].

3.5. Lymphocyte Function

Like phagocytes, B- and T-lymphocytes accumulate vitamin C to high levels via SVCT [192,193]. The role of vitamin C within these cells is less clear, although antioxidant protection has been suggested [194]. In vitro studies have indicated that incubation of vitamin C with lymphocytes promotes proliferation [76,77], resulting in enhanced antibody generation [78], and also provides resistance to various cell death stimuli [195]. Furthermore, vitamin C appears to have an important role in developmental differentiation and maturation of immature T-cells (Table 1) [76,79]. Similar proliferative and differentiation/maturation effects have been observed with mature and immature natural killer cells, respectively [196].

Early studies in guinea pigs showed enhanced mitotic activity of isolated peripheral blood lymphocytes following intraperitoneal vitamin C treatment, and enhanced humoral antibody levels during immunization [82–85]. Although one human intervention study has reported positive associations between antibody levels (immunoglobulin (Ig)M, (Ig)G, (Ig)A) and vitamin C supplementation [85], another has not [62]. Instead, Anderson and coworkers showed that oral and intravenous supplementation of low gram doses of vitamin C to children with asthma and healthy volunteers enhanced lymphocyte transformation, an ex vivo measure of mitogen-induced proliferation and enlargement of T-lymphocytes (Table 1) [62,63,81]. Administration of vitamin C to elderly people was also shown to enhance ex vivo lymphocyte proliferation [80], a finding confirmed using combinations of vitamin C with vitamins A and/or E [148,197]. Exposure to toxic chemicals can affect lymphocyte function, and both natural killer cell activity and lymphocyte blastogenic responses to T- and B-cell mitogens were restored to normal levels following vitamin C supplementation [198]. Although the human studies mentioned above are encouraging, it is apparent that more human intervention studies are needed to confirm these findings.

Recent research in wild-type and Gulo knockout mice indicated that parenteral administration of 200 mg/kg vitamin C modulated the immunosuppression of regulatory T-cells (Tregs) observed in sepsis [89]. Vitamin C administration enhanced Treg proliferation and inhibited the negative immunoregulation of Tregs by inhibiting the expression of specific transcription factors, antigens, and cytokines [89]. The mechanisms involved likely rely on the gene regulatory effects of vitamin C [79,89,199,200]. For example, recent research has implicated vitamin C in epigenetic regulation through its action as a cofactor for the iron-containing dioxygenases which hydroxylate methylated DNA and histones [22,201]. The ten-eleven translocation (TET) enzymes hydroxylate methylcytosine residues, which may act as epigenetic marks in their own right, and also facilitate removal of the methylated residues, an important process in epigenetic regulation [202]. Preliminary evidence indicates that vitamin C can regulate T-cell maturation via epigenetic mechanisms involving the TETs and histone demethylation [79,199,200]. It is likely that the cell signaling and gene regulatory functions of vitamin C, via regulation of transcription factors and epigenetic marks, play major roles in its immune-regulating functions.

3.6. Inflammatory Mediators

Cytokines are important cell signaling molecules secreted by a variety of immune cells, both innate and adaptive, in response to infection and inflammation [1]. They comprise a broad range of molecules, including chemokines, interferons (IFNs), ILs, lymphokines, and TNFs, which modulate both humoral and cell-based immune responses, and regulate the maturation, growth, and responsiveness of specific cell populations. Cytokines can elicit pro-inflammatory or anti-inflammatory responses, and vitamin C appears to modulate systemic and leukocyte-derived cytokines in a complex manner.

Incubation of vitamin C with peripheral blood lymphocytes decreased lipopolysaccharide (LPS)-induced generation of the pro-inflammatory cytokines TNF-α and IFN-γ, and increased anti-inflammatory IL-10 production, while having no effect on IL-1β levels [77]. Furthermore, in vitro addition of vitamin C to peripheral blood monocytes isolated from pneumonia patients decreased the generation of the pro-inflammatory cytokines TNF-α and IL-6 [86]. However, another study found that in vitro treatment of peripheral blood monocytes with vitamin C and/or vitamin E enhanced LPS-stimulated TNF-α generation, but did not affect IL-1β generation [87]. Furthermore, incubation of vitamin C with virus-infected human and murine fibroblasts enhanced generation of antiviral IFN [91–93]. Supplementation of healthy human volunteers with 1 g/day vitamin C (with and without vitamin E) was shown to enhance peripheral blood mononuclear cell-derived IL-10, IL-1, and TNF-α following stimulation with LPS [87,94]. Thus, the effect of vitamin C on cytokine generation appears to depend on the cell type and/or the inflammatory stimulant. Recent research has indicated that vitamin C treatment of microglia, resident myeloid-derived macrophages in the central nervous system, attenuates activation of the cells and synthesis of the pro-inflammatory cytokines TNF, IL-6, and IL-1β [90]. This is indicative of an anti-inflammatory phenotype.

Preclinical studies using Gluo knockout mice have highlighted the cytokine-modulating effects of vitamin C. Vitamin C-deficient Gulo knockout mice infected with influenza virus showed enhanced synthesis of the pro-inflammatory cytokines TNF-α and IL-1α/β in their lungs, and decreased production of the anti-viral cytokine IFN-α/β [88]. Administration of vitamin C to Gulo mice with polymicrobial peritonitis resulted in decreased synthesis of the pro-inflammatory cytokines TNF-α and IL-1β by isolated neutrophils [75]. Another study in septic Gulo mice administered 200 mg/kg parenteral vitamin C has shown decreased secretion of the inhibitory cytokines TGF-β and IL-10 by Tregs [89]. In this study, attenuated IL-4 secretion and augmented IFN-γ secretion was also observed, suggesting immune-modulating effects of vitamin C in sepsis. Overall, vitamin C appears to normalize cytokine generation, likely through its gene-regulating effects.

Histamine is an immune mediator produced by basophils, eosinophils, and mast cells during the immune response to pathogens and stress. Histamine stimulates vasodilation and increased capillary permeability, resulting in the classic allergic symptoms of runny nose and eyes. Studies using guinea pigs, a vitamin C-requiring animal model, have indicated that vitamin C depletion is associated with enhanced circulating histamine levels, and that supplementation of the animals with vitamin C resulted in decreased histamine levels [56,95–98]. Enhanced histamine generation was found to increase the utilization of vitamin C in these animals [96]. Consistent with the animal studies, human intervention studies with oral vitamin C (125 mg/day to 2 g/day) and intravenous vitamin C (7.5 g infusion) have reported decreased histamine levels [61,99–101], which was more apparent in patients with allergic compared with infectious diseases [101]. Although vitamin C has been proposed to 'detoxify' histamine [96,97], the precise mechanisms responsible for the in vivo decrease in histamine levels following vitamin C administration are currently unknown. Furthermore, effects of vitamin C supplementation on histamine levels are not observed in all studies [203].

4. Vitamin C Insufficiency Conditions

Numerous environmental and health conditions can have an impact on vitamin C status. In this section we discuss examples which also have a link with impaired immunity and increased susceptibility to infection. For example, exposure to air pollution containing oxidants, such as ozone and nitrogen dioxide, can upset the oxidant-antioxidant balance within the body and cause oxidative stress [204]. Oxidative stress can also occur if antioxidant defenses are impaired, which may be the case when vitamin C levels are insufficient [205]. Air pollution can damage respiratory tract lining fluid and increase the risk of respiratory disease, particularly in children and the elderly [204,206] who are at risk of both impaired immunity and vitamin C insufficiency [14,204]. Vitamin C is a free-radical scavenger that can scavenge superoxide and peroxyl radicals, hydrogen peroxide, hypochlorous acid, and oxidant air pollutants [207,208]. The antioxidant properties of vitamin C enable it to protect lung cells exposed to oxidants and oxidant-mediated damage caused by various pollutants, heavy metals, pesticides, and xenobiotics [204,209].

Tobacco smoke is an underestimated pollutant in many parts of the world. Both smokers and passive smokers have lower plasma and leukocyte vitamin C levels than non-smokers [10,210,211], partly due to increased oxidative stress and to both a lower intake and a higher metabolic turnover of vitamin C compared to non-smokers [10,211–213]. Mean serum concentrations of vitamin C in adults who smoke have been found to be one-third lower than those of non-smokers, and it has been recommended that smokers should consume an additional 35 mg/day of vitamin C to ensure there is sufficient ascorbic acid to repair oxidant damage [10,14]. Vitamin C levels are also lower in children and adolescents exposed to environmental tobacco smoke [214]. Research in vitamin C-deficient guinea pigs exposed to tobacco smoke has indicated that vitamin C can protect against protein damage and lipid peroxidation [213,215]. In passive smokers exposed to environmental tobacco smoke, vitamin C supplementation significantly reduced plasma F_2-isoprostane concentrations, a measure of oxidative stress [216]. Tobacco use increases susceptibility to bacterial and viral infections [217,218], in which vitamin C may play a role. For example, in a population-based study the risk of developing obstructive airways disease was significantly higher in those with the lowest plasma vitamin C concentrations (26 µmol/L) compared to never smokers, a risk that decreased with increasing vitamin C concentration [219].

Individuals with diabetes are at greater risk of common infections, including influenza, pneumonia, and foot infections, which are associated with increased morbidity and mortality [220,221]. Several immune-related changes are observed in obesity that contribute towards the development of type 2 diabetes. A major factor is persistent low-grade inflammation of adipose tissue in obese subjects, which plays a role in the progression to insulin resistance and type 2 diabetes, and which is not present in the adipose tissue of lean subjects [222,223]. The adipose tissue is infiltrated by pro-inflammatory macrophages and T-cells, leading to the accumulation of pro-inflammatory cytokines such as interleukins and TNF-α [224,225]. A decrease in plasma vitamin C levels has been observed in studies of type 2 diabetes [18,226], and a major cause of increased need for vitamin C in type 2 diabetes is thought to be the high level of oxidative stress caused by hyperglycemia [10,227,228]. Inverse correlations have been reported between plasma vitamin C concentrations and the risk of diabetes, hemoglobin A1c concentrations (an index of glucose tolerance), fasting and postprandial blood glucose, and oxidative stress [219,229–232]. Meta-analysis of interventional studies has indicted that supplementation with vitamin C can improve glycemic control in type 2 diabetes [233].

Elderly people are particularly susceptible to infections due to immunosenescence and decreased immune cell function [234]. For example, common viral infections such as respiratory illnesses, that are usually self-limiting in healthy young people, can lead to the development of complications such as pneumonia, resulting in increased morbidity and mortality in elderly people. A lower mean vitamin C status has been observed in free-living or institutionalized elderly people, indicated by lowered plasma and leukocyte concentrations [10,235,236], which is of concern because low vitamin C concentrations (<17 µmol/L) in older people (aged 75–82 years) are strongly predictive of all-cause mortality [237]. Acute and chronic diseases that are prevalent in this age group may also play an important part in the reduction of vitamin C reserves [238–240]. Institutionalization in particular is an aggravating factor in this age group, resulting in even lower plasma vitamin C levels than in non-institutionalized elderly people. It is noteworthy that elderly hospitalized patients with acute respiratory infections have been shown to fare significantly better with vitamin C supplementation than those not receiving the vitamin [241]. Decreased immunological surveillance in individuals older than 60 years also results in greater risk of cancer, and patients with cancer, particularly those undergoing cancer treatments, have compromised immune systems, decreased vitamin C status, and enhanced risk of developing sepsis [242,243]. Hospitalized patients, in general, have lower vitamin C status than the general population [244].

5. Vitamin C and Infection

A major symptom of the vitamin C deficiency disease scurvy is the marked susceptibility to infections, particularly of the respiratory tract, with pneumonia being one of the most frequent complications of scurvy and a major cause of death [7]. Patients with acute respiratory infections, such as pulmonary tuberculosis and pneumonia, have decreased plasma vitamin C concentrations relative to control subjects [245]. Administration of vitamin C to patients with acute respiratory infections returns their plasma vitamin C levels to normal and ameliorates the severity of the respiratory symptoms [246]. Cases of acute lung infections have shown rapid clearance of chest X-rays following administration of intravenous vitamin C [247,248]. This vitamin C-dependent clearance of neutrophils from infected lungs could conceivably be due to enhanced apoptosis and subsequent phagocytosis and clearance of the spent neutrophils by macrophages [73]. Pre-clinical studies of animals with sepsis-induced lung injury have indicated that vitamin C administration can increase alveolar fluid clearance, enhance bronchoalveolar epithelial barrier function, and attenuate sequestration of neutrophils [74], all essential factors for normal lung function.

Meta-analysis has indicated that vitamin C supplementation with doses of 200 mg or more daily is effective in ameliorating the severity and duration of the common cold, and the incidence of the common cold if also exposed to physical stress [249]. Supplementation of individuals who had an inadequate vitamin C status (i.e., <45 µmol/L) also decreased the incidence of the common cold [203]. Surprisingly, few studies have assessed vitamin C status during the common cold [250]. Significant decreases in both leukocyte vitamin C levels, and urinary excretion of the vitamin, have been reported to occur during common cold episodes, with levels returning to normal following the infection [251–254]. These changes indicate that vitamin C is utilized during the common cold infection. Administration of gram doses of vitamin C during the common cold episode ameliorated the decline in leukocyte vitamin C levels, suggesting that administration of vitamin C may be beneficial for the recovery process [251].

Beneficial effects of vitamin C on recovery have been noted in pneumonia. In elderly people hospitalized because of pneumonia, who were determined to have very low vitamin C levels, administration of vitamin C reduced the respiratory symptom score in the more severe patients [246]. In other pneumonia patients, low-dose vitamin C (0.25–0.8 g/day) reduced the hospital stay by 19% compared with no vitamin C supplementation, whereas the higher-dose group (0.5–1.6 g/day) reduced the duration by 36% [255]. There was also a positive effect on the normalization of chest X-ray, temperature, and erythrocyte sedimentation rate [255]. Since prophylactic vitamin C administration also appears to decrease the risk of developing more serious respiratory infections, such as pneumonia [256], it is likely that the low vitamin C levels observed during respiratory infections are both a cause and a consequence of the disease.

6. Conclusions

Overall, vitamin C appears to exert a multitude of beneficial effects on cellular functions of both the innate and adaptive immune system. Although vitamin C is a potent antioxidant protecting the body against endogenous and exogenous oxidative challenges, it is likely that its action as a cofactor for numerous biosynthetic and gene regulatory enzymes plays a key role in its immune-modulating effects. Vitamin C stimulates neutrophil migration to the site of infection, enhances phagocytosis and oxidant generation, and microbial killing. At the same time, it protects host tissue from excessive damage by enhancing neutrophil apoptosis and clearance by macrophages, and decreasing neutrophil necrosis and NETosis. Thus, it is apparent that vitamin C is necessary for the immune system to mount and sustain an adequate response against pathogens, whilst avoiding excessive damage to the host.

Vitamin C appears to be able to both prevent and treat respiratory and systemic infections by enhancing various immune cell functions. Prophylactic prevention of infection requires dietary vitamin C intakes that provide at least adequate, if not saturating plasma levels (i.e., 100–200 mg/day), which optimize cell and tissue levels. In contrast, treatment of established infections requires significantly higher (gram) doses of the vitamin to compensate for the increased metabolic demand.

Epidemiological studies indicate that hypovitaminosis C is still relatively common in Western populations, and vitamin C deficiency is the fourth leading nutrient deficiency in the United States. Reasons include reduced intake combined with limited body stores. Increased needs occur due to pollution and smoking, fighting infections, and diseases with oxidative and inflammatory components, e.g., type 2 diabetes, etc. Ensuring adequate intake of vitamin C through the diet or via supplementation, especially in groups such as the elderly or in individuals exposed to risk factors for vitamin C insufficiency, is required for proper immune function and resistance to infections.

Acknowledgments: Thanks are given to Mark Hampton for critically reviewing the manuscript and Deborah Nock (Medical WriteAway, Norwich, UK) for medical writing support and editorial assistance on behalf of Bayer Consumer Care Ltd. A.C.C. is the recipient of a Health Research Council of New Zealand Sir Charles Hercus Health Research Fellowship.

Author Contributions: A.C.C. and S.M. conceived and wrote the review, and A.C.C. had primary responsibility for the final content.

References

1. Parkin, J.; Cohen, B. An overview of the immune system. *Lancet* **2001**, *357*, 1777–1789. [CrossRef]
2. Maggini, S.; Wintergerst, E.S.; Beveridge, S.; Hornig, D.H. Selected vitamins and trace elements support immune function by strengthening epithelial barriers and cellular and humoral immune responses. *Br. J. Nutr.* **2007**, *98*, S29–S35. [CrossRef] [PubMed]
3. Webb, A.L.; Villamor, E. Update: Effects of antioxidant and non-antioxidant vitamin supplementation on immune function. *Nutr. Rev.* **2007**, *65*, 181. [CrossRef] [PubMed]
4. Burns, J.J. Missing step in man, monkey and guinea pig required for the biosynthesis of L-ascorbic acid. *Nature* **1957**, *180*, 553. [CrossRef] [PubMed]
5. Nishikimi, M.; Fukuyama, R.; Minoshima, S.; Shimizu, N.; Yagi, K. Cloning and chromosomal mapping of the human nonfunctional gene for L-gulono-gamma-lactone oxidase, the enzyme for L-ascorbic acid biosynthesis missing in man. *J. Biol. Chem.* **1994**, *269*, 13685–13688. [PubMed]
6. Sauberlich, H.E. A history of scurvy and vitamin C. In *Vitamin C in Health and Disease*; Packer, L., Fuchs, J., Eds.; Marcel Dekker: New York, NY, USA, 1997; pp. 1–24.
7. Hemila, H. Vitamin C and Infections. *Nutrients* **2017**, *9*, 339. [CrossRef] [PubMed]
8. Carr, A.C.; McCall, C. The role of vitamin C in the treatment of pain: New insights. *J. Transl. Med.* **2017**, *15*, 77. [CrossRef] [PubMed]
9. Krebs, H.A. The Sheffield Experiment on the vitamin C requirement of human adults. *Proc. Nutr. Soc.* **1953**, *12*, 237–246. [CrossRef]
10. Institute of Medicine Panel on Dietary Antioxidants and Related Compounds. *Dietary Reference Intakes for Vitamin C, Vitamin E, Selenium, and Carotenoids*; National Academies Press: Washington, DC, USA, 2000.
11. Levine, M.; Dhariwal, K.R.; Welch, R.W.; Wang, Y.; Park, J.B. Determination of optimal vitamin C requirements in humans. *Am. J. Clin. Nutr.* **1995**, *62*, 1347S–1356S. [PubMed]
12. Carr, A.C.; Frei, B. Toward a new recommended dietary allowance for vitamin C based on antioxidant and health effects in humans. *Am. J. Clin. Nutr.* **1999**, *69*, 1086–1087. [PubMed]

13. Schleicher, R.L.; Carroll, M.D.; Ford, E.S.; Lacher, D.A. Serum vitamin C and the prevalence of vitamin C deficiency in the United States: 2003–2004 National Health and Nutrition Examination Survey (NHANES). *Am. J. Clin. Nutr.* **2009**, *90*, 1252–1263. [CrossRef] [PubMed]

14. US Centers for Disease Control and Prevention. *Second National Report on Biochemical Indicators of Diet and Nutrition in the US Population 2012*; National Center for Environmental Health: Atlanta, GA, USA, 2012.

15. Maggini, S.; Beveridge, S.; Sorbara, J.; Senatore, G. Feeding the immune system: The role of micronutrients in restoring resistance to infections. *CAB Rev.* **2008**, *3*, 1–21. [CrossRef]

16. Huskisson, E.; Maggini, S.; Ruf, M. The role of vitamins and minerals in energy metabolism and well-being. *J. Int. Med. Res.* **2007**, *35*, 277–289. [CrossRef] [PubMed]

17. Carr, A.; Frei, B. Does vitamin C act as a pro-oxidant under physiological conditions? *FASEB J.* **1999**, *13*, 1007–1024. [PubMed]

18. Mandl, J.; Szarka, A.; Banhegyi, G. Vitamin C: Update on physiology and pharmacology. *Br. J. Pharmacol.* **2009**, *157*, 1097–1110. [CrossRef] [PubMed]

19. Englard, S.; Seifter, S. The biochemical functions of ascorbic acid. *Annu. Rev. Nutr.* **1986**, *6*, 365–406. [CrossRef] [PubMed]

20. Carr, A.C.; Shaw, G.M.; Fowler, A.A.; Natarajan, R. Ascorbate-dependent vasopressor synthesis: A rationale for vitamin C administration in severe sepsis and septic shock? *Crit. Care* **2015**, *19*, e418. [CrossRef] [PubMed]

21. Kuiper, C.; Vissers, M.C. Ascorbate as a co-factor for Fe- and 2-oxoglutarate dependent dioxygenases: Physiological activity in tumor growth and progression. *Front. Oncol.* **2014**, *4*, 359. [CrossRef] [PubMed]

22. Young, J.I.; Zuchner, S.; Wang, G. Regulation of the epigenome by vitamin C. *Annu. Rev. Nutr.* **2015**, *35*, 545–564. [CrossRef] [PubMed]

23. Pullar, J.M.; Carr, A.C.; Vissers, M.C.M. The roles of vitamin C in skin health. *Nutrients* **2017**, *9*, 866. [CrossRef] [PubMed]

24. Rhie, G.; Shin, M.H.; Seo, J.Y.; Choi, W.W.; Cho, K.H.; Kim, K.H.; Park, K.C.; Eun, H.C.; Chung, J.H. Aging- and photoaging-dependent changes of enzymic and nonenzymic antioxidants in the epidermis and dermis of human skin in vivo. *J. Investig. Dermatol.* **2001**, *117*, 1212–1217. [CrossRef] [PubMed]

25. Shindo, Y.; Witt, E.; Han, D.; Epstein, W.; Packer, L. Enzymic and non-enzymic antioxidants in epidermis and dermis of human skin. *J. Investig. Dermatol.* **1994**, *102*, 122–124. [CrossRef] [PubMed]

26. McArdle, F.; Rhodes, L.E.; Parslew, R.; Jack, C.I.; Friedmann, P.S.; Jackson, M.J. UVR-induced oxidative stress in human skin in vivo: Effects of oral vitamin C supplementation. *Free Radic. Biol. Med.* **2002**, *33*, 1355–1362. [CrossRef]

27. Steiling, H.; Longet, K.; Moodycliffe, A.; Mansourian, R.; Bertschy, E.; Smola, H.; Mauch, C.; Williamson, G. Sodium-dependent vitamin C transporter isoforms in skin: Distribution, kinetics, and effect of UVB-induced oxidative stress. *Free Radic. Biol. Med.* **2007**, *43*, 752–762. [CrossRef] [PubMed]

28. Hodges, R.E.; Baker, E.M.; Hood, J.; Sauberlich, H.E.; March, S.C. Experimental scurvy in man. *Am. J. Clin. Nutr.* **1969**, *22*, 535–548. [PubMed]

29. Hodges, R.E.; Hood, J.; Canham, J.E.; Sauberlich, H.E.; Baker, E.M. Clinical manifestations of ascorbic acid deficiency in man. *Am. J. Clin. Nutr.* **1971**, *24*, 432–443. [PubMed]

30. Kivirikko, K.I.; Myllyla, R.; Pihlajaniemi, T. Protein hydroxylation: Prolyl 4-hydroxylase, an enzyme with four cosubstrates and a multifunctional subunit. *FASEB J.* **1989**, *3*, 1609–1617. [PubMed]

31. Geesin, J.C.; Darr, D.; Kaufman, R.; Murad, S.; Pinnell, S.R. Ascorbic acid specifically increases type I and type III procollagen messenger RNA levels in human skin fibroblast. *J. Investig. Dermatol.* **1988**, *90*, 420–424. [CrossRef] [PubMed]

32. Kishimoto, Y.; Saito, N.; Kurita, K.; Shimokado, K.; Maruyama, N.; Ishigami, A. Ascorbic acid enhances the expression of type 1 and type 4 collagen and SVCT2 in cultured human skin fibroblasts. *Biochem. Biophys. Res. Commun.* **2013**, *430*, 579–584. [CrossRef] [PubMed]

33. Nusgens, B.V.; Humbert, P.; Rougier, A.; Colige, A.C.; Haftek, M.; Lambert, C.A.; Richard, A.; Creidi, P.; Lapiere, C.M. Topically applied vitamin C enhances the mRNA level of collagens I and III, their processing enzymes and tissue inhibitor of matrix metalloproteinase 1 in the human dermis. *J. Investig. Dermatol.* **2001**, *116*, 853–859. [CrossRef] [PubMed]

34. Tajima, S.; Pinnell, S.R. Ascorbic acid preferentially enhances type I and III collagen gene transcription in human skin fibroblasts. *J. Dermatol. Sci.* **1996**, *11*, 250–253. [CrossRef]

35. Davidson, J.M.; LuValle, P.A.; Zoia, O.; Quaglino, D., Jr.; Giro, M. Ascorbate differentially regulates elastin and collagen biosynthesis in vascular smooth muscle cells and skin fibroblasts by pretranslational mechanisms. *J. Biol. Chem.* **1997**, *272*, 345–352. [CrossRef] [PubMed]

36. Fuchs, J.; Kern, H. Modulation of UV-light-induced skin inflammation by D-alpha-tocopherol and L-ascorbic acid: A clinical study using solar simulated radiation. *Free Radic. Biol. Med.* **1998**, *25*, 1006–1012. [CrossRef]

37. Lauer, A.C.; Groth, N.; Haag, S.F.; Darvin, M.E.; Lademann, J.; Meinke, M.C. Dose-dependent vitamin C uptake and radical scavenging activity in human skin measured with in vivo electron paramagnetic resonance spectroscopy. *Skin Pharmacol. Physiol.* **2013**, *26*, 147–154. [CrossRef] [PubMed]

38. Valacchi, G.; Sticozzi, C.; Belmonte, G.; Cervellati, F.; Demaude, J.; Chen, N.; Krol, Y.; Oresajo, C. Vitamin C compound mixtures prevent ozone-induced oxidative damage in human keratinocytes as initial assessment of pollution protection. *PLoS ONE* **2015**, *10*, e0131097. [CrossRef] [PubMed]

39. Valacchi, G.; Muresan, X.M.; Sticozzi, C.; Belmonte, G.; Pecorelli, A.; Cervellati, F.; Demaude, J.; Krol, Y.; Oresajo, C. Ozone-induced damage in 3D-skin model is prevented by topical vitamin C and vitamin E compound mixtures application. *J. Dermatol. Sci.* **2016**, *82*, 209–212. [CrossRef] [PubMed]

40. Lin, J.Y.; Selim, M.A.; Shea, C.R.; Grichnik, J.M.; Omar, M.M.; Monteiro-Riviere, N.A.; Pinnell, S.R. UV photoprotection by combination topical antioxidants vitamin C and vitamin E. *J. Am. Acad. Dermatol.* **2003**, *48*, 866–874. [CrossRef] [PubMed]

41. Pasonen-Seppanen, S.; Suhonen, T.M.; Kirjavainen, M.; Suihko, E.; Urtti, A.; Miettinen, M.; Hyttinen, M.; Tammi, M.; Tammi, R. Vitamin C enhances differentiation of a continuous keratinocyte cell line (REK) into epidermis with normal stratum corneum ultrastructure and functional permeability barrier. *Histochem. Cell Biol.* **2001**, *116*, 287–297. [CrossRef] [PubMed]

42. Savini, I.; Catani, M.V.; Rossi, A.; Duranti, G.; Melino, G.; Avigliano, L. Characterization of keratinocyte differentiation induced by ascorbic acid: Protein kinase C involvement and vitamin C homeostasis. *J. Investig. Dermatol.* **2002**, *118*, 372–379. [CrossRef] [PubMed]

43. Ponec, M.; Weerheim, A.; Kempenaar, J.; Mulder, A.; Gooris, G.S.; Bouwstra, J.; Mommaas, A.M. The formation of competent barrier lipids in reconstructed human epidermis requires the presence of vitamin C. *J. Investig. Dermatol.* **1997**, *109*, 348–355. [CrossRef] [PubMed]

44. Uchida, Y.; Behne, M.; Quiec, D.; Elias, P.M.; Holleran, W.M. Vitamin C stimulates sphingolipid production and markers of barrier formation in submerged human keratinocyte cultures. *J. Investig. Dermatol.* **2001**, *117*, 1307–1313. [CrossRef] [PubMed]

45. Kim, K.P.; Shin, K.O.; Park, K.; Yun, H.J.; Mann, S.; Lee, Y.M.; Cho, Y. Vitamin C stimulates epidermal ceramide production by regulating its metabolic enzymes. *Biomol. Ther.* **2015**, *23*, 525–530. [CrossRef] [PubMed]

46. Mohammed, B.M.; Fisher, B.J.; Kraskauskas, D.; Ward, S.; Wayne, J.S.; Brophy, D.F.; Fowler, A.A., III; Yager, D.R.; Natarajan, R. Vitamin C promotes wound healing through novel pleiotropic mechanisms. *Int. Wound J.* **2016**, *13*, 572–584. [CrossRef] [PubMed]

47. Duarte, T.L.; Cooke, M.S.; Jones, G.D. Gene expression profiling reveals new protective roles for vitamin C in human skin cells. *Free Radic. Biol. Med.* **2009**, *46*, 78–87. [CrossRef] [PubMed]

48. Desneves, K.J.; Todorovic, B.E.; Cassar, A.; Crowe, T.C. Treatment with supplementary arginine, vitamin C and zinc in patients with pressure ulcers: A randomised controlled trial. *Clin. Nutr.* **2005**, *24*, 979–987. [CrossRef] [PubMed]

49. Taylor, T.V.; Rimmer, S.; Day, B.; Butcher, J.; Dymock, I.W. Ascorbic acid supplementation in the treatment of pressure-sores. *Lancet* **1974**, *2*, 544–546. [CrossRef]

50. Stankova, L.; Gerhardt, N.B.; Nagel, L.; Bigley, R.H. Ascorbate and phagocyte function. *Infect. Immun.* **1975**, *12*, 252–256. [PubMed]

51. Winterbourn, C.C.; Vissers, M.C. Changes in ascorbate levels on stimulation of human neutrophils. *Biochim. Biophys. Acta* **1983**, *763*, 175–179. [CrossRef]

52. Parker, A.; Cuddihy, S.L.; Son, T.G.; Vissers, M.C.; Winterbourn, C.C. Roles of superoxide and myeloperoxidase in ascorbate oxidation in stimulated neutrophils and $H_{(2)}O_{(2)}$-treated HL60 cells. *Free Radic. Biol. Med.* **2011**, *51*, 1399–1405. [CrossRef] [PubMed]

53. Oberritter, H.; Glatthaar, B.; Moser, U.; Schmidt, K.H. Effect of functional stimulation on ascorbate content in phagocytes under physiological and pathological conditions. *Int. Arch. Allergy Appl. Immunol.* **1986**, *81*, 46–50. [CrossRef] [PubMed]

54. Goldschmidt, M.C. Reduced bactericidal activity in neutrophils from scorbutic animals and the effect of ascorbic acid on these target bacteria in vivo and in vitro. *Am. J. Clin. Nutr.* **1991**, *54*, 1214S–1220S. [PubMed]

55. Goldschmidt, M.C.; Masin, W.J.; Brown, L.R.; Wyde, P.R. The effect of ascorbic acid deficiency on leukocyte phagocytosis and killing of actinomyces viscosus. *Int. J. Vitam. Nutr. Res.* **1988**, *58*, 326–334. [PubMed]

56. Johnston, C.S.; Huang, S.N. Effect of ascorbic acid nutriture on blood histamine and neutrophil chemotaxis in guinea pigs. *J. Nutr.* **1991**, *121*, 126–130. [PubMed]

57. Rebora, A.; Dallegri, F.; Patrone, F. Neutrophil dysfunction and repeated infections: Influence of levamisole and ascorbic acid. *Br. J. Dermatol.* **1980**, *102*, 49–56. [CrossRef] [PubMed]

58. Patrone, F.; Dallegri, F.; Bonvini, E.; Minervini, F.; Sacchetti, C. Disorders of neutrophil function in children with recurrent pyogenic infections. *Med. Microbiol. Immunol.* **1982**, *171*, 113–122. [CrossRef] [PubMed]

59. Boura, P.; Tsapas, G.; Papadopoulou, A.; Magoula, I.; Kountouras, G. Monocyte locomotion in anergic chronic brucellosis patients: The in vivo effect of ascorbic acid. *Immunopharmacol. Immunotoxicol.* **1989**, *11*, 119–129. [CrossRef] [PubMed]

60. Anderson, R.; Theron, A. Effects of ascorbate on leucocytes: Part III. In vitro and in vivo stimulation of abnormal neutrophil motility by ascorbate. *S. Afr. Med. J.* **1979**, *56*, 429–433. [PubMed]

61. Johnston, C.S.; Martin, L.J.; Cai, X. Antihistamine effect of supplemental ascorbic acid and neutrophil chemotaxis. *J. Am. Coll. Nutr.* **1992**, *11*, 172–176. [PubMed]

62. Anderson, R.; Oostiuuizen, R.; Maritz, R.; Theron, A.; Van Rensburg, A.J. The effects of increasing weekly doses of ascorbate on certain cellular and humoral immune functions in normal volunteers. *Am. J. Clin. Nutr.* **1980**, *33*, 71–76. [PubMed]

63. Anderson, R. Ascorbate-mediated stimulation of neutrophil motility and lymphocyte transformation by inhibition of the peroxidase/H_2O_2/halide system in vitro and in vivo. *Am. J. Clin. Nutr.* **1981**, *34*, 1906–1911. [PubMed]

64. Ganguly, R.; Durieux, M.F.; Waldman, R.H. Macrophage function in vitamin C-deficient guinea pigs. *Am. J. Clin. Nutr.* **1976**, *29*, 762–765. [PubMed]

65. Corberand, J.; Nguyen, F.; Fraysse, B.; Enjalbert, L. Malignant external otitis and polymorphonuclear leukocyte migration impairment. Improvement with ascorbic acid. *Arch. Otolaryngol.* **1982**, *108*, 122–124. [CrossRef] [PubMed]

66. Levy, R.; Schlaeffer, F. Successful treatment of a patient with recurrent furunculosis by vitamin C: Improvement of clinical course and of impaired neutrophil functions. *Int. J. Dermatol.* **1993**, *32*, 832–834. [CrossRef] [PubMed]

67. Levy, R.; Shriker, O.; Porath, A.; Riesenberg, K.; Schlaeffer, F. Vitamin C for the treatment of recurrent furunculosis in patients with imparied neutrophil functions. *J. Infect. Dis.* **1996**, *173*, 1502–1505. [CrossRef] [PubMed]

68. Nungester, W.J.; Ames, A.M. The relationship between ascorbic acid and phagocytic activity. *J. Infect. Dis.* **1948**, *83*, 50–54. [CrossRef] [PubMed]

69. Shilotri, P.G. Phagocytosis and leukocyte enzymes in ascorbic acid deficient guinea pigs. *J. Nutr.* **1977**, *107*, 1513–1516. [PubMed]

70. Shilotri, P.G. Glycolytic, hexose monophosphate shunt and bactericidal activities of leukocytes in ascorbic acid deficient guinea pigs. *J. Nutr.* **1977**, *107*, 1507–1512. [PubMed]

71. Sharma, P.; Raghavan, S.A.; Saini, R.; Dikshit, M. Ascorbate-mediated enhancement of reactive oxygen species generation from polymorphonuclear leukocytes: Modulatory effect of nitric oxide. *J. Leukoc. Biol.* **2004**, *75*, 1070–1078. [CrossRef] [PubMed]

72. Rebora, A.; Crovato, F.; Dallegri, F.; Patrone, F. Repeated staphylococcal pyoderma in two siblings with defective neutrophil bacterial killing. *Dermatologica* **1980**, *160*, 106–112. [CrossRef] [PubMed]

73. Vissers, M.C.; Wilkie, R.P. Ascorbate deficiency results in impaired neutrophil apoptosis and clearance and is associated with up-regulation of hypoxia-inducible factor 1alpha. *J. Leukoc. Biol.* **2007**, *81*, 1236–1244. [CrossRef] [PubMed]

74. Fisher, B.J.; Kraskauskas, D.; Martin, E.J.; Farkas, D.; Wegelin, J.A.; Brophy, D.; Ward, K.R.; Voelkel, N.F.; Fowler, A.A., III; Natarajan, R. Mechanisms of attenuation of abdominal sepsis induced acute lung injury by ascorbic acid. *Am. J. Physiol. Lung Cell. Mol. Physiol.* **2012**, *303*, L20–L32. [CrossRef] [PubMed]

75. Mohammed, B.M.; Fisher, B.J.; Kraskauskas, D.; Farkas, D.; Brophy, D.F.; Fowler, A.A.; Natarajan, R. Vitamin C: A novel regulator of neutrophil extracellular trap formation. *Nutrients* **2013**, *5*, 3131–3151. [CrossRef] [PubMed]

76. Huijskens, M.J.; Walczak, M.; Koller, N.; Briede, J.J.; Senden-Gijsbers, B.L.; Schnijderberg, M.C.; Bos, G.M.; Germeraad, W.T. Technical advance: Ascorbic acid induces development of double-positive T cells from human hematopoietic stem cells in the absence of stromal cells. *J. Leukoc. Biol.* **2014**, *96*, 1165–1175. [CrossRef] [PubMed]

77. Molina, N.; Morandi, A.C.; Bolin, A.P.; Otton, R. Comparative effect of fucoxanthin and vitamin C on oxidative and functional parameters of human lymphocytes. *Int. Immunopharmacol.* **2014**, *22*, 41–50. [CrossRef] [PubMed]

78. Tanaka, M.; Muto, N.; Gohda, E.; Yamamoto, I. Enhancement by ascorbic acid 2-glucoside or repeated additions of ascorbate of mitogen-induced IgM and IgG productions by human peripheral blood lymphocytes. *Jpn. J. Pharmacol.* **1994**, *66*, 451–456. [CrossRef] [PubMed]

79. Manning, J.; Mitchell, B.; Appadurai, D.A.; Shakya, A.; Pierce, L.J.; Wang, H.; Nganga, V.; Swanson, P.C.; May, J.M.; Tantin, D.; et al. Vitamin C promotes maturation of T-cells. *Antioxid. Redox Signal.* **2013**, *19*, 2054–2067. [CrossRef] [PubMed]

80. Kennes, B.; Dumont, I.; Brohee, D.; Hubert, C.; Neve, P. Effect of vitamin C supplements on cell-mediated immunity in old people. *Gerontology* **1983**, *29*, 305–310. [CrossRef] [PubMed]

81. Anderson, R.; Hay, I.; van Wyk, H.; Oosthuizen, R.; Theron, A. The effect of ascorbate on cellular humoral immunity in asthmatic children. *S. Afr. Med. J.* **1980**, *58*, 974–977. [PubMed]

82. Fraser, R.C.; Pavlovic, S.; Kurahara, C.G.; Murata, A.; Peterson, N.S.; Taylor, K.B.; Feigen, G.A. The effect of variations in vitamin C intake on the cellular immune response of guinea pigs. *Am. J. Clin. Nutr.* **1980**, *33*, 839–847. [PubMed]

83. Feigen, G.A.; Smith, B.H.; Dix, C.E.; Flynn, C.J.; Peterson, N.S.; Rosenberg, L.T.; Pavlovic, S.; Leibovitz, B. Enhancement of antibody production and protection against systemic anaphylaxis by large doses of vitamin C. *Res. Commun. Chem. Pathol. Pharmacol.* **1982**, *38*, 313–333. [CrossRef]

84. Prinz, W.; Bloch, J.; Gilich, G.; Mitchell, G. A systematic study of the effect of vitamin C supplementation on the humoral immune response in ascorbate-dependent mammals. I. The antibody response to sheep red blood cells (a T-dependent antigen) in guinea pigs. *Int. J. Vitam. Nutr. Res.* **1980**, *50*, 294–300. [PubMed]

85. Prinz, W.; Bortz, R.; Bregin, B.; Hersch, M. The effect of ascorbic acid supplementation on some parameters of the human immunological defence system. *Int. J. Vitam. Nutr. Res.* **1977**, *47*, 248–257. [PubMed]

86. Chen, Y.; Luo, G.; Yuan, J.; Wang, Y.; Yang, X.; Wang, X.; Li, G.; Liu, Z.; Zhong, N. Vitamin C mitigates oxidative stress and tumor necrosis factor-alpha in severe community-acquired pneumonia and LPS-induced macrophages. *Mediators Inflamm.* **2014**, *2014*, 426740. [CrossRef] [PubMed]

87. Jeng, K.C.; Yang, C.S.; Siu, W.Y.; Tsai, Y.S.; Liao, W.J.; Kuo, J.S. Supplementation with vitamins C and E enhances cytokine production by peripheral blood mononuclear cells in healthy adults. *Am. J. Clin. Nutr.* **1996**, *64*, 960–965. [PubMed]

88. Kim, Y.; Kim, H.; Bae, S.; Choi, J.; Lim, S.Y.; Lee, N.; Kong, J.M.; Hwang, Y.I.; Kang, J.S.; Lee, W.J. Vitamin C is an essential factor on the anti-viral immune responses through the production of interferon-a/b at the initial stage of influenza A virus (H_3N_2) infection. *Immune Netw.* **2013**, *13*, 70–74. [CrossRef] [PubMed]

89. Gao, Y.L.; Lu, B.; Zhai, J.H.; Liu, Y.C.; Qi, H.X.; Yao, Y.; Chai, Y.F.; Shou, S.T. The parenteral vitamin C improves sepsis and sepsis-induced multiple organ dysfunction syndrome via preventing cellular immunosuppression. *Mediat. Inflamm.* **2017**, *2017*, 4024672. [CrossRef] [PubMed]

90. Portugal, C.C.; Socodato, R.; Canedo, T.; Silva, C.M.; Martins, T.; Coreixas, V.S.; Loiola, E.C.; Gess, B.; Rohr, D.; Santiago, A.R.; et al. Caveolin-1-mediated internalization of the vitamin C transporter SVCT2 in microglia triggers an inflammatory phenotype. *Sci. Signal.* **2017**, *10*. [CrossRef] [PubMed]

91. Dahl, H.; Degre, M. The effect of ascorbic acid on production of human interferon and the antiviral activity in vitro. *Acta Pathol. Microbiol. Scand. B* **1976**, *84b*, 280–284. [CrossRef] [PubMed]

92. Karpinska, T.; Kawecki, Z.; Kandefer-Szerszen, M. The influence of ultraviolet irradiation, L-ascorbic acid and calcium chloride on the induction of interferon in human embryo fibroblasts. *Arch. Immunol. Ther. Exp.* **1982**, *30*, 33–37.

93. Siegel, B.V. Enhancement of interferon production by poly(rI)-poly(rC) in mouse cell cultures by ascorbic acid. *Nature* **1975**, *254*, 531–532. [CrossRef] [PubMed]

94. Canali, R.; Natarelli, L.; Leoni, G.; Azzini, E.; Comitato, R.; Sancak, O.; Barella, L.; Virgili, F. Vitamin C supplementation modulates gene expression in peripheral blood mononuclear cells specifically upon an inflammatory stimulus: A pilot study in healthy subjects. *Genes Nutr.* **2014**, *9*, 390. [CrossRef] [PubMed]

95. Dawson, W.; West, G.B. The influence of ascorbic acid on histamine metabolism in guinea-pigs. *Br. J. Pharmacol. Chemother.* **1965**, *24*, 725–734. [CrossRef] [PubMed]

96. Nandi, B.K.; Subramanian, N.; Majumder, A.K.; Chatterjee, I.B. Effect of ascorbic acid on detoxification of histamine under stress conditions. *Biochem. Pharmacol.* **1974**, *23*, 643–647. [CrossRef]

97. Subramanian, N.; Nandi, B.K.; Majumder, A.K.; Chatterjee, I.B. Role of L-ascorbic acid on detoxification of histamine. *Biochem. Pharmacol.* **1973**, *22*, 1671–1673. [CrossRef]

98. Chatterjee, I.B.; Gupta, S.D.; Majumder, A.K.; Nandi, B.K.; Subramanian, N. Effect of ascorbic acid on histamine metabolism in scorbutic guinea-pigs. *J. Physiol.* **1975**, *251*, 271–279. [CrossRef] [PubMed]

99. Clemetson, C.A. Histamine and ascorbic acid in human blood. *J. Nutr.* **1980**, *110*, 662–668. [PubMed]

100. Johnston, C.S.; Solomon, R.E.; Corte, C. Vitamin C depletion is associated with alterations in blood histamine and plasma free carnitine in adults. *J. Am. Coll. Nutr.* **1996**, *15*, 586–591. [CrossRef] [PubMed]

101. Hagel, A.F.; Layritz, C.M.; Hagel, W.H.; Hagel, H.J.; Hagel, E.; Dauth, W.; Kressel, J.; Regnet, T.; Rosenberg, A.; Neurath, M.F.; et al. Intravenous infusion of ascorbic acid decreases serum histamine concentrations in patients with allergic and non-allergic diseases. *Naunyn Schmiedebergs Arch. Pharmacol.* **2013**, *386*, 789–793. [CrossRef] [PubMed]

102. Bruno, R.S.; Leonard, S.W.; Atkinson, J.; Montine, T.J.; Ramakrishnan, R.; Bray, T.M.; Traber, M.G. Faster plasma vitamin E disappearance in smokers is normalized by vitamin C supplementation. *Free Radic. Biol. Med.* **2006**, *40*, 689–697. [CrossRef] [PubMed]

103. Parsons, K.K.; Maeda, N.; Yamauchi, M.; Banes, A.J.; Koller, B.H. Ascorbic acid-independent synthesis of collagen in mice. *Am. J. Physiol. Endocrinol. Metab.* **2006**, *290*, E1131–E1139. [CrossRef] [PubMed]

104. Ross, R.; Benditt, E.P. Wound healing and collagen formation. II. Fine structure in experimental scurvy. *J. Cell Biol.* **1962**, *12*, 533–551. [CrossRef] [PubMed]

105. Fukushima, R.; Yamazaki, E. Vitamin C requirement in surgical patients. *Curr. Opin. Clin. Nutr. Metab. Care* **2010**, *13*, 669–676. [CrossRef] [PubMed]

106. Blass, S.C.; Goost, H.; Tolba, R.H.; Stoffel-Wagner, B.; Kabir, K.; Burger, C.; Stehle, P.; Ellinger, S. Time to wound closure in trauma patients with disorders in wound healing is shortened by supplements containing antioxidant micronutrients and glutamine: A PRCT. *Clin. Nutr.* **2012**, *31*, 469–475. [CrossRef] [PubMed]

107. Cereda, E.; Gini, A.; Pedrolli, C.; Vanotti, A. Disease-specific, versus standard, nutritional support for the treatment of pressure ulcers in institutionalized older adults: A randomized controlled trial. *J. Am. Geriatr. Soc.* **2009**, *57*, 1395–1402. [CrossRef] [PubMed]

108. Martin, P.; Leibovich, S.J. Inflammatory cells during wound repair: The good, the bad and the ugly. *Trends Cell Biol.* **2005**, *15*, 599–607. [CrossRef] [PubMed]

109. Wilgus, T.A.; Roy, S.; McDaniel, J.C. Neutrophils and Wound Repair: Positive Actions and Negative Reactions. *Adv. Wound Care* **2013**, *2*, 379–388. [CrossRef] [PubMed]

110. Wong, S.L.; Demers, M.; Martinod, K.; Gallant, M.; Wang, Y.; Goldfine, A.B.; Kahn, C.R.; Wagner, D.D. Diabetes primes neutrophils to undergo NETosis, which impairs wound healing. *Nat. Med.* **2015**, *21*, 815–819. [CrossRef] [PubMed]

111. Washko, P.; Rotrosen, D.; Levine, M. Ascorbic acid transport and accumulation in human neutrophils. *J. Biol. Chem.* **1989**, *264*, 18996–19002. [PubMed]

112. Bergsten, P.; Amitai, G.; Kehrl, J.; Dhariwal, K.R.; Klein, H.G.; Levine, M. Millimolar concentrations of ascorbic acid in purified human mononuclear leukocytes. Depletion and reaccumulation. *J. Biol. Chem.* **1990**, *265*, 2584–2587. [PubMed]

113. Evans, R.M.; Currie, L.; Campbell, A. The distribution of ascorbic acid between various cellular components of blood, in normal individuals, and its relation to the plasma concentration. *Br. J. Nutr.* **1982**, *47*, 473–482. [CrossRef] [PubMed]

114. Levine, M.; Conry-Cantilena, C.; Wang, Y.; Welch, R.W.; Washko, P.W.; Dhariwal, K.R.; Park, J.B.; Lazarev, A.; Graumlich, J.F.; King, J.; et al. Vitamin C pharmacokinetics in healthy volunteers: Evidence for a recommended dietary allowance. *Proc. Natl. Acad. Sci. USA* **1996**, *93*, 3704–3709. [CrossRef] [PubMed]

115. Levine, M.; Wang, Y.; Padayatty, S.J.; Morrow, J. A new recommended dietary allowance of vitamin C for healthy young women. *Proc. Natl. Acad. Sci. USA* **2001**, *98*, 9842–9846. [CrossRef] [PubMed]

116. Carr, A.C.; Bozonet, S.M.; Pullar, J.M.; Simcock, J.W.; Vissers, M.C. Human skeletal muscle ascorbate is highly responsive to changes in vitamin C intake and plasma concentrations. *Am. J. Clin. Nutr.* **2013**, *97*, 800–807. [CrossRef] [PubMed]

117. Vissers, M.C.; Bozonet, S.M.; Pearson, J.F.; Braithwaite, L.J. Dietary ascorbate intake affects steady state tissue concentrations in vitamin C-deficient mice: Tissue deficiency after suboptimal intake and superior bioavailability from a food source (kiwifruit). *Am. J. Clin. Nutr.* **2011**, *93*, 292–301. [CrossRef] [PubMed]

118. Corpe, C.P.; Lee, J.H.; Kwon, O.; Eck, P.; Narayanan, J.; Kirk, K.L.; Levine, M. 6-Bromo-6-deoxy-l-ascorbic acid: An ascorbate analog specific for Na^+-dependent vitamin C transporter but not glucose transporter pathways. *J. Biol. Chem.* **2005**, *280*, 5211–5220. [CrossRef] [PubMed]

119. Washko, P.W.; Wang, Y.; Levine, M. Ascorbic acid recycling in human neutrophils. *J. Biol. Chem.* **1993**, *268*, 15531–15535. [PubMed]

120. Buettner, G.R. The pecking order of free radicals and antioxidants: Lipid peroxidation, alpha-tocopherol, and ascorbate. *Arch. Biochem. Biophys.* **1993**, *300*, 535–543. [CrossRef] [PubMed]

121. Sen, C.K.; Packer, L. Antioxidant and redox regulation of gene transcription. *FASEB J.* **1996**, *10*, 709–720. [PubMed]

122. Li, N.; Karin, M. Is NF-kappaB the sensor of oxidative stress? *Faseb J.* **1999**, *13*, 1137–1143. [PubMed]

123. Macdonald, J.; Galley, H.F.; Webster, N.R. Oxidative stress and gene expression in sepsis. *Br. J. Anaesth.* **2003**, *90*, 221–232. [CrossRef] [PubMed]

124. Tan, P.H.; Sagoo, P.; Chan, C.; Yates, J.B.; Campbell, J.; Beutelspacher, S.C.; Foxwell, B.M.; Lombardi, G.; George, A.J. Inhibition of NF-kappa B and oxidative pathways in human dendritic cells by antioxidative vitamins generates regulatory T cells. *J. Immunol.* **2005**, *174*, 7633–7644. [CrossRef] [PubMed]

125. Winterbourn, C.C.; Hampton, M.B. Thiol chemistry and specificity in redox signaling. *Free Radic. Biol. Med.* **2008**, *45*, 549–561. [CrossRef] [PubMed]

126. Griffiths, H.R.; Willetts, R.S.; Grant, M.M.; Mistry, N.; Lunec, J.; Bevan, R.J. In vivo vitamin C supplementation increases phosphoinositol transfer protein expression in peripheral blood mononuclear cells from healthy individuals. *Br. J. Nutr.* **2009**, *101*, 1432–1439. [CrossRef] [PubMed]

127. Grant, M.M.; Mistry, N.; Lunec, J.; Griffiths, H.R. Dose-dependent modulation of the T cell proteome by ascorbic acid. *Br. J. Nutr.* **2007**, *97*, 19–26. [CrossRef] [PubMed]

128. Lammermann, T. In the eye of the neutrophil swarm-navigation signals that bring neutrophils together in inflamed and infected tissues. *J. Leukoc. Biol.* **2016**, *100*, 55–63. [CrossRef] [PubMed]

129. Demaret, J.; Venet, F.; Friggeri, A.; Cazalis, M.A.; Plassais, J.; Jallades, L.; Malcus, C.; Poitevin-Later, F.; Textoris, J.; Lepape, A.; et al. Marked alterations of neutrophil functions during sepsis-induced immunosuppression. *J. Leukoc. Biol.* **2015**, *98*, 1081–1090. [CrossRef] [PubMed]

130. Arraes, S.M.; Freitas, M.S.; da Silva, S.V.; de Paula Neto, H.A.; Alves-Filho, J.C.; Auxiliadora Martins, M.; Basile-Filho, A.; Tavares-Murta, B.M.; Barja-Fidalgo, C.; Cunha, F.Q. Impaired neutrophil chemotaxis in sepsis associates with GRK expression and inhibition of actin assembly and tyrosine phosphorylation. *Blood* **2006**, *108*, 2906–2913. [CrossRef] [PubMed]

131. Chishti, A.D.; Shenton, B.K.; Kirby, J.A.; Baudouin, S.V. Neutrophil chemotaxis and receptor expression in clinical septic shock. *Intensive Care Med.* **2004**, *30*, 605–611. [CrossRef] [PubMed]

132. Tavares-Murta, B.M.; Zaparoli, M.; Ferreira, R.B.; Silva-Vergara, M.L.; Oliveira, C.H.; Murta, E.F.; Ferreira, S.H.; Cunha, F.Q. Failure of neutrophil chemotactic function in septic patients. *Crit. Care Med.* **2002**, *30*, 1056–1061. [CrossRef] [PubMed]

133. Hotchkiss, R.S.; Monneret, G.; Payen, D. Sepsis-induced immunosuppression: From cellular dysfunctions to immunotherapy. *Nat. Rev. Immunol.* **2013**, *13*, 862–874. [CrossRef] [PubMed]

134. Vohra, K.; Khan, A.J.; Telang, V.; Rosenfeld, W.; Evans, H.E. Improvement of neutrophil migration by systemic vitamin C in neonates. *J. Perinatol.* **1990**, *10*, 134–136. [PubMed]

135. Roos, D. Chronic granulomatous disease. *Br. Med. Bull.* **2016**, *118*, 50–63. [CrossRef] [PubMed]

136. Introne, W.; Boissy, R.E.; Gahl, W.A. Clinical, molecular, and cell biological aspects of Chediak-Higashi syndrome. *Mol. Genet. Metab.* **1999**, *68*, 283–303. [CrossRef] [PubMed]

137. Anderson, R.; Dittrich, O.C. Effects of ascorbate on leucocytes: Part IV. Increased neutrophil function and clinical improvement after oral ascorbate in 2 patients with chronic granulomatous disease. *S. Afr. Med. J.* **1979**, *56*, 476–480. [PubMed]

138. Anderson, R. Assessment of oral ascorbate in three children with chronic granulomatous disease and defective neutrophil motility over a 2-year period. *Clin. Exp. Immunol.* **1981**, *43*, 180–188. [PubMed]

139. Anderson, R. Effects of ascorbate on normal and abnormal leucocyte functions. *Int. J. Vitam. Nutr. Res. Suppl.* **1982**, *23*, 23–34. [PubMed]

140. Gallin, J.I.; Elin, R.J.; Hubert, R.T.; Fauci, A.S.; Kaliner, M.A.; Wolff, S.M. Efficacy of ascorbic acid in Chediak-Higashi syndrome (CHS): Studies in humans and mice. *Blood* **1979**, *53*, 226–234. [PubMed]

141. Boxer, L.A.; Watanabe, A.M.; Rister, M.; Besch, H.R., Jr.; Allen, J.; Baehner, R.L. Correction of leukocyte function in Chediak-Higashi syndrome by ascorbate. *N. Engl. J. Med.* **1976**, *295*, 1041–1045. [CrossRef] [PubMed]

142. Yegin, O.; Sanal, O.; Yeralan, O.; Gurgey, A.; Berkel, A.I. Defective lymphocyte locomotion in Chediak-Higashi syndrome. *Am. J. Dis. Child.* **1983**, *137*, 771–773. [PubMed]

143. Weening, R.S.; Schoorel, E.P.; Roos, D.; van Schaik, M.L.; Voetman, A.A.; Bot, A.A.; Batenburg-Plenter, A.M.; Willems, C.; Zeijlemaker, W.P.; Astaldi, A. Effect of ascorbate on abnormal neutrophil, platelet and lymphocytic function in a patient with the Chediak-Higashi syndrome. *Blood* **1981**, *57*, 856–865. [PubMed]

144. Boxer, L.A.; Vanderbilt, B.; Bonsib, S.; Jersild, R.; Yang, H.H.; Baehner, R.L. Enhancement of chemotactic response and microtubule assembly in human leukocytes by ascorbic acid. *J. Cell. Physiol.* **1979**, *100*, 119–126. [CrossRef] [PubMed]

145. Boxer, L.A.; Albertini, D.F.; Baehner, R.L.; Oliver, J.M. Impaired microtubule assembly and polymorphonuclear leucocyte function in the Chediak-Higashi syndrome correctable by ascorbic acid. *Br. J. Haematol.* **1979**, *43*, 207–213. [CrossRef] [PubMed]

146. Parker, W.H.; Rhea, E.M.; Qu, Z.C.; Hecker, M.R.; May, J.M. Intracellular ascorbate tightens the endothelial permeability barrier through Epac1 and the tubulin cytoskeleton. *Am. J. Physiol. Cell Physiol.* **2016**, *311*, C652–C662. [CrossRef] [PubMed]

147. Bozonet, S.M.; Carr, A.C.; Pullar, J.M.; Vissers, M.C.M. Enhanced human neutrophil vitamin C status, chemotaxis and oxidant generation following dietary supplementation with vitamin C-rich SunGold kiwifruit. *Nutrients* **2015**, *7*, 2574–2588. [CrossRef] [PubMed]

148. De la Fuente, M.; Ferrandez, M.D.; Burgos, M.S.; Soler, A.; Prieto, A.; Miquel, J. Immune function in aged women is improved by ingestion of vitamins C and E. *Can. J. Physiol. Pharmacol.* **1998**, *76*, 373–380. [CrossRef] [PubMed]

149. Winterbourn, C.C.; Kettle, A.J.; Hampton, M.B. Reactive oxygen species and neutrophil function. *Annu. Rev. Biochem.* **2016**, *85*, 765–792. [CrossRef] [PubMed]

150. Patrone, F.; Dallegri, F.; Bonvini, E.; Minervini, F.; Sacchetti, C. Effects of ascorbic acid on neutrophil function. Studies on normal and chronic granulomatous disease neutrophils. *Acta Vitaminol. Enzymol.* **1982**, *4*, 163–168. [PubMed]

151. Foroozanfar, N.; Lucas, C.F.; Joss, D.V.; Hugh-Jones, K.; Hobbs, J.R. Ascorbate (1 g/day) does not help the phagocyte killing defect of X-linked chronic granulomatous disease. *Clin. Exp. Immunol.* **1983**, *51*, 99–102. [PubMed]

152. Hampton, M.B.; Kettle, A.J.; Winterbourn, C.C. Inside the neutrophil phagosome: Oxidants, myeloperoxidase, and bacterial killing. *Blood* **1998**, *92*, 3007–3017. [PubMed]

153. Wenisch, C.; Graninger, W. Are soluble factors relevant for polymorphonuclear leukocyte dysregulation in septicemia? *Clin. Diagn. Lab. Immunol.* **1995**, *2*, 241–245. [PubMed]

154. Danikas, D.D.; Karakantza, M.; Theodorou, G.L.; Sakellaropoulos, G.C.; Gogos, C.A. Prognostic value of phagocytic activity of neutrophils and monocytes in sepsis. Correlation to CD64 and CD14 antigen expression. *Clin. Exp. Immunol.* **2008**, *154*, 87–97. [CrossRef] [PubMed]

155. Stephan, F.; Yang, K.; Tankovic, J.; Soussy, C.J.; Dhonneur, G.; Duvaldestin, P.; Brochard, L.; Brun-Buisson, C.; Harf, A.; Delclaux, C. Impairment of polymorphonuclear neutrophil functions precedes nosocomial infections in critically ill patients. *Crit. Care Med.* **2002**, *30*, 315–322. [CrossRef] [PubMed]

156. McGovern, N.N.; Cowburn, A.S.; Porter, L.; Walmsley, S.R.; Summers, C.; Thompson, A.A.; Anwar, S.; Willcocks, L.C.; Whyte, M.K.; Condliffe, A.M.; et al. Hypoxia selectively inhibits respiratory burst activity and killing of Staphylococcus aureus in human neutrophils. *J. Immunol.* **2011**, *186*, 453–463. [CrossRef] [PubMed]

157. Drifte, G.; Dunn-Siegrist, I.; Tissieres, P.; Pugin, J. Innate immune functions of immature neutrophils in patients with sepsis and severe systemic inflammatory response syndrome. *Crit. Care Med.* **2013**, *41*, 820–832. [CrossRef] [PubMed]

158. Bass, D.A.; Olbrantz, P.; Szejda, P.; Seeds, M.C.; McCall, C.E. Subpopulations of neutrophils with increased oxidative product formation in blood of patients with infection. *J. Immunol.* **1986**, *136*, 860–866. [PubMed]

159. Pillay, J.; Ramakers, B.P.; Kamp, V.M.; Loi, A.L.; Lam, S.W.; Hietbrink, F.; Leenen, L.P.; Tool, A.T.; Pickkers, P.; Koenderman, L. Functional heterogeneity and differential priming of circulating neutrophils in human experimental endotoxemia. *J. Leukoc. Biol.* **2010**, *88*, 211–220. [CrossRef] [PubMed]

160. Wenisch, C.; Fladerer, P.; Patruta, S.; Krause, R.; Horl, W. Assessment of neutrophil function in patients with septic shock: Comparison of methods. *Clin. Diagn. Lab. Immunol.* **2001**, *8*, 178–180. [CrossRef] [PubMed]

161. Fox, S.; Leitch, A.E.; Duffin, R.; Haslett, C.; Rossi, A.G. Neutrophil apoptosis: Relevance to the innate immune response and inflammatory disease. *J. Innate Immun.* **2010**, *2*, 216–227. [CrossRef] [PubMed]

162. Hampton, M.B.; Fadeel, B.; Orrenius, S. Redox regulation of the caspases during apoptosis. *Ann. N. Y. Acad. Sci.* **1998**, *854*, 328–335. [CrossRef] [PubMed]

163. Fadeel, B.; Ahlin, A.; Henter, J.I.; Orrenius, S.; Hampton, M.B. Involvement of caspases in neutrophil apoptosis: Regulation by reactive oxygen species. *Blood* **1998**, *92*, 4808–4818. [PubMed]

164. Wilkie, R.P.; Vissers, M.C.; Dragunow, M.; Hampton, M.B. A functional NADPH oxidase prevents caspase involvement in the clearance of phagocytic neutrophils. *Infect. Immun.* **2007**, *75*, 3256–3263. [CrossRef] [PubMed]

165. Keel, M.; Ungethum, U.; Steckholzer, U.; Niederer, E.; Hartung, T.; Trentz, O.; Ertel, W. Interleukin-10 counterregulates proinflammatory cytokine-induced inhibition of neutrophil apoptosis during severe sepsis. *Blood* **1997**, *90*, 3356–3363. [PubMed]

166. Jimenez, M.F.; Watson, R.W.; Parodo, J.; Evans, D.; Foster, D.; Steinberg, M.; Rotstein, O.D.; Marshall, J.C. Dysregulated expression of neutrophil apoptosis in the systemic inflammatory response syndrome. *Arch. Surg.* **1997**, *132*, 1263–1269. [CrossRef] [PubMed]

167. Harter, L.; Mica, L.; Stocker, R.; Trentz, O.; Keel, M. Mcl-1 correlates with reduced apoptosis in neutrophils from patients with sepsis. *J. Am. Coll. Surg.* **2003**, *197*, 964–973. [CrossRef] [PubMed]

168. Taneja, R.; Parodo, J.; Jia, S.H.; Kapus, A.; Rotstein, O.D.; Marshall, J.C. Delayed neutrophil apoptosis in sepsis is associated with maintenance of mitochondrial transmembrane potential and reduced caspase-9 activity. *Crit. Care Med.* **2004**, *32*, 1460–1469. [CrossRef] [PubMed]

169. Fotouhi-Ardakani, N.; Kebir, D.E.; Pierre-Charles, N.; Wang, L.; Ahern, S.P.; Filep, J.G.; Milot, E. Role for myeloid nuclear differentiation antigen in the regulation of neutrophil apoptosis during sepsis. *Am. J. Respir. Crit. Care Med.* **2010**, *182*, 341–350. [CrossRef] [PubMed]

170. Paunel-Gorgulu, A.; Flohe, S.; Scholz, M.; Windolf, J.; Logters, T. Increased serum soluble Fas after major trauma is associated with delayed neutrophil apoptosis and development of sepsis. *Crit. Care* **2011**, *15*, R20. [CrossRef] [PubMed]

171. Paunel-Gorgulu, A.; Kirichevska, T.; Logters, T.; Windolf, J.; Flohe, S. Molecular mechanisms underlying delayed apoptosis in neutrophils from multiple trauma patients with and without sepsis. *Mol. Med.* **2012**, *18*, 325–335. [CrossRef] [PubMed]

172. Tamayo, E.; Gomez, E.; Bustamante, J.; Gomez-Herreras, J.I.; Fonteriz, R.; Bobillo, F.; Bermejo-Martin, J.F.; Castrodeza, J.; Heredia, M.; Fierro, I.; et al. Evolution of neutrophil apoptosis in septic shock survivors and nonsurvivors. *J. Crit. Care* **2012**, *27*, 415. [CrossRef] [PubMed]

173. Fialkow, L.; Fochesatto Filho, L.; Bozzetti, M.C.; Milani, A.R.; Rodrigues Filho, E.M.; Ladniuk, R.M.; Pierozan, P.; de Moura, R.M.; Prolla, J.C.; Vachon, E.; et al. Neutrophil apoptosis: A marker of disease severity in sepsis and sepsis-induced acute respiratory distress syndrome. *Crit. Care* **2006**, *10*, R155. [CrossRef] [PubMed]

174. Ertel, W.; Keel, M.; Infanger, M.; Ungethum, U.; Steckholzer, U.; Trentz, O. Circulating mediators in serum of injured patients with septic complications inhibit neutrophil apoptosis through up-regulation of protein-tyrosine phosphorylation. *J. Trauma* **1998**, *44*, 767–775. [CrossRef] [PubMed]

175. Parlato, M.; Souza-Fonseca-Guimaraes, F.; Philippart, F.; Misset, B.; Adib-Conquy, M.; Cavaillon, J.M. CD24-triggered caspase-dependent apoptosis via mitochondrial membrane depolarization and reactive oxygen species production of human neutrophils is impaired in sepsis. *J. Immunol.* **2014**, *192*, 2449–2459. [CrossRef] [PubMed]

176. Colotta, F.; Re, F.; Polentarutti, N.; Sozzani, S.; Mantovani, A. Modulation of granulocyte survival and programmed cell death by cytokines and bacterial products. *Blood* **1992**, *80*, 2012–2020. [PubMed]

177. Mikirova, N.; Riordan, N.; Casciari, J. Modulation of Cytokines in Cancer Patients by Intravenous Ascorbate Therapy. *Med. Sci. Monit.* **2016**, *22*, 14–25. [CrossRef] [PubMed]

178. Ferron-Celma, I.; Mansilla, A.; Hassan, L.; Garcia-Navarro, A.; Comino, A.M.; Bueno, P.; Ferron, J.A. Effect of vitamin C administration on neutrophil apoptosis in septic patients after abdominal surgery. *J. Surg. Res.* **2009**, *153*, 224–230. [CrossRef] [PubMed]

179. Pechous, R.D. With Friends like These: The Complex Role of Neutrophils in the Progression of Severe Pneumonia. *Front. Cell. Infect. Microbiol.* **2017**, *7*, 160. [CrossRef] [PubMed]

180. Zawrotniak, M.; Rapala-Kozik, M. Neutrophil extracellular traps (NETs)—Formation and implications. *Acta Biochim. Pol.* **2013**, *60*, 277–284. [PubMed]

181. Fuchs, T.A.; Abed, U.; Goosmann, C.; Hurwitz, R.; Schulze, I.; Wahn, V.; Weinrauch, Y.; Brinkmann, V.; Zychlinsky, A. Novel cell death program leads to neutrophil extracellular traps. *J. Cell Biol.* **2007**, *176*, 231–241. [CrossRef] [PubMed]

182. Brinkmann, V.; Reichard, U.; Goosmann, C.; Fauler, B.; Uhlemann, Y.; Weiss, D.S.; Weinrauch, Y.; Zychlinsky, A. Neutrophil extracellular traps kill bacteria. *Science* **2004**, *303*, 1532–1535. [CrossRef] [PubMed]

183. Parker, H.; Albrett, A.M.; Kettle, A.J.; Winterbourn, C.C. Myeloperoxidase associated with neutrophil extracellular traps is active and mediates bacterial killing in the presence of hydrogen peroxide. *J. Leukoc. Biol.* **2012**, *91*, 369–376. [CrossRef] [PubMed]

184. Czaikoski, P.G.; Mota, J.M.; Nascimento, D.C.; Sonego, F.; Castanheira, F.V.; Melo, P.H.; Scortegagna, G.T.; Silva, R.L.; Barroso-Sousa, R.; Souto, F.O.; et al. Neutrophil extracellular traps induce organ damage during experimental and clinical sepsis. *PLoS ONE* **2016**, *11*, e0148142. [CrossRef] [PubMed]

185. Camicia, G.; Pozner, R.; de Larranaga, G. Neutrophil extracellular traps in sepsis. *Shock* **2014**, *42*, 286–294. [CrossRef] [PubMed]

186. Silk, E.; Zhao, H.; Weng, H.; Ma, D. The role of extracellular histone in organ injury. *Cell Death Dis.* **2017**, *8*, e2812. [CrossRef] [PubMed]

187. Margraf, S.; Logters, T.; Reipen, J.; Altrichter, J.; Scholz, M.; Windolf, J. Neutrophil-derived circulating free DNA (cf-DNA/NETs): A potential prognostic marker for posttraumatic development of inflammatory second hit and sepsis. *Shock* **2008**, *30*, 352–358. [CrossRef] [PubMed]

188. Natarajan, R.; Fisher, B.J.; Syed, A.A.; Fowler, A.A. Impact of intravenous ascorbic acid infusion on novel biomarkers in patients with severe sepsis. *J. Pulm. Respir. Med.* **2014**, *4*, 8. [CrossRef]

189. Elks, P.M.; van Eeden, F.J.; Dixon, G.; Wang, X.; Reyes-Aldasoro, C.C.; Ingham, P.W.; Whyte, M.K.; Walmsley, S.R.; Renshaw, S.A. Activation of hypoxia-inducible factor-1alpha (Hif-1alpha) delays inflammation resolution by reducing neutrophil apoptosis and reverse migration in a zebrafish inflammation model. *Blood* **2011**, *118*, 712–722. [CrossRef] [PubMed]

190. Hirota, K.; Semenza, G.L. Regulation of hypoxia-inducible factor 1 by prolyl and asparaginyl hydroxylases. *Biochem. Biophys. Res. Commun.* **2005**, *338*, 610–616. [CrossRef] [PubMed]

191. McInturff, A.M.; Cody, M.J.; Elliott, E.A.; Glenn, J.W.; Rowley, J.W.; Rondina, M.T.; Yost, C.C. Mammalian target of rapamycin regulates neutrophil extracellular trap formation via induction of hypoxia-inducible factor 1 alpha. *Blood* **2012**, *120*, 3118–3125. [CrossRef] [PubMed]

192. Hong, J.M.; Kim, J.H.; Kang, J.S.; Lee, W.J.; Hwang, Y.I. Vitamin C is taken up by human T cells via sodium-dependent vitamin C transporter 2 (SVCT2) and exerts inhibitory effects on the activation of these cells in vitro. *Anat. Cell Biol.* **2016**, *49*, 88–98. [CrossRef] [PubMed]

193. Bergsten, P.; Yu, R.; Kehrl, J.; Levine, M. Ascorbic acid transport and distribution in human B lymphocytes. *Arch. Biochem. Biophys.* **1995**, *317*, 208–214. [CrossRef] [PubMed]

194. Lenton, K.J.; Therriault, H.; Fulop, T.; Payette, H.; Wagner, J.R. Glutathione and ascorbate are negatively correlated with oxidative DNA damage in human lymphocytes. *Carcinogenesis* **1999**, *20*, 607–613. [CrossRef] [PubMed]

195. Campbell, J.D.; Cole, M.; Bunditrutavorn, B.; Vella, A.T. Ascorbic acid is a potent inhibitor of various forms of T cell apoptosis. *Cell. Immunol.* **1999**, *194*, 1–5. [CrossRef] [PubMed]

196. Huijskens, M.J.; Walczak, M.; Sarkar, S.; Atrafi, F.; Senden-Gijsbers, B.L.; Tilanus, M.G.; Bos, G.M.; Wieten, L.; Germeraad, W.T. Ascorbic acid promotes proliferation of natural killer cell populations in culture systems applicable for natural killer cell therapy. *Cytotherapy* **2015**, *17*, 613–620. [CrossRef] [PubMed]

197. Penn, N.D.; Purkins, L.; Kelleher, J.; Heatley, R.V.; Mascie-Taylor, B.H.; Belfield, P.W. The effect of dietary supplementation with vitamins A, C and E on cell-mediated immune function in elderly long-stay patients: A randomized controlled trial. *Age Ageing* **1991**, *20*, 169–174. [CrossRef] [PubMed]

198. Heuser, G.; Vojdani, A. Enhancement of natural killer cell activity and T and B cell function by buffered vitamin C in patients exposed to toxic chemicals: The role of protein kinase-C. *Immunopharmacol. Immunotoxicol.* **1997**, *19*, 291–312. [CrossRef] [PubMed]

199. Sasidharan Nair, V.; Song, M.H.; Oh, K.I. Vitamin C Facilitates Demethylation of the Foxp3 Enhancer in a Tet-Dependent Manner. *J. Immunol.* **2016**, *196*, 2119–2131. [CrossRef] [PubMed]

200. Nikolouli, E.; Hardtke-Wolenski, M.; Hapke, M.; Beckstette, M.; Geffers, R.; Floess, S.; Jaeckel, E.; Huehn, J. Alloantigen-Induced Regulatory T Cells Generated in Presence of Vitamin C Display Enhanced Stability of Foxp3 Expression and Promote Skin Allograft Acceptance. *Front. Immunol.* **2017**, *8*, 748. [CrossRef] [PubMed]

201. Monfort, A.; Wutz, A. Breathing-in epigenetic change with vitamin C. *EMBO Rep.* **2013**, *14*, 337–346. [CrossRef] [PubMed]

202. Song, C.X.; He, C. Potential functional roles of DNA demethylation intermediates. *Trends Biochem. Sci.* **2013**, *38*, 480–484. [CrossRef] [PubMed]

203. Johnston, C.S.; Barkyoumb, G.M.; Schumacher, S.S. Vitamin C supplementation slightly improves physical activity levels and reduces cold incidence in men with marginal vitamin C status: A randomized controlled trial. *Nutrients* **2014**, *6*, 2572–2583. [CrossRef] [PubMed]

204. Haryanto, B.; Suksmasari, T.; Wintergerst, E.; Maggini, S. Multivitamin supplementation supports immune function and ameliorates conditions triggered by reduced air quality. *Vitam. Miner.* **2015**, *4*, 1–15.

205. Romieu, I.; Castro-Giner, F.; Kunzli, N.; Sunyer, J. Air pollution, oxidative stress and dietary supplementation: A review. *Eur. Respir. J.* **2008**, *31*, 179–196. [CrossRef] [PubMed]

206. Kelly, F.; Dunster, C.; Mudway, I. Air pollution and the elderly: Oxidant/antioxidant issues worth consideration. *Eur. Respir. J.* **2003**, *21*, 70s–75s. [CrossRef]

207. Marmot, A.; Eley, J.; Stafford, M.; Stansfeld, S.; Warwick, E.; Marmot, M. Building health: An epidemiological study of "sick building syndrome" in the Whitehall II study. *Occup. Environ. Med.* **2006**, *63*, 283–289. [CrossRef] [PubMed]

208. Pozzer, A.; Zimmermann, P.; Doering, U.; van Aardenne, J.; Tost, H.; Dentener, F.; Janssens-Maenhout, G.; Lelieveld, J. Effects of business-as-usual anthropogenic emissions on air quality. *Atmos. Chem. Phys.* **2012**, *12*, 6915–6937. [CrossRef]

209. Sram, R.J.; Binkova, B.; Rossner, P., Jr. Vitamin C for DNA damage prevention. *Mutat. Res.* **2012**, *733*, 39–49. [CrossRef] [PubMed]

210. Tribble, D.; Giuliano, L.; Fortmann, S. Reduced plasma ascorbic acid concentrations in nonsmokers regularly exposed to environmental tobacco smoke. *Am. J. Clin. Nutr.* **1993**, *58*, 886–890. [PubMed]

211. Valkonen, M.; Kuusi, T. Passive smoking induces atherogenic changes in low-density lipoprotein. *Circulation* **1998**, *97*, 2012–2016. [CrossRef] [PubMed]

212. Schectman, G.; Byrd, J.C.; Hoffmann, R. Ascorbic acid requirements for smokers: Analysis of a population survey. *Am. J. Clin. Nutr.* **1991**, *53*, 1466–1470. [PubMed]

213. Preston, A.M.; Rodriguez, C.; Rivera, C.E.; Sahai, H. Influence of environmental tobacco smoke on vitamin C status in children. *Am. J. Clin. Nutr.* **2003**, *77*, 167–172. [PubMed]

214. Strauss, R. Environmental tobacco smoke and serum vitamin C levels in children. *Pediatrics* **2001**, *107*, 540–542. [CrossRef] [PubMed]

215. Panda, K.; Chattopadhyay, R.; Chattopadhyay, D.J.; Chatterjee, I.B. Vitamin C prevents cigarette smoke-induced oxidative damage in vivo. *Free Radic. Biol. Med.* **2000**, *29*, 115–124. [CrossRef]

216. Dietrich, M.; Block, G.; Benowitz, N.; Morrow, J.; Hudes, M.; Jacob, P., III; Norkus, E.; Packer, L. Vitamin C supplementation decreases oxidative stress biomarker f2-isoprostanes in plasma of nonsmokers exposed to environmental tobacco smoke. *Nutr. Cancer* **2003**, *45*, 176–184. [CrossRef] [PubMed]

217. Bagaitkar, J.; Demuth, D.; Scott, D. Tobacco use increases susceptibility to bacterial infection. *Tob. Induc. Dis.* **2008**, *4*, 12. [CrossRef] [PubMed]

218. Arcavi, L.; Benowitz, N.L. Cigarette smoking and infection. *Arch. Intern. Med.* **2004**, *164*, 2206–2216. [CrossRef] [PubMed]

219. Sargeant, L.; Jaeckel, A.; Wareham, N. Interaction of vitamin C with the relation between smoking and obstructive airways disease in EPIC Norfolk. European Prospective Investigation into Cancer and Nutrition. *Eur. Respir. J.* **2000**, *16*, 397–403. [CrossRef] [PubMed]

220. Peleg, A.Y.; Weerarathna, T.; McCarthy, J.S.; Davis, T.M. Common infections in diabetes: Pathogenesis, management and relationship to glycaemic control. *Diabetes Metab. Res. Rev.* **2007**, *23*, 3–13. [CrossRef] [PubMed]

221. Narayan, K.M.V.; Williams, D.; Gregg, E.W.; Cowie, C.C. (Eds.) *Diabetes Public Health: From Data to Policy*; Oxford University Press: Oxford, UK, 2011.

222. Pirola, L.; Ferraz, J. Role of pro- and anti-inflammatory phenomena in the physiopathology of type 2 diabetes and obesity. *World J. Biol. Chem.* **2017**, *8*, 120–128. [CrossRef] [PubMed]

223. Donath, M. Targeting inflammation in the treatment of type 2 diabetes: Time to start. *Nat. Rev. Drug Discov.* **2014**, *13*, 465–476. [CrossRef] [PubMed]

224. Ferrante, A.W., Jr. Macrophages, fat, and the emergence of immunometabolism. *J. Clin. Investig.* **2013**, *123*, 4992–4993. [CrossRef] [PubMed]

225. Osborn, O.; Olefsky, J.M. The cellular and signaling networks linking the immune system and metabolism in disease. *Nat. Med.* **2012**, *18*, 363–374. [CrossRef] [PubMed]

226. Wilson, R.; Willis, J.; Gearry, R.; Skidmore, P.; Fleming, E.; Frampton, C.; Carr, A. Inadequate vitamin C status in prediabetes and type 2 diabetes mellitus: Associations with glycaemic control, obesity, and smoking. *Nutrients* **2017**, *9*, 997. [CrossRef] [PubMed]

227. Maggini, S.; Wenzlaff, S.; Hornig, D. Essential role of vitamin C and zinc in child immunity and health. *J. Int. Med. Res.* **2010**, *38*, 386–414. [CrossRef] [PubMed]

228. Wintergerst, E.; Maggini, S.; Hornig, D. Immune-enhancing role of vitamin C and zinc and effect on clinical conditions. *Ann. Nutr. Metab.* **2006**, *50*, 85–94. [CrossRef] [PubMed]

229. Harding, A.H.; Wareham, N.J.; Bingham, S.A.; Khaw, K.; Luben, R.; Welch, A.; Forouhi, N.G. Plasma vitamin C level, fruit and vegetable consumption, and the risk of new-onset type 2 diabetes mellitus: The European prospective investigation of cancer—Norfolk prospective study. *Arch. Intern. Med.* **2008**, *168*, 1493–1499. [CrossRef] [PubMed]

230. Kositsawat, J.; Freeman, V.L. Vitamin C and A1c relationship in the National Health and Nutrition Examination Survey (NHANES) 2003–2006. *J. Am. Coll. Nutr.* **2011**, *30*, 477–483. [CrossRef] [PubMed]

231. Carter, P.; Gray, L.J.; Talbot, D.; Morris, D.H.; Khunti, K.; Davies, M.J. Fruit and vegetable intake and the association with glucose parameters: A cross-sectional analysis of the Let's Prevent Diabetes Study. *Eur. J. Clin. Nutr.* **2013**, *67*, 12–17. [CrossRef] [PubMed]

232. Mazloom, Z.; Hejazi, N.; Dabbaghmanesh, M.H.; Tabatabaei, H.R.; Ahmadi, A.; Ansar, H. Effect of vitamin C supplementation on postprandial oxidative stress and lipid profile in type 2 diabetic patients. *Pak. J. Biol. Sci.* **2011**, *14*, 900–904. [PubMed]

233. Ashor, A.W.; Werner, A.D.; Lara, J.; Willis, N.D.; Mathers, J.C.; Siervo, M. Effects of vitamin C supplementation on glycaemic control: A systematic review and meta-analysis of randomised controlled trials. *Eur. J. Clin. Nutr.* **2017**. [CrossRef] [PubMed]

234. Hajishengallis, G. Too old to fight? Aging and its toll on innate immunity. *Mol. Oral Microbiol.* **2010**, *25*, 25–37. [CrossRef] [PubMed]

235. Cheng, L.; Cohen, M.; Bhagavan, H. Vitamin C and the elderly. In *CRC Handbook of Nutrition in the Aged*; Watson, R., Ed.; CRC Press Inc.: Boca Raton, FL, USA, 1985; pp. 157–185.

236. Simon, J.; Hudes, E.; Tice, J. Relation of serum ascorbic acid to mortality among US adults. *J. Am. Coll. Nutr.* **2001**, *20*, 255–263. [CrossRef] [PubMed]

237. Fletcher, A.; Breeze, E.; Shetty, P. Antioxidant vitamins and mortality in older persons: Findings from the nutrition add-on study to the Medical Research Council Trial of Assessment and Management of Older People in the Community. *Am. J. Clin. Nutr.* **2003**, *78*, 999–1010. [PubMed]

238. Thurman, J.; Mooradian, A. Vitamin supplementation therapy in the elderly. *Drugs Aging* **1997**, *11*, 433–449. [CrossRef] [PubMed]

239. Hanck, A. Vitamin C in the elderly. *Int. J. Vitam. Nutr. Res. Suppl.* **1983**, *24*, 257–269. [PubMed]

240. Schorah, C.J. The level of vitamin C reserves required in man: Towards a solution to the controversy. *Proc. Nutr. Soc.* **1981**, *40*, 147–154. [CrossRef] [PubMed]

241. Hunt, C.; Chakravorty, N.; Annan, G. The clinical and biochemical effects of vitamin C supplementation in short-stay hospitalized geriatric patients. *Int. J. Vitam. Nutr. Res.* **1984**, *54*, 65–74. [PubMed]

242. Mayland, C.R.; Bennett, M.I.; Allan, K. Vitamin C deficiency in cancer patients. *Palliat. Med.* **2005**, *19*, 17–20. [CrossRef] [PubMed]

243. Danai, P.A.; Moss, M.; Mannino, D.M.; Martin, G.S. The epidemiology of sepsis in patients with malignancy. *Chest* **2006**, *129*, 1432–1440. [CrossRef] [PubMed]

244. Gan, R.; Eintracht, S.; Hoffer, L.J. Vitamin C deficiency in a university teaching hospital. *J. Am. Coll. Nutr.* **2008**, *27*, 428–433. [CrossRef] [PubMed]

245. Bakaev, V.V.; Duntau, A.P. Ascorbic acid in blood serum of patients with pulmonary tuberculosis and pneumonia. *Int. J. Tuberc. Lung Dis.* **2004**, *8*, 263–266. [PubMed]

246. Hunt, C.; Chakravorty, N.K.; Annan, G.; Habibzadeh, N.; Schorah, C.J. The clinical effects of vitamin C supplementation in elderly hospitalised patients with acute respiratory infections. *Int. J. Vitam. Nutr. Res.* **1994**, *64*, 212–219. [PubMed]

247. Bharara, A.; Grossman, C.; Grinnan, D.; Syed, A.A.; Fisher, B.J.; DeWilde, C.; Natarajan, R.; Fowler, A.A. Intravenous vitamin C administered as adjunctive therapy for recurrent acute respiratory distress syndrome. *Case Rep. Crit. Care* **2016**, *2016*, 8560871. [CrossRef] [PubMed]

248. Fowler, A.A.; Kim, C.; Lepler, L.; Malhotra, R.; Debesa, O.; Natarajan, R.; Fisher, B.J.; Syed, A.; DeWilde, C.; Priday, A.; et al. Intravenous vitamin C as adjunctive therapy for enterovirus/rhinovirus induced acute respiratory distress syndrome. *World J. Crit. Care Med.* **2017**, *6*, 85–90. [CrossRef] [PubMed]

249. Hemila, H.; Chalker, E. Vitamin C for preventing and treating the common cold. *Cochrane Database Syst. Rev.* **2013**, *1*, CD000980.

250. Hemila, H. Vitamin C and the common cold. *Br. J. Nutr.* **1992**, *67*, 3–16. [CrossRef] [PubMed]

251. Hume, R.; Weyers, E. Changes in leucocyte ascorbic acid during the common cold. *Scott. Med. J.* **1973**, *18*, 3–7. [CrossRef] [PubMed]

252. Wilson, C.W. Ascorbic acid function and metabolism during colds. *Ann. N. Y. Acad. Sci.* **1975**, *258*, 529–539. [CrossRef] [PubMed]

253. Schwartz, A.R.; Togo, Y.; Hornick, R.B.; Tominaga, S.; Gleckman, R.A. Evaluation of the efficacy of ascorbic acid in prophylaxis of induced rhinovirus 44 infection in man. *J. Infect. Dis.* **1973**, *128*, 500–505. [CrossRef] [PubMed]

254. Davies, J.E.; Hughes, R.E.; Jones, E.; Reed, S.E.; Craig, J.W.; Tyrrell, D.A. Metabolism of ascorbic acid (vitamin C) in subjects infected with common cold viruses. *Biochem. Med.* **1979**, *21*, 78–85. [CrossRef]

255. Mochalkin, N. Ascorbic acid in the complex therapy of acute pneumonia. *Voen. Med. Zhurnal* **1970**, *9*, 17–21. Available online: http://www.mv.helsinki.fi/home/hemila/T5.pdf (accessed on 5 December 2014).

256. Hemila, H.; Louhiala, P. Vitamin C for preventing and treating pneumonia. *Cochrane Database Syst. Rev.* **2013**, *8*, CD005532.

13

Systematic Review of Intravenous Ascorbate in Cancer Clinical Trials

Gina Nauman [1], Javaughn Corey Gray [2], Rose Parkinson [2], Mark Levine [1] and Channing J. Paller [2,*

[1] National Institutes of Health, National Institute of Diabetes and Digestive and Kidney Diseases, Clinical Nutrition Section, Bethesda, MD 20892, USA; gn157@georgetown.edu (G.N.); markl@bdg8.niddk.nih.gov (M.L.)

[2] Sidney Kimmel Comprehensive Cancer Center, Johns Hopkins Medical Institutions, Baltimore, MD 21287, USA; corey.gray@jhmi.edu (J.C.G.); rparkin1@jhmi.edu (R.P.)

* Correspondence: cpaller1@jhmi.edu

Abstract: Background: Ascorbate (vitamin C) has been evaluated as a potential treatment for cancer as an independent agent and in combination with standard chemotherapies. This review assesses the evidence for safety and clinical effectiveness of intravenous (IV) ascorbate in treating various types of cancer. Methods: Single arm and randomized Phase I/II trials were included in this review. The PubMed, MEDLINE, and Cochrane databases were searched. Results were screened by three of the authors (GN, RP, and CJP) to determine if they met inclusion criteria, and then summarized using a narrative approach. Results: A total of 23 trials involving 385 patients met the inclusion criteria. Only one trial, in ovarian cancer, randomized patients to receive vitamin C or standard of care (chemotherapy). That trial reported an 8.75 month increase in progression-free survival (PFS) and an improved trend in overall survival (OS) in the vitamin C treated arm. Conclusion: Overall, vitamin C has been shown to be safe in nearly all patient populations, alone and in combination with chemotherapies. The promising results support the need for randomized placebo-controlled trials such as the ongoing placebo-controlled trials of vitamin C and chemotherapy in prostate cancer.

Keywords: intravenous; ascorbate; vitamin C; clinical trials; cancer; patients

1. Introduction

Ascorbate (vitamin C) was proposed to have anticancer effects as early as the 1950s [1,2] However, the earliest effort to using high-dose vitamin C—both intravenously (IV) and orally—as a cancer treatment occurred in the 1970s, by Scottish surgeon Ewan Cameron and his colleague Allan Campbell. For comparison purposes, in 1974, the recommended dietary allowance of vitamin C was 0.045 g (45 mg) daily [3]. Cameron and Campbell treated 50 patients with various types of advanced cancers with high doses of oral ascorbate, IV ascorbate, or both. Several responses were observed following this treatment [4–6]. These findings led to a collaboration between Cameron and Nobel Prize winning chemist Linus Pauling on the evaluation of two case series of cancer patients [5,7]. The data obtained from these cancer patients suggested that there was a potential survival benefit when their treatment was supplemented with oral and IV vitamin C [7,8]. Limitations of these findings have subsequently been described [9], including that the findings were retrospective, without controls or blinding, and that studied patients may have been at risk for endemic vitamin C deficiency.

To test ascorbate prospectively, two randomized, placebo-controlled prospective trials were conducted at the Mayo Clinic, in which cancer patients received either placebo or 10 g of oral ascorbate. Each study noted no significant difference between the ascorbate-treated and placebo-treated groups [2,10]. Based on these results, ascorbates role in cancer treatment was dismissed [11,12].

However, there was renewed interest in the use of vitamin C as a cancer treatment, based on the discovery that intravenous ascorbate produced plasma ascorbate concentrations that were much higher than those from oral ascorbate, and were not possible from oral ascorbate [9,13,14]. Although Cameron's subjects received both intravenous and oral ascorbate, subjects in the two randomized placebo-controlled trials at Mayo Clinic received only oral ascorbate. The significance of this key difference was not previously recognized until ascorbate pharmacokinetic studies in healthy subjects revealed the importance of the route of administration.

Subsequently, emerging preclinical and clinical studies led to a revival of interest into the clinical potential of intravenous ascorbate as a cancer chemotherapeutic agent, specifically its synergy with chemotherapy and amelioration of chemotherapy-induced side effects [15]. Additional studies on the efficacy of vitamin C as a therapeutic have shown that intravenous administration achieves high plasma concentrations that are not achievable through oral administration [13,16–18]. Specifically, oral administration of vitamin C at a dose of 1.25 g achieved a maximum plasma concentration of 134.8 ± 20.6 µmol/L (µM), while IV administration of vitamin C achieved a maximum plasma concentration of 885 ± 201.2 µmol/L [13,16]. In the text that follows, we refer to plasma ascorbate concentrations as pharmacologic when they can only be achieved by intravenous administration in humans, and as parenteral (intravenous or intraperitoneal) administration in rodents.

The role of intravenous vitamin C in combination with chemotherapy as a cancer treatment is still being examined and various trials into this subject matter are ongoing. This systematic review summarizes the clinical trials of IV ascorbate to date which were primarily composed of single-arm trials examining dose-limiting toxicities, progression-free survival, and overall survival.

1.1. Clinical Pharmacokinetics of Vitamin C

Clinical data show that intravenous and oral administration of ascorbate yield differing plasma concentrations. When ascorbate is given orally, fasting plasma concentrations are maintained at <100 µM [13] but when oral doses exceed 200 mg, the percentage of the absorbed dose decreases, with a decrease in ascorbate bioavailability, and renal excretion increases [13,19]. In contrast, intravenous administration bypasses the intestinal absorption system. This allows plasma concentrations to be elevated to pharmacologic concentrations (mmol/L [mM] values) that are unachievable via oral administration [20]. In healthy humans, plasma vitamin C concentrations were significantly higher following IV administration compared to oral dosing, and the difference in plasma concentration increased according to the dose delivered. It was found that the mean peak values from IV administration were 6.6-fold higher than the mean peak values from oral administration at a dose of 1.25 g vitamin C [16]. IV ascorbate can be administered by either bolus or continuous infusion. Bolus infusion can be considered as dosing based on pharmacokinetics that occurs over a defined period of time, usually 1.5–2 h [17,21,22]. Continuous infusion is usually considered over periods of time >12 h. Bolus administration of ascorbate has been used more commonly than continuous administration. With a dose of 1 g/kg, bolus administration produces peak plasma ascorbate concentrations of approximately 25 mM, with concentrations maintained above 10 mM for approximately 4 h and return to baseline (<0.1 mM) after approximately 12 h [18]. Following IV administration of pharmacologic ascorbate doses, the plasma half-life is as rapid as 0.5–1 h. With 10 g administered continuously over 24 h, steady-state plasma concentrations can be estimated to be approximately 1–2 mM [19,23]. When oral ascorbate intake stops, the plasma half-life is approximately 8–20 days, due to the action of renal transporters reabsorbing filtered ascorbate [9,18,24,25].

Additionally, some but not all preclinical data indicate that ascorbate can accumulate in solid tumors at higher concentrations than surrounding normal tissue [26–28]. This suggests that cancerous cells are especially affected by vitamin C, which favors the clinical potential of high-dose intravenous vitamin C as a cancer therapeutic [20].

1.2. Possible Mechanisms of Anti-Tumor Effects of Vitamin C

Several major mechanisms have been proposed to explain why only pharmacologic ascorbate concentrations have cytotoxic effects on some but not all cancer cells. Two mechanisms include increased pro-oxidant damage that is irreparable by tumor cells, and oxidation of ascorbate into dehydroascorbic acid (DHA), which is an unstable metabolite and can be cytotoxic [20]. Most data indicate that the first pathway predominates, specifically by generation of extracellular hydrogen peroxide (H_2O_2) by pharmacologic ascorbate and a trace transition metal, usually iron [29,30]. Hydrogen peroxide is cell permeant, and, in the presence of pharmacologic ascorbate, H_2O_2 reactive oxygen species (ROS) are formed extracellularly and/or intracellularly [31]. These ROS have multiple downstream targets, including but not limited to DNA damage, mitochondrial damage, and stimulation of apoptotic pathways [29,32,33].

To learn experimentally whether extracellular H_2O_2 is essential, the enzyme catalase is added. At concentrations used by nearly all laboratories, catalase is a non-permeant protein that dismutates H_2O_2 to water and oxygen. The great majority of in vitro work shows that cell death is blunted or eliminated by catalase addition, pointing to the key role of H_2O_2. The second pathway involves dehydroascorbic acid (DHA), the reversible oxidized form of ascorbate. This pathway is based on findings that tumor cells transport DHA and then internally reduce it to ascorbate. In specifically engineered cells, this reduction triggers scavenging of glutathione (GSH), induces oxidative stress, inactivates glyceraldehyde 3-phosphate dehydrogenase (GAPDH), inhibits glycolytic flux, and leads to an energy crisis that triggers cell death [34,35]. DHA findings are attractive, but have several limitations, including that extracellular H_2O_2 may still be the initial driver of ascorbate oxidation to DHA, and that DHA does not cause cell death in a variety of unmodified cancer cells that do respond to ascorbate [29,30,36,37].

Two additional mechanisms of ascorbate action in cancer are based on ascorbate's activity as a cofactor for Fe (II) 2-oxoglutarate dioxygenase enzymes. As a co-factor, ascorbate modulates DNA demethylation and epigenetic marks through interaction with the ten eleven translocation (TET) enzyme family [38,39]. Ascorbate binds to the catalytic domain facilitating TET-mediated DNA demethylation [38,40]. This reverses the hypermethylation triggered in oncogenic states and subsequently activates tumor suppressor genes [40,41]. Reactivation of tumor suppressor genes allows for anti-tumor mechanisms to become active and increases chemosensitivity. Ascorbate action on TET may have promise in preventing tumor development especially in myelodysplastic syndrome [3,42]. Similarly, ascorbate acts as a co-factor for hypoxia-inducible transcription factors (HIFs) prolyl-4-hydroxylase domain (PHD) enzymes. Prolyl-4-hydroxylation is necessary for targeting of HIFs for proteolytic degradation [43–45]. In solid tumors, HIF-1 helps tumor cells shift from aerobic metabolism to anaerobic metabolism increasing flux through glycolysis to maintain energy production [43]. This activity in tumor cells creates a state that is dependent on glycolytic metabolites. It is possible that the DHA mechanism discussed above works in tandem with the HIF mechanism to cause global disruption of metabolic functioning in the tumor cell triggering cell death. For both TET-mediated and HIF-mediated mechanisms, ascorbate action at physiologically relevant concentrations may prevent cancer development. For cancer treatment, only pharmacologic ascorbate was found to be effective [30].

For the majority of cancer cells in vitro, ascorbate concentrations less than 5 mM are sufficient to induce a 50% decrease in cell survival. In contrast, many non-cancerous cells are capable of tolerating ascorbate concentrations of 20 mM, indicating less sensitivity [36]. Note that in vitro there is some heterogeneity in response to ascorbate in tumor and non-tumor cells alike. Perhaps 10–15% of cancer cells are insensitive to 20 mM ascorbate. Moreover, the death of cancer cells is thought to be selectively induced by extracellular ascorbate, and not intracellular ascorbate [17,36,46,47].

1.3. Synergy with Chemotherapy

Translational synergy of pharmacologic ascorbate with chemotherapy was first demonstrated using cell and mouse pancreatic cancer models [48]. Ascorbate was synergistic with gemcitabine both in vitro and in vivo, without apparent harm. The synergy of ascorbate with conventional chemotherapy is the subject of many clinical studies (Tables 1 and 2). Further, ascorbate was permissive for dose reductions of gemcitabine in these pre-clinical studies. These findings have clinical promise, but to date only individual cases have been reported, without data for failure rates [49]. Ascorbate synergy with conventional chemotherapy was also rigorously investigated in ovarian cancer models. The combination of ascorbic acid and conventional chemotherapeutic agents synergistically inhibited ovarian cancer cell lines and xenografts in mice [50]. Ma et al. exposed ovarian cancer cell lines (OVCAR5, OVCAR8, and SHIN3) to ascorbate and carboplatin in varying molar ratios, using HIO-80 cells, a nontumorigenic ovarian cell line, as a control. The results of this preclinical study demonstrated that the combination of ascorbate and carboplatin induced greater cell death in all cancer cell lines compared to either drug individually [50]. The HIO-80 ovarian epithelial cell line was shown to be equally sensitive to carboplatin alone, and the ascorbate-carboplatin combination. The SHIN3 cell line was implanted into athymic mice to further test the synergistic effect. Ascorbate and carboplatin were shown to be more effective at reducing tumor burden compared to either ascorbate or carboplatin alone. Clinically, multiple trials have demonstrated the safety of ascorbic acid when combined with chemotherapy in the treatment of several cancers including multiple myeloma, ovarian and pancreatic cancer [21,50–52].

2. Materials and Methods

This review's protocol was developed by the authors and was designed to summarize the results of clinical trials in which cancer patients are treated with intravenous vitamin C, either as a single agent or in combination with standard therapies. The population of interest for this review included patients with a current diagnosis of cancer of any type and stage. The intervention of interest was treatment with intravenous ascorbate alone or in combination with standard cancer therapies. Uncontrolled studies or controlled studies that included comparisons against no treatment, placebo, or other standard of care therapies were of interest. Outcomes of interest included Common Terminology Criteria for Adverse Events (CTCAE) adverse events or other measured toxicities, quality of life, progression free survival and overall survival. Randomized controlled trials were of primary interest, but all study designs were included in the initial search.

An electronic literature search was conducted in the PubMed, MEDLINE, and Cochrane databases. PubMed served as an interface for searching MEDLINE (Figure 1). The exact search term combination used in the PubMed search was: "Ascorbate OR Vitamin C AND Cancer NOT Bowel Preparation AND Clinical Trial". The exact search term combination used in the Cochrane database search was: "cancer" "vitamin c" "clinical trial". Following retrieval of the studies, three authors screened the studies (GN, RP, and CJP), eliminated duplicates, and removed all studies that were not clinical trials or not relevant to the subject matter. These authors then screened the remaining studies a second time, removing trials that examined oral ascorbate, and trials that were terminated prematurely and/or had no results. After the second screening, the remaining studies were summarized using a narrative approach.

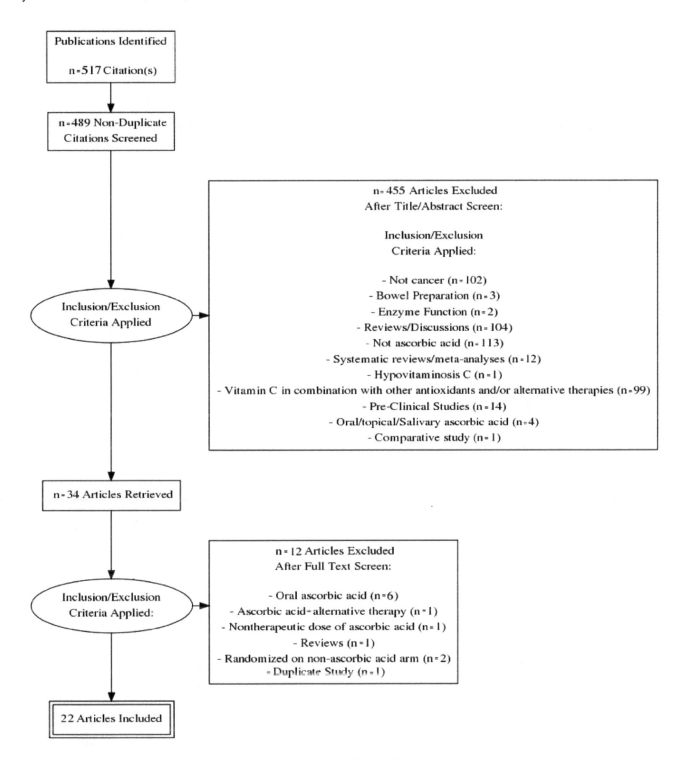

Figure 1. Prisma Flow Diagram.

Study Characteristics

A total of 22 articles (containing 23 trials) that included 401 patients evaluated IV ascorbate (Tables 1–3). Of these trials, eleven trials evaluated arsenic trioxide in combination with intravenous ascorbic acid clinical trials, nine evaluated intravenous ascorbic acid in combination with non-redox cycling agents, and three trials evaluated intravenous ascorbic acid alone. The median sample size of these studies was 17 (range, 3–65) and the IV dose of ascorbate ranged from 1 g daily to 1.5 g/kg thrice weekly.

Table 1. Low dose IV ascorbate + arsenic trioxide trials—Phase I and II trials.

Reference	n	Patient Diagnosis	Trial Design	IV AA Treatment Type and Frequency	Concurrent Treatment Dose	Toxicity	Reported Outcomes/Conclusions
[52]	22	Refractory multiple myeloma	Single Arm	1 g on days 1, 4, 8, and 11 of a 21-day cycle for a maximum of 8 cycles	Bortezomib and Arsenic Trioxide	One occurrence of grade 4 thrombocytopenia was observed in a patient receiving high-dose bortezomib	Objective responses were observed in 27% of patients (2 partial and 4 minor). Median progression-free survival was 5 months and overall survival had not been reached.
[53]	65	Relapsed or refractory multiple myeloma	Single Arm	1 g on days 1–4 of week 1 and twice weekly during weeks 2–5 of a 6 week cycle.	Melphalan and Arsenic Trioxide	Grade 3/4 hematological (3%) or cardiac adverse events occurred infrequently, but grade 3/4 adverse events fever/chills (15%), pain (8%), and fatigue (6%) were reported.	Objective responses occurred in 48% of patients, including complete, partial, and minor responses. Median progression-free survival and overall survival were 7 and 19 months respectively.
[54]	20	Multiple myeloma, relapsed and refractory	Single Arm	1000 mg for 5 consecutive days during week 1, followed by twice weekly during weeks 2–12	Dexamethasone and Arsenic Trioxide	Grade 3 events in 45% and grade 4 events in 5%	30% complete and partial response. Overall median survival was 962 days. 10 patients developed grade 3/4 toxicity to combination treatment.
[55]	17	Lymphoid malignancies, relapsed and refractory.	Single Arm	1000 mg for 5 days during week 1 followed by twice weekly during weeks 2–6	Arsenic Trioxide	1 cardiac death, multiple grade 3 and 4 events	Overall median survival was 7.6 months 6% complete and partial response. Study closed at first interim analysis.
[56]	11	Advanced melanoma	Single Arm	1000 mg for 5 days during week 0, and then twice weekly for an 8 week cycle.	Temozolomide and Arsenic Trioxide	Multiple grade 1 and 2 events.	No responses seen in the first 10 evaluable patients leading to early closure of study.
[57]	5	Refractory metastatic colorectal carcinoma	Single Arm	1000 mg/day for 5 days a week for 5 weeks	Arsenic Trioxide	Grade 3 nausea, vomiting, diarrhea, thrombocytopenia, and anemia	No complete or partial remission observed. CT scans showed stable or progressive disease.
[58]	20	Multiple myeloma, relapsed and refractory	Single Arm	1 mg (one dose during the first week, twice weekly during weeks 2–4)	Dexamethasone and Arsenic Trioxide	Multiple grade 3 and 4 events	Clinical response was observed in 40% of patients (including partial and minor). Median progression free survival = 4 months and median overall survival = 11 months. Authors state that it was difficult to assess activity of each individual agent.
[59]	11	Non-acute promyelocytic leukemia; acute myeloid leukemia (non-APL AML)	Single Arm	1 g/day for 5 days a week for 5 weeks	Arsenic Trioxide	Few grade 3 or 4 adverse effects and the most common grade 3 toxicity was infection though possibly related to the leukemia	One patient achieved a complete response; another achieved a complete remission with incomplete hematologic recovery. Authors concluded that arsenic trioxide + ascorbic acid had limited clinical meaning in non-APL AML patients.
[60]	6	Relapsed or refractory myeloma	Single Arm	1000 mg/day for 25 days over 35 days total.	Arsenic Trioxide	One episode of grade 3 hematologic toxicity (leukopenia) was observed.	Two patients had partial responses; four had stable disease.

Table 1. *Cont.*

Reference	n	Patient Diagnosis	Trial Design	IV AA Treatment Type and Frequency	Concurrent Treatment Dose	Toxicity	Reported Outcomes/Conclusions
[61]	10	Relapsed/refractory multiple myeloma	Single Arm	1 g daily for 3 days of week 1, then twice weekly for a 3-week cycle.	Arsenic Trioxide and Bortezomib	No dose limiting adverse effects.	40% response rate with one patient achieving a durable partial response.
[62]	13	Myelodysplastic Syndrome and Acute Myeloid Leukemia (concurrent diagnoses)	Single Arm	1 g for 5 days during week following each dose of IV Arsenic Trioxide and then once weekly thereafter	Decitabine and Arsenic Trioxide	Grade 3 and 4 events; two patient deaths occurred not related to treatment	One morphologic complete remission was observed. Five patients had stable disease after recovery. 0.2 mg/kg identified as maximum tolerated dose of arsenic in combination with Decitabine and Ascorbic Acid.

Note: This table illustrates the eleven clinical trials that evaluated intravenous ascorbate in combination with arsenic trioxide.

Table 2. High dose IV ascorbate + standard therapies—Phase I and II Trials.

Reference	n	Patient Diagnosis	Trial Design	IV AA Treatment Type and Frequency	Concurrent Treatment Dose	Toxicity	Reported Outcomes/Conclusions
[63]	17	Advanced tumors	Single Arm	Five cohorts treated with 30, 50, 70, 90, and 110 g/m² for 4 consecutive days for 4 weeks.	Multivitamin and Eicosapentaenoic acid	Grade 3 and grade 4 hyponatremia, hyperkalemia	3 patients had stable disease, 13 had progressive disease. Recommended dose is 70–80 g/m². This translates to approximately 125 g because the average patient has a body surface area of 1.6–1.9 m².
[64]	3	Relapsed lymphoma	Single Arm	75 g twice weekly	Rituximab, cyclophosphamide, cytarabine, etoposide, dexamethasone	Grade 3 neutropenia, anemia, thrombocytopenia	The authors concluded that 75 g was a safe dose.
[51]	11	Advanced pancreatic adenocarcinoma	Single Arm	15–125 g twice weekly	Gemcitabine	No dose limiting adverse effects	Mean plasma ascorbate levels were significantly higher than baseline. Mean survival time of subjects completing 8 weeks of therapy was 13 ± 2 months.
[21]	14	Pancreatic adenocarcinoma, stage IV	Single Arm	50, 75, and 100 g per infusion (3 cohorts) thrice weekly for 8 weeks	Gemcitabine and Erlotinib	Multiple toxicities, all grades, thought to not be related to AA; grade 4 adverse event included two patients with pulmonary embolism	50% of patients had stable disease. Survival analysis excluded 5 patients who progressed quickly (3 died). Overall mean survival was 182 days.

Table 2. *Cont.*

Reference	n	Patient Diagnosis	Trial Design	IV AA Treatment Type and Frequency	Concurrent Treatment Dose	Toxicity	Reported Outcomes/Conclusions
[50]	25	Stage 3/4 ovarian cancer	Randomized	75 or 100 g twice weekly for 12 months (target plasma concentration 20–23 mM)	Carboplatin and paclitaxel	Ascorbate did not increase grade 3/4; grade 1 and 2 toxicities were substantially decreased	8.75 month increase in PFS in AA-treated arm. Trend to improved OS in AA group; no numerical data reported.
[22]	16	Various cancer types (lung, rectum, colon, bladder, ovary, cervix, tonsil, breast, biliary tract)	Single Arm	1.5 g/kg body weight infused three times (at least one day apart) on week days during weeks when chemotherapy was administered (but not on the same day as intravenous chemotherapy) and any two days at least one day apart during weeks when no chemotherapy was given.	Standard care chemotherapy.	Increased thirst and increased urinary flow; these adverse symptoms did not appear to be caused by the ascorbate molecule	Patients experienced unexpected transient stable disease, increased energy, and functional improvement.
[30] Phase I study	13	Glioblastoma	Single Arm	Radiation phase: radiation (61.2 Gy in 34 fractions), temozolomide (75 mg/m^2 daily for a maximum of 49 days), ascorbate (doses ranging from 15–125 g, 3 times per week for 7 weeks) Adjuvant phase: 6 cycles of 28 days; treatment with temozolomide (1 dose-escalation to 200 mg/m^2 if no toxicity in cycle 1), ascorbate (2 times per week, dose-escalation until 20 mM plasma concentration, around ~85 g infusion).	Ascorbate with radiation and temozolomide	Radiation phase toxicity: Grade 2 and 3 fatigue and nausea; grade 2 infection; grade 3 vomiting Adjuvant phase toxicity: grade 2 fatigue and nausea; grade 1 vomiting; grade 3 leukopenia; and grade 3 neutropenia.	Progression-free survival 13.3 months; average overall survival 21.5 months.
[30] Phase II study	14	Advanced stage non-small cell lung cancer	Single Arm	1 cycle is 21 days; IV carboplatin (AUC 6, 4 cycles), IV paclitaxel (200 mg/m^2, 4 cycles), IV pharmacological ascorbate (two 75 g infusions per week, up to 4 cycles)	Carboplatin, paclitaxel, and ascorbate	No grade 3 or 4 toxicities related to ascorbate	Imaging confirmed partial responses to therapy ($n = 4$), stable disease ($n = 9$), disease progression ($n = 1$)
[65]	14	Locally advanced or metastatic prostate cancer	Single Arm	Phase I: Escalating dose of IVC from 25 g to 100 g and gemcitabine alone at 1000 mg/m^2 (week 3) with a few patients receiving reduced doses and gemcitabine with IVC (week 4) Phase IIa: no gemcitabine for 1 week and then continuous treatment of gemcitabine until disease progression or unacceptable toxicity and IVC 3 times per week	IVC and gemcitabine	Low toxicity; Increased thirst and nausea were caused by IVC	Patients experienced a mix of stable disease, partial response and disease progression.

Note: This table illustrates the nine clinical trials that evaluated intravenous ascorbate in combination with non-redox cycling chemotherapy agents.

Table 3. High dose IV ascorbate only—Phase I and II trials.

Reference	n	Cancer Type	Trial Design	IV AA Treatment Type and Frequency	Toxicity	Reported Outcomes/Conclusions
				Phase I		
[18]	24	Advanced cancer or hematologic malignancy	Single Arm	1.5 g/kg body weight three times weekly	No dose limiting adverse effects.	Two patients had unexpectedly stable disease.
				Phase II		
[66]	23	Castration-resistant prostate cancer	Single Arm	5 g during weekly week 1, 30 g weekly during week 2, and 60 g weekly during weeks 3–12	Multiple grade 3 events including hypertension and anemia; two patients experienced pulmonary embolism.	Adverse events were thought to be more likely related to disease progression than ascorbic acid.
[23]	11	Late stage terminal cancer patients	Single Arm	150–710 mg/kg/day for up to eight weeks	Two Grade 3 adverse events: one patient with a history of renal calculi developed a kidney stone after thirteen days of treatment and another patient experienced hypokalemia after six weeks of treatment.	One patient had stable disease and continued the treatment for forty-eight weeks. Intravenous vitamin C was deemed relatively safe so long as the patient does not have a history of kidney stone formation.

Note: This table illustrates the three IV ascorbate-only trials evaluated in this review. These trials evaluated IV ascorbate as a single intervention.

3. Results

3.1. Trials Evaluating Low-Dose Intravenous Ascorbic Acid in Combination with Arsenic Trioxide

Out of the 23 clinical trials included in this paper, 11 trials with a total of 200 patients used low dose intravenous ascorbic acid in combination with arsenic trioxide (As_2O_3) (Table 1). In the study design of trials such as these, ascorbic acid does not act as an anti-cancer therapy in its own right. The dose used in such studies (one gram per day) is not considered a pharmacologic or effective dose. The justification for selecting this dose is that when given orally it saturates plasma and ascorbate tissue ascorbate concentrations. However, in most studies, ascorbate was administered intravenously, for unclear reasons [29]. Ascorbate was added as a redox cycling compound to facilitate the anti-cancer activity of As_2O_3. Thus, for these trials, the main source of anti-cancer activity is As_2O_3 and all of the effects produced in these trials should be attributed to As_2O_3 [29].

Berenson et al. reported two phase II trials [52,53] in patients with refractory/multiple myeloma that included low dose IV ascorbic acid. In the 2006 study, patients ($n = 65$) received IV ascorbic acid (1 g on Days 1–4) and As_2O_3 and melphalan. A response rate of 48% was observed with a progression-free survival of seven months and overall survival of 19 months [53]. In the 2007 study, patients ($n = 22$) were treated with IV ascorbate (1 g on Days 1, 4, 8, and 11 of a 21-day cycle for a maximum of eight cycles) in combination with Bortezomib and As_2O_3 [52]. A response rate of 27% was observed and median progression-free survival was five months. Both studies reported grade 3/4 adverse events. Because of the trial design and types of toxicities, adverse events were likely related to chemotherapy.

Two As_2O_3 trials examined the benefits of IV ascorbate in combination with chemotherapy used response rate as the primary outcome [54,55]. Abou-Jawade et al. reported a single arm study of IV ascorbate (1000 mg daily for five days and then twice weekly for nine weeks) in combination with Dexamethasone and As_2O_3 for patients of relapsed and refractory myeloma ($n = 20$). The authors reported an overall response rate of 30%, which included both partial and complete response. Ten patients developed grade 3 or 4 toxicity to this treatment combination, although toxicity due to ascorbate was not defined. Chang et al. reported a similar phase II trial in which patients with lymphoid malignancies ($n = 17$) were treated with IV ascorbate (1000 mg daily for five days then twice weekly) alongside As_2O_3. An overall response rate of 6% was reported and severe toxicities (multiple grade 3, 4, and 5 events) were observed. The trial was closed after the first interim analysis due to lack of activity. Similarly, in a phase II trial by Bael et al. in patients with advanced melanoma ($n = 11$) being treated with IV ascorbate (1000 mg for five days for one week, then twice weekly for an additional eight weeks) in combination with Temozolomide and As_2O_3, no responses were seen in the first 10 evaluable patients leading to early closure of the study [56].

Three trials examined the benefit of IV ascorbate (1000 mg/day for five days) in combination with As_2O_3 only [57–59]. Subbarayan et al. reported a study in which patients of refractory metastatic colorectal carcinoma ($n = 5$) were treated with this combination, and multiple grade 3 events were reported (nausea, vomiting, diarrhea, thrombocytopenia, and anemia), although no complete or partial remission was observed [57]. Wu et al. reported a similar trial with patients of relapsed/refractory multiple myeloma ($n = 20$), but this study was reported in a letter format only [58]. A median survival time of 11 months was observed. In the 2014 study by Aldoss et al., however, intravenous AA was evaluated in combination with As_2O_3, which is highly effective in acute promyelocytic leukemia (APL), but, despite its multiple mechanisms of action, it has no activity in acute myeloid leukemia (AML) that excludes APL (non-APL AML). The patient population ($n = 11$) in this study were all diagnosed with non-APL AML and were administered intravenous As_2O_3 (0.25 mg/kg/day over 1–4 h) with intravenous AA (1 g/day over 30 min after As_2O_3) for five days a week for five weeks (25 doses). Among 10 evaluable patients, one achieved a complete response, one achieved a partial remission with incomplete hematologic recovery, and four patients had disappearance of blasts from peripheral blood and bone marrow. The observed As_2O_3 toxicity was mild; very few grade 3 or 4 adverse effects and the most common grade 3 toxicity was infection, although possibly related to the leukemia. The authors concluded that combination of As_2O_3 and AA had limited clinical meaningful anti-leukemia activity in patients with non-APL AML [59].

Bahlis et al. reported a study using As_2O_3 in combination with IV ascorbate to ascertain dosing of As_2O_3. Patients of refractory myeloma ($n = 6$) were treated with IV ascorbate dose of 1000 mg/day for 25 days over 35 days total, and 0.25 mg/kg per day of As_2O_3 was defined as an appropriate dose [60]. A partial response rate of 36% was observed and no toxicities above grade 2 were reported. It is unclear if these toxicities were due to the addition of ascorbic acid, increased As_2O_3, the schedule, or duration of treatment. Held et al. reported a similar phase I trial that also aimed to estimate the maximum tolerated dose of As_2O_3 and bortezomib that can be used in combination with IV ascorbate (1 g daily for three days of Week 1, then twice weekly for a three-week cycle) in patients with relapsed/refractory multiple myeloma ($n = 10$) [61]. No dose-limiting toxicities were reported and a 40% response rate was reported. Welch et al. reported a trial with patients of myelodysplastic syndrome and acute myeloid leukemia ($n = 13$) being treated with Decitabine and As_2O_3 and IV ascorbate (1000 mg for five days during Week 1 following each dose of IV As_2O_3 and then once weekly thereafter) [62]. Five patients had stable disease after recovery and multiple grade 3 and 4 events were reported; the authors stated that these adverse events were expected given the patient population and type of chemotherapy but did not clarify if the addition of ascorbate was a contributing factor.

3.2. Trials Evaluating High-Dose Intravenous Ascorbic Acid with Standard Chemo- and Radiotherapy Agents

Stephenson et al. reported a phase I trial with patients with advanced malignancies ($n = 17$) being treated with IV ascorbate 70–80 g/m^2 (this translates to approximately 125 g because the average patient has body surface of 1.6–1.9 m^2) [67] 3–4 times a week to obtain optimal peak plasma concentrations in combination with multivitamin and eicosapentaenoic acid treatment [63]. Only two patients completed the entire four-week study period, and stable disease rate and progressive disease rate of 19% and 81% were reported, respectively. Grade 3 and 4 metabolic toxicities (hypernatremia and hypokalemia) related to ascorbate was observed. Kawada et al. reported a similar study in patients with relapsed lymphoma ($n = 3$) that were treated with rituximab, cyclophosphamide, cytarabine, etoposide, and dexamethasone alongside IV ascorbate (75 g twice weekly) [64]. Grade 3 neutropenia, anemia, and thrombocytopenia were observed, but no obvious side effects due to ascorbic acid were observed, leading the authors to conclude that 75 g of IV ascorbate is a safe dose. It is likely that hypernatremia and hyperkalemia, reported by Stephenson et al., was secondary to the approximately two-fold higher ascorbate dose that patients received in comparison to other trials.

Two phase I trials examined the benefits of IV ascorbate in combination with gemcitabine in patients with advanced pancreas adenocarcinoma [21,51]. Both Welsh et al. ($n = 13$) and Monti et al. ($n = 14$) reported toxicity in patients related to gemcitabine and not secondary to ascorbate [21,51]. Response rates and survival duration in both studies were reported only for patients who did not progress within the first month of treatment and are thus not representative of standard clinical reporting. Monti et al. reported that seven of nine patients had stable disease with a mean overall survival of 155 ± 182 days and Welsh et al. reported a 13 ± 2-month mean survival in the nine patients that were analyzed.

Ma et al. reported a trial of patients with stage 3 and 4 ovarian cancer ($n = 25$) receiving carboplatin and paclitaxel chemotherapy [50]. Patients were randomized to either IV ascorbate (75 g or 100 g twice weekly for 12 months) with chemotherapy ($n = 13$) or chemotherapy alone ($n = 12$). The trial was not blinded and the primary outcome was toxicity. The ascorbate group was observed to have fewer grade 1/2 adverse events per encounter as compared to the group that received only chemotherapy. A trend toward improvement in median overall-survival was reported, although no numerical data were reported. Median time for disease progression/relapse was reported as 25.5 months in the ascorbate arm and 16.75 in the chemotherapy arm. This trial also demonstrated key information related to the safety profile of ascorbate as patients were treated for more than a year with minimal adverse effects.

Hoffer et al. (2015) reported a study with patients of various cancer types ($n = 16$) treated with IV ascorbate. Patients were administered ascorbate at a dose of 1.5 g/kg three times on weekdays during weeks when chemotherapy was administered, and at least one day apart during weeks when no chemotherapy was given). This was given in combination with standard care chemotherapy, which was not defined [22]. Adverse effects included increased thirst and urinary flow. Transient stable disease, increased energy, and functional improvement were observed in patients.

Schoenfeld et al. (2017) reported a phase I study with glioblastoma (GBM) patients ($n = 13$) receiving pharmacological ascorbate with radiation and temozolomide [30]. The study had two phases: the radiation phase (which started on Day 1 of the radiation phase and ended on Cycle 1, Day 1 of the adjuvant period) and the adjuvant phase (which began on Cycle 1, Day 1 until Cycle 6, Day 28) [30]. The participants in the radiation phase received radiation (61.2 Gy in 34 fractions), temozolomide (75 mg/m^2 daily for a maximum of 49 days) and ascorbate (dose cohorts ranging from 15–125 g, three times per week for seven weeks) [30]. In the adjuvant phase, participants received temozolomide (Days 1–5 of a 28-day cycle and one dose-escalation to 200 mg/m^2 took place if Cycle 1 was tolerable) and ascorbate (infusions took place two times per week and dose was increased over two infusions until a plasma concentration of 20 mM was reached, which was achieved with an 87.5 g infusion) for about 28 weeks [30]. Adverse effects in the radiation phase included grade 2 and 3 fatigue and nausea, grade 2 infection, and grade 3 vomiting. In the adjuvant phase, patients experienced grade 2 fatigue and nausea, grade 1 vomiting, grade 3 leukopenia, and neutropenia. At the time of publishing in 2017, the average PFS with Schoenfeld et al.'s therapy was 13.3 months as compared to PFS of seven months in Stupp et al. (2005) [61] which treated GBM patients with similar characteristics with concurrent radiation and temozolomide or radiation only. Average overall survival was 21.5 months as compared to 14 months in Stupp et al., 2005 [30].

Schoenfeld et al. (2017) also reported a phase II study with advanced stage non-small-cell-lung carcinoma (NSCLC) patients ($n = 14$) treated with carboplatin, paclitaxel and pharmacological ascorbate [30]. Participants were administered IV carboplatin (AUC 6, four cycles), IV paclitaxel (200 mg/m^2, four cycles), and IV pharmacological ascorbate (75 g per infusion, two infusions per week, up to four cycles); one cycle was 28 days [30]. No grade 3 or 4 toxicities related to ascorbate were noted. Imaging-confirmed partial responses to therapy in patients who completed the trial ($n = 4$), stable disease ($n = 9$), and new lesion development ($n = 1$) indicating disease progression despite the patient having a stable target lesion [30].

Polireddy et al. (2017) reported a Phase I/IIa trial with locally advanced or metastatic prostate cancer patients ($n = 14$) who were not eligible for surgical resection with high-dose IVC and gemcitabine chemotherapy [62]. Phase I initially enrolled 14 patients but only 12 patients completed a pharmacokinetic evaluation of IVC and gemcitabine alone. IVC dose escalated from 25 g to 100 g and gemcitabine dose at 1000 mg/m^2, with a few patients receiving reduced doses as determined by the treating oncologist give from Week 1 to Week 4 and subsequently in combination during Week 4. In Phase IIa, the 12 patients were given IVC three-times weekly at doses determined by the treating oncologist and gemcitabine following a rest week after two consecutive weeks of a determined dose and then treatment until tumor progression or patient withdrawal. Overall survival was 15.1 months with 5 of 12 patients not surviving over one year, 6 of 12 patients surviving over one year, and 1 of 12 surviving more than two decades after diagnosis. Over the course of treatment, one patient with Stage III pancreatic ductal carcinoma experienced tumor shrinkage/stabilization and tumor margins becoming more distinct, making the patient eligible for surgery. Grade 1 nausea and thirst related to IVC were the only adverse events noted. The study showed IVC has low toxicity and does not alter gemcitabine pharmacokinetics significantly.

3.3. IV Ascorbate Only Trials

Hoffer et al. (2008) reported a phase I trial in patients with advanced cancer or hematologic malignancy ($n = 24$) treated with up to 1.5 g/kg body weight of IV ascorbate three times weekly.

No dose limiting adverse effects were reported and two patients had unexpectedly stable disease [18]. Nielsen et al. (2017) reported a similar study in patients with castration-resistant prostate cancer (n = 23) treated with IV ascorbate 5 g once during Week 1, 30 g weekly during Week 2, and 60 g once weekly during Weeks 3–12 [34]. Multiple grade 3 events were reported including hypertension and anemia; two patients experienced a pulmonary embolism; however, the authors stated that treatment-induced toxicity was limited and the two episodes of pulmonary embolism can likely be attributed to the fact that cancer is known to increase the risk of thromboembolic events. However, without a placebo-controlled trial, attribution to disease or ascorbate cannot be definitely proven. Both studies reported no anticancer response or disease remission.

Lastly, Riordan et al. reported a trial in which late stage terminal cancer patients (n = 11) were given continuous infusions of 150–710 mg/kg/day for up to eight weeks. Intravenous infusions increased plasma ascorbate concentrations to a mean of 1.1 mM. Two Grade 3 adverse events to the agent were reported: one patient with a history of renal calculi developed a kidney stone after thirteen days of treatment and another patient experienced hypokalemia after six weeks of treatment; the authors state that these adverse events could possibly be related to ascorbic acid, but it remains unclear. One patient had stable disease and continued the treatment for forty-eight weeks. The authors concluded that intravenous vitamin C administered continuously is relatively safe so long as the patient does not have a history of kidney stone formation [23].

3.4. Potential of Benefit and Current Limitations

Clinical trials that have examined the use of IV ascorbate in cancer patient populations have yielded results that suggest its potential to produce various beneficial effects. In one trial, IV ascorbate was used in elderly patients with advanced cancer who had failed all other therapies. Two of the patients had unexpected stable disease after eight weeks of ascorbic acid treatment [18]. A phase I trial in patients with metastatic stage 4 pancreatic cancer who were treated with gemcitabine and IV ascorbate as primary therapy until tumor progression showed few toxicities associated with the treatment [51]. The nine patients had a tripling of disease free interval compared to literature controls and a doubling of survival compared to retrospective controls. Some patients were treated for longer durations, for instance over a year in the Ma et al. trial [50], and had substantially decreased grade 1 and 2 adverse events when compared to the group not receiving ascorbate.

Similarly, a trial of patients with metastatic stage 4 pancreatic cancer illustrated benefit as eight of nine patients experienced tumor shrinkage after eight weeks of primary therapy (gemcitabine and erlotinib) and pharmacological ascorbate as measure by CT scans [21]. The results of these trials and others discussed in this article suggest that IV ascorbate is useful as a single agent or combined with a primary therapy. It has the benefit of being a non-toxic treatment modality and reducing toxicity of chemotherapeutics when combined with conventional therapies. In one randomized ovarian cancer trial, patients receiving IV ascorbic acid reported lower levels of low-grade gastrointestinal, hepatobiliary, dermatological, immune/infection, pulmonary and renal toxicities commonly associated with carboplatin and paclitaxel treatment [50]. One retrospective cohort study [68] compared breast cancer patients who received IV ascorbic acid to those who did not, at a dose of 7.5 g weekly without blinding. In the first year following surgery, patients who received ascorbate when compared to a control group had significant reductions in nausea (p = 0.022), loss of appetite (p = 0.005), fatigue (p = 0.023), dizziness (p = 0.004) and hemorrhagic diathesis (p = 0.032). Limitations of this study are the absence of blinding, the non-therapeutic dosing and once weekly frequency of ascorbate administration. Even so, the results suggest that IV ascorbate could induce reduction in toxicities, perhaps via mechanisms that are different than those that target cancer cells. To definitively associate IV ascorbate with clinical benefit and/or toxicity, more rigorous randomized-placebo trials must be conducted. Many of the clinical studies conducted to date do not contain a control group, which makes determining efficacy difficult.

In addition to examining efficacy, there is need for a determination of IV AA dosing amount, dosing frequency, and duration of treatment alone or in combination with other therapies. Currently, there is no consensus on these parameters. For dosing of intravenous ascorbate, doses used most frequently are based on one of a few regimens suggested by Riordan and colleagues. The goal was to achieve a plasma concentration of approximately 22 mM, which was effective in a hollow-fiber tumor model [69]. This dosing amount translates as approximately 1 g/kg. For dosing frequency, a regimen of 2–3 times weekly was empiric, with patient ability and/or willingness to receive treatment being limiting factors. Considering dosing amount and frequency together, therapy less than twice weekly, with dosing less than 1 g/kg, appears to be therapeutically ineffective [66], while dosing at 1 g/kg at least twice weekly has promise [21,51]. For duration needed to assess responsiveness, clinically detectable ascorbate action is relatively slow compared to many other cancer therapies. In most reports, a minimum 2–3-month time frame was needed to assess response [17,21,51,69,70]. Due to unknowns about concomitant administration with standard chemotherapies, ascorbate most often has been administered alone, without other chemotherapy on the same day. When ascorbate was administered on the same day as chemotherapy in a series of cases, the clinical response was seemingly enhanced by ascorbate [66,70]. Unfortunately, in this case series, only minimal information was provided about adverse events and non-responders. Based on the totality of available evidence and our experience, some recommendations can be made for future studies. These recommendations include that ascorbate dosing should be 1 g/kg, at a minimum frequency of twice weekly, and with a minimum of a two-month and preferably three-month trial period before efficacy is assessed. However, further research into the potential benefit of IV AA is necessary before well-defined clinical recommendations can be made.

4. Future Directions

Thus far, a total of 185 cancer patients have been treated with IV vitamin C within the clinical trials discussed in this review, excluding those treated with low-dose vitamin C (redox coupling mechanism) (Figure 2). Moreover, there are 11 studies in progress that aim to investigate the clinical efficacy of pharmacological IV ascorbate (Table 4) including a total of 405 patients. There are two randomized studies (NCT03175341 and NCT02516670) and two non-randomized studies (NCT01852890 and NCT01752491). Both hematological and solid organ malignancies are being evaluated. Note that, even though all studies using ascorbate are included, ascorbate dosing may be well below that considered pharmacologic dosing.

In the Phase I trials, the safety of high dose ascorbate is being tested in combination with gemcitabine and radiation therapy (NCT01852890), temozolomide, and radiation therapy (NCT01752491), and gemcitabine, cisplatin, and nab-paclitaxel (NCT03410030). These studies aim to further determine the safety and toxicity of high dose ascorbate, in addition to establishing a pharmacokinetic profile, elucidating the biological responsiveness, and determining its efficacy in reducing side effects of chemotherapy.

In the Phase II trials, ascorbate is being tested in combination with gemcitabine and nab-paclitaxel (NCT02905578), temozolomide and radiation therapy (NCT02344355). The randomized Phase II trials, such as *Docetaxel with or without Ascorbic Acid in Treating Patients with Metastatic Prostate Cancer (NCT02516670)*, provide a vehicle for assessing the clinical effectiveness of ascorbate in a high-quality, placebo-controlled setting. These kinds of trials have the potential to further elucidate any synergistic anticancer effects that IV ascorbate might have when used in combination with chemotherapeutic agents. This has the potential to provide patients with additional treatment options.

Table 4. Upcoming and active interventional trials utilizing pharmacological IV ascorbate.

Phase	Trial Title	Trial Design	IV AA Treatment Type and Frequency	Interventions	Status	Enrollment	NCT Identifier
Phase I	Gemcitabine, Ascorbate, Radiation Therapy for Pancreatic Cancer	Single Arm	50 g–100 g during radiation therapy for 5–6 weeks; escalating dose based on tolerance	Ascorbate Gemcitabine Radiation Therapy	Ongoing, closed to accrual	16	NCT01852890
Phase I	High-Dose Ascorbate in Glioblastoma Multiforme	Single Arm	15 g–87.5 g by IV 3×/week for 12 weeks	Ascorbate Temozolomide Radiation Therapy	Ongoing, closed to accrual	13	NCT01752491
Phase I	High Dose Ascorbic Acid (AA) + Nanoparticle Paclitaxel Protein Bound + Cisplatin + Gemcitabine (AA NABPLAGEM) in Patients Who Have No Prior Therapy for Their Metastatic Pancreatic Cancer	Single Arm	No dosing information provided	Ascorbic Acid Nab-paclitaxel Cisplatin Gemcitabine	Ongoing, actively recruiting participants	36	NCT03410030
Phase II	High-dose Ascorbate for Pancreatic Cancer (PACMAN 2.1)	Single Arm	75 g by IV 3×/week for 4 weeks	Ascorbate Gemcitabine Nab-paclitaxel	Accrual began 28 May 2018	30	NCT02905578
Phase II	High-Dose Ascorbate in Stage IV Non-Small Cell Lung Cancer	Single Arm	75 g by IV 2×/week for up to 12 weeks	Ascorbic Acid Carboplatin Paclitaxel	Ongoing, actively recruiting participants	57	NCT02420314
Phase II	High-Dose Ascorbate in Glioblastoma Multiforme	Single Arm	87.5 g by IV 3×/week during radiation therapy After radiation ascorbate 2×/week	Temozolomide Ascorbic Acid Radiation Therapy	Ongoing, actively recruiting participants	90	NCT0344355
Phase II	Adding Ascorbate to Chemotherapy and Radiation Therapy for NSCLC (XACT-LUNG)	Single Arm	Concurrent phase: 75 g by IV 3×/week for up to 7 weeks Consolidation phase: 75 g by IV 2×/week for two cycles (42 days)	Paclitaxel Carboplatin Ascorbate Radiation Therapy	Ongoing, actively recruiting participants	46	NCT02905591
Phase II	Docetaxel with or Without Ascorbic Acid in Treating Patients with Metastatic Prostate Cancer	Randomized	1 g/kg 3× per week	Docetaxel Ascorbic Acid or Placebo	Ongoing, actively recruiting participants	69	NCT02516670

Table 4. *Cont.*

Phase	Trial Title	Trial Design	IV AA Treatment Type and Frequency	Interventions	Status	Enrollment	NCT Identifier
Phase I/II	Randomized Study to Evaluate the Role of Intravenous Ascorbic Acid Supplementation to Conventional Neoadjuvant Chemotherapy in Women with Breast Cancer	Randomized	1.5 g on day 1 followed by 0.75 g on day 2–4 at each chemotherapy cycle	Ascorbic Acid Placebo	Status Unknown	30	NCT03175341
Phase I/II	Evaluating the Safety and Tolerability of Vitamin C in Patients with Intermediate or High Risk Myelodysplastic Syndrome with TET2 Mutations	Single Arm	50 gm CIVI/24 h x 5 days every 4 week	Ascorbic acid	Accrual begins 26 June 2018	18	NCT03433781

Note: This table illustrates the current and upcoming trials listed on clinicaltrials.gov that are utilizing standard of care chemotherapeutics in combination with pharmacological IV ascorbate.

In addition to these clinical studies, laboratory research has attempted to elucidate the mechanism of action of vitamin C in cancer cells. Yun et al. showed that high dose vitamin C selectively killed KRAS and BRAF mutants in colorectal cancer cells by inducing increased uptake of oxidized vitamin C and targeting the glycolytic pathway [34], although these findings have not been confirmed by others [30,36,48]. Nevertheless, potential remains to identify subtypes of cancer that might benefit from IV pharmacological ascorbate in a clinical setting.

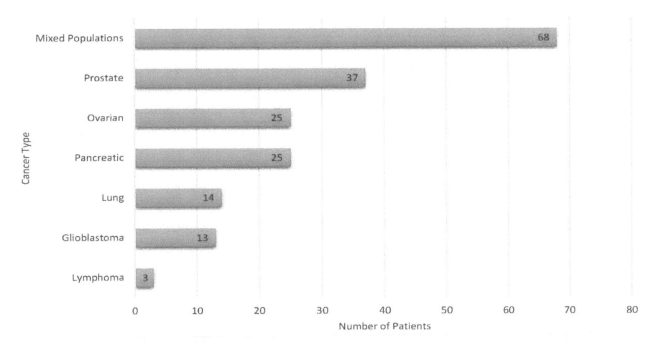

Figure 2. This figure represents the total number of cancer patients ($n = 185$) that were treated with intravenous ascorbic acid within the clinical trials summarized in this paper. This figure does not include patients who were enrolled in trials that used arsenic trioxide.

5. Conclusions

Evidence supporting the existence of an anticancer effect of intravenous ascorbate is mixed, whether it is given a single agent or in combination with other concurrent standard therapies. In single-arm trials that used IV ascorbate in combination with concurrent standard therapies, it is unclear which agent delivered which effects. Only one randomized clinical trial has been reported, showing a trend toward overall survival, a significant 8.5 week increase in progression-free survival, and decreased adverse events in the IV ascorbate arm in ovarian cancer patients.

Current research indicates that IV ascorbate is well tolerated and has reported some positive results. However, high-quality placebo-controlled trials such as those being offered in prostate (NCT02516670) and breast cancer (NCT03175341) are needed to strengthen the present evidence base to support continuation of IV ascorbate being offered as a treatment by practitioners. Until these trials are completed, patients should be informed of the investigational status of IV ascorbate as a cancer treatment.

Acknowledgments: C.J.P. was supported by NIH P30 CA006973, K23 CA197526 and the Marcus Foundation. M.L. was supported by the Intramural Research Program, NIDDK, NIH DK053212-12.

Abbreviations

AA	Ascorbic Acid
AML	Acute Myeloid Leukemia
APL	Acute Promyelocytic Leukemia
As_2O_3	Arsenic Trioxide
CT	Computed Tomography
CTCAE	Common Terminology Criteria for Adverse Events
DHA	Dehydroascorbic acid
DNA	Deoxyribonucleic acid
GBM	Glioblastoma
GADPH	Glyceraldehyde 3-phosphate dehydrogenase
GSH	Glutathione
HIF	Hypoxia inducible factors
H_2O_2	Hydrogen Peroxide
IV	Intravenous
IVC	Intravenous vitamin C
mM	Millimolar
NSCLC	Non-small cell lung cancer
OS	Overall survival
PFS	Progression free survival
PHD	Prolyl-4-hydroxylase domain
ROS	Reactive oxygen species
TET	Ten eleven translocation

References

1. McCormick, W. Cancer: The preconditioning factor in pathogenesis; a new etiologic approach. *Arch. Pediatr.* **1954**, *71*, 313–322. [PubMed]
2. Moertel, C.G.; Fleming, T.R.; Creagan, E.T.; Rubin, J.; O'Connell, M.J.; Ames, M.M. High-dose vitamin C versus placebo in the treatment of patients with advanced cancer who have had no prior chemotherapy. A randomized double-blind comparison. *N. Engl. J. Med.* **1985**, *312*, 137–141. [CrossRef] [PubMed]
3. Cimmino, L.; Dolgalev, I.; Wang, Y.; Yoshimi, A.; Martin, G.H.; Wang, J.; Ng, V.; Xia, B.; Witkowski, M.T.; Mitchell-Flack, M.; et al. Restoration of TET2 Function Blocks Aberrant Self-Renewal and Leukemia Progression. *Cell* **2017**, *170*, 1079–1095. [CrossRef] [PubMed]
4. Cameron, E.; Pauling, L. The orthomolecular treatment of cancer. I. The role of ascorbic acid in host resistance. *Chem. Biol. Interact.* **1974**, *9*, 273–283. [CrossRef]
5. Cameron, E.; Campbell, A. The orthomolecular treatment of cancer. II. Clinical trial of high-dose ascorbic acid supplements in advanced human cancer. *Chem. Biol. Interact.* **1974**, *9*, 285–315. [CrossRef]
6. Cameron, E.; Campbell, A.; Jack, T. The orthomolecular treatment of cancer. III. Reticulum cell sarcoma: Double complete regression induced by high-dose ascorbic acid therapy. *Chem. Biol. Interact.* **1975**, *11*, 387–393. [CrossRef]
7. Cameron, E.; Pauling, L. Supplemental ascorbate in the supportive treatment of cancer: Prolongation of survival times in terminal human cancer. *Proc. Natl. Acad. Sci. USA* **1976**, *73*, 3685–3689. [CrossRef] [PubMed]
8. Cameron, E.; Pauling, L. Supplemental ascorbate in the supportive treatment of cancer: Reevaluation of prolongation of survival times in terminal human cancer. *Proc. Natl. Acad. Sci. USA* **1978**, *75*, 4538–4542. [CrossRef] [PubMed]
9. Padayatty, S.J.; Levine, M. Reevaluation of ascorbate in cancer treatment: Emerging evidence, open minds and serendipity. *J. Am. Coll. Nutr.* **2000**, *19*, 423–425. [CrossRef] [PubMed]
10. Creagan, E.T.; Moertel, C.G.; O'Fallon, J.R.; Schutt, A.J.; O'Connell, M.J.; Rubin, J.; Frytak, S. Failure of high-dose vitamin C (ascorbic acid) therapy to benefit patients with advanced cancer. A controlled trial. *N. Engl. J. Med.* **1979**, *301*, 687–690. [CrossRef] [PubMed]

11. Jacobs, C.; Hutton, B.; Ng, T.; Shorr, R.; Clemons, M. Is there a role for oral or intravenous ascorbate (vitamin C) in treating patients with cancer? A systematic review. *Oncologist* **2015**, *20*, 210–223. [CrossRef] [PubMed]

12. Wittes, R.E. Vitamin C and cancer. *N. Engl. J. Med.* **1985**, *312*, 178–179. [CrossRef] [PubMed]

13. Levine, M.; Conry-Cantilena, C.; Wang, Y.; Welch, R.W.; Washko, P.W.; Dhariwal, K.R.; Park, J.B.; Lazarev, A.; Graumlich, J.F.; King, J.; et al. Vitamin C pharmacokinetics in healthy volunteers: Evidence for a recommended dietary allowance. *Proc. Natl. Acad. Sci. USA* **1996**, *93*, 3704–3709. [CrossRef] [PubMed]

14. Levine, M.; Wang, Y.; Padayatty, S.J.; Morrow, J. A new recommended dietary allowance of vitamin C for healthy young women. *Proc. Natl. Acad. Sci. USA* **2001**, *98*, 9842–9846. [CrossRef] [PubMed]

15. Du, J.; Cullen, J.J.; Buettner, G.R. Ascorbic acid: Chemistry, biology and the treatment of cancer. *Biochim. Biophys. Acta* **2012**, *1826*, 443–457. [CrossRef] [PubMed]

16. Padayatty, S.J.; Sun, H.; Wang, Y.; Riordan, H.D.; Hewitt, S.M.; Katz, A.; Wesley, R.A.; Levine, M. Vitamin C pharmacokinetics: Implications for oral and intravenous use. *Ann. Intern. Med.* **2004**, *140*, 533–537. [CrossRef] [PubMed]

17. Chen, Q.; Espey, M.G.; Sun, A.Y.; Pooput, C.; Kirk, K.L.; Krishna, M.C.; Khosh, D.B.; Drisko, J.; Levine, M. Pharmacologic doses of ascorbate act as a prooxidant and decrease growth of aggressive tumor xenografts in mice. *Proc. Natl. Acad. Sci. USA* **2008**, *105*, 11105–11109. [CrossRef] [PubMed]

18. Hoffer, L.J.; Levine, M.; Assouline, S.; Melnychuk, D.; Padayatty, S.J.; Rosadiuk, K.; Rousseau, C.; Robitaille, L.; Miller, W.H., Jr. Phase I clinical trial of i.v. ascorbic acid in advanced malignancy. *Ann. Oncol.* **2008**, *19*, 1969–1974. [CrossRef] [PubMed]

19. Graumlich, J.F.; Ludden, T.M.; Conry-Cantilena, C.; Cantilena, L.R., Jr.; Wang, Y.; Levine, M. Pharmacokinetic model of ascorbic acid in healthy male volunteers during depletion and repletion. *Pharm. Res.* **1997**, *14*, 1133–1139. [CrossRef] [PubMed]

20. Ohno, S.; Ohno, Y.; Suzuki, N.; Soma, G.; Inoue, M. High-dose vitamin C (ascorbic acid) therapy in the treatment of patients with advanced cancer. *Anticancer Res.* **2009**, *29*, 809–815. [PubMed]

21. Monti, D.A.; Mitchell, E.; Bazzan, A.J.; Littman, S.; Zabrecky, G.; Yeo, C.J.; Pillai, M.V.; Newberg, A.B.; Deshmukh, S.; Levine, M. Phase I evaluation of intravenous ascorbic acid in combination with gemcitabine and erlotinib in patients with metastatic pancreatic cancer. *PLoS ONE* **2012**, *7*, e29794. [CrossRef] [PubMed]

22. Hoffer, L.J.; Robitaille, L.; Zakarian, R.; Melnychuk, D.; Kavan, P.; Agulnik, J.; Cohen, V.; Small, D.; Miller, W.H., Jr. High-dose intravenous vitamin C combined with cytotoxic chemotherapy in patients with advanced cancer: A phase I-II clinical trial. *PLoS ONE* **2015**, *10*, e0120228. [CrossRef] [PubMed]

23. Riordan, H.D.; Casciari, J.J.; Gonzalez, M.J.; Riordan, N.H.; Miranda-Massari, J.R.; Taylor, P.; Jackson, J.A. A pilot clinical study of continuous intravenous ascorbate in terminal cancer patients. *P. R. Health Sci. J.* **2005**, *24*, 269–276. [PubMed]

24. Duconge, J.; Miranda-Massari, J.R.; Gonzalez, M.J.; Jackson, J.A.; Warnock, W.; Riordan, N.H. Pharmacokinetics of vitamin C: Insights into the oral and intravenous administration of ascorbate. *P. R. Health Sci. J.* **2008**, *27*, 7–19. [PubMed]

25. Pauling, L. Are recommended daily allowances for vitamin C adequate? *Proc. Natl. Acad. Sci. USA* **1974**, *71*, 4442–4446. [CrossRef] [PubMed]

26. Langemann, H.; Torhorst, J.; Kabiersch, A.; Krenger, W.; Honegger, C.G. Quantitative determination of water- and lipid-soluble antioxidants in neoplastic and non-neoplastic human breast tissue. *Int. J. Cancer* **1989**, *43*, 1169–1173. [CrossRef] [PubMed]

27. Honegger, C.G.; Torhorst, J.; Langemann, H.; Kabiersch, A.; Krenger, W. Quantitative determination of water-soluble scavengers in neoplastic and non-neoplastic human breast tissue. *Int. J. Cancer* **1988**, *41*, 690–694. [CrossRef] [PubMed]

28. Agus, D.B.; Vera, J.C.; Golde, D.W. Stromal cell oxidation: A mechanism by which tumors obtain vitamin C. *Cancer Res.* **1999**, *59*, 4555–4558. [PubMed]

29. Violet, P.C.; Levine, M. Pharmacologic Ascorbate in Myeloma Treatment: Doses Matter. *EBioMedicine* **2017**, *18*, 9–10. [CrossRef] [PubMed]

30. Schoenfeld, J.D.; Sibenaller, Z.A.; Mapuskar, K.A.; Wagner, B.A.; Cramer-Morales, K.L.; Furqan, M.; Sandhu, S.; Carlisle, T.L.; Smith, M.C.; Abu Hejleh, T.; et al. $O_2^{\bullet-}$ and H_2O_2-Mediated Disruption of Fe Metabolism Causes the Differential Susceptibility of NSCLC and GBM Cancer Cells to Pharmacological Ascorbate. *Cancer Cell* **2017**, *31*, 487–500. [CrossRef] [PubMed]

31. Antunes, F.; Cadenas, E. Estimation of H_2O_2 gradients across biomembranes. *FEBS Lett.* **2000**, *475*, 121–126. [CrossRef]

32. Hyslop, P.A.; Hinshaw, D.B.; Halsey, W.A., Jr.; Schraufstatter, I.U.; Sauerheber, R.D.; Spragg, R.G.; Jackson, J.H.; Cochrane, C.G. Mechanisms of oxidant-mediated cell injury. The glycolytic and mitochondrial pathways of ADP phosphorylation are major intracellular targets inactivated by hydrogen peroxide. *J. Biol. Chem.* **1988**, *263*, 1665–1675. [PubMed]

33. Ahmad, I.M.; Aykin-Burns, N.; Sim, J.E.; Walsh, S.A.; Higashikubo, R.; Buettner, G.R.; Venkataraman, S.; Mackey, M.A.; Flanagan, S.W.; Oberley, L.W.; et al. Mitochondrial O^{2-} and H_2O_2 mediate glucose deprivation-induced stress in human cancer cells. *J. Biol. Chem.* **2005**, *280*, 4254–4263. [CrossRef] [PubMed]

34. Yun, J.; Mullarky, E.; Lu, C.; Bosch, K.N.; Kavalier, A.; Rivera, K.; Roper, J.; Chio, I.I.; Giannopoulou, E.G.; Rago, C.; et al. Vitamin C selectively kills KRAS and BRAF mutant colorectal cancer cells by targeting GAPDH. *Science* **2015**, *350*, 1391–1396. [CrossRef] [PubMed]

35. Van der Reest, J.; Gottlieb, E. Anti-cancer effects of vitamin C. revisited. *Cell Res.* **2016**, *26*, 269–270. [CrossRef] [PubMed]

36. Chen, Q.; Espey, M.G.; Krishna, M.C.; Mitchell, J.B.; Corpe, C.P.; Buettner, G.R.; Shacter, E.; Levine, M. Pharmacologic ascorbic acid concentrations selectively kill cancer cells: Action as a pro-drug to deliver hydrogen peroxide to tissues. *Proc. Natl. Acad. Sci. USA* **2005**, *102*, 13604–13609. [CrossRef] [PubMed]

37. Chen, S.; Roffey, D.M.; Dion, C.A.; Arab, A.; Wai, E.K. Effect of Perioperative Vitamin C Supplementation on Postoperative Pain and the Incidence of Chronic Regional Pain Syndrome: A Systematic Review and Meta-Analysis. *Clin. J. Pain* **2016**, *32*, 179–185. [CrossRef] [PubMed]

38. Blaschke, K.; Ebata, K.T.; Karimi, M.M.; Zepeda-Martinez, J.A.; Goyal, P.; Mahapatra, S.; Tam, A.; Laird, D.J.; Hirst, M.; Rao, A.; et al. Vitamin C induces Tet-dependent DNA demethylation and a blastocyst-like state in ES cells. *Nature* **2013**, *500*, 222–226. [CrossRef] [PubMed]

39. Minor, E.A.; Court, B.L.; Young, J.I.; Wang, G. Ascorbate induces ten-eleven translocation (Tet) methylcytosine dioxygenase-mediated generation of 5-hydroxymethylcytosine. *J. Biol. Chem.* **2013**, *288*, 13669–13674. [CrossRef] [PubMed]

40. Shenoy, N.; Bhagat, T.; Nieves, E.; Stenson, M.; Lawson, J.; Choudhary, G.S.; Habermann, T.; Nowakowski, G.; Singh, R.; Wu, X.; et al. Upregulation of TET activity with ascorbic acid induces epigenetic modulation of lymphoma cells. *Blood Cancer J.* **2017**, *7*, e587. [CrossRef] [PubMed]

41. Wu, X.; Zhang, Y. TET-mediated active DNA demethylation: Mechanism, function and beyond. *Nat. Rev. Genet.* **2017**, *18*, 517–534. [CrossRef] [PubMed]

42. Agathocleous, M.; Meacham, C.E.; Burgess, R.J.; Piskounova, E.; Zhao, Z.; Crane, G.M.; Cowin, B.L.; Bruner, E.; Murphy, M.M.; Chen, W.; et al. Ascorbate regulates haematopoietic stem cell function and leukaemogenesis. *Nature* **2017**, *549*, 476–481. [CrossRef] [PubMed]

43. Masoud, G.N.; Li, W. HIF-1alpha pathway: Role, regulation and intervention for cancer therapy. *Acta Pharm. Sin. B* **2015**, *5*, 378–389. [CrossRef] [PubMed]

44. Campbell, E.J.; Vissers, M.C.; Bozonet, S.; Dyer, A.; Robinson, B.A.; Dachs, G.U. Restoring physiological levels of ascorbate slows tumor growth and moderates HIF-1 pathway activity in $Gulo^{-/-}$ mice. *Cancer Med.* **2015**, *4*, 303–314. [CrossRef] [PubMed]

45. Carr, A.C.; Vissers, M.C.; Cook, J.S. The effect of intravenous vitamin C on cancer- and chemotherapy-related fatigue and quality of life. *Front. Oncol.* **2014**, *4*, 283. [CrossRef] [PubMed]

46. Chen, Q.; Espey, M.G.; Sun, A.Y.; Lee, J.H.; Krishna, M.C.; Shacter, E.; Choyke, P.L.; Pooput, C.; Kirk, K.L.; Buettner, G.R.; et al. Ascorbate in pharmacologic concentrations selectively generates ascorbate radical and hydrogen peroxide in extracellular fluid in vivo. *Proc. Natl. Acad. Sci. USA* **2007**, *104*, 8749–8754. [CrossRef] [PubMed]

47. Chen, P.; Yu, J.; Chalmers, B.; Drisko, J.; Yang, J.; Li, B.; Chen, Q. Pharmacological ascorbate induces cytotoxicity in prostate cancer cells through ATP depletion and induction of autophagy. *Anticancer Drugs* **2012**, *23*, 437–444. [CrossRef] [PubMed]

48. Espey, M.G.; Chen, P.; Chalmers, B.; Drisko, J.; Sun, A.Y.; Levine, M.; Chen, Q. Pharmacologic ascorbate synergizes with gemcitabine in preclinical models of pancreatic cancer. *Free Radic. Biol. Med.* **2011**, *50*, 1610–1619. [CrossRef] [PubMed]

49. Ong, C.P. High Dose Vitamin C and Low Dose Chemo Treatment. *J. Cancer Sci.* **2018**, *5*, 4.

50. Ma, Y.; Chapman, J.; Levine, M.; Polireddy, K.; Drisko, J.; Chen, Q. High-dose parenteral ascorbate enhanced chemosensitivity of ovarian cancer and reduced toxicity of chemotherapy. *Sci. Transl. Med.* **2014**, *6*, 222ra18. [CrossRef] [PubMed]

51. Welsh, J.L.; Wagner, B.A.; van't Erve, T.J.; Zehr, P.S.; Berg, D.J.; Halfdanarson, T.R.; Yee, N.S.; Bodeker, K.L.; Du, J.; Roberts, L.J., 2nd; et al. Pharmacological ascorbate with gemcitabine for the control of metastatic and node-positive pancreatic cancer (PACMAN): Results from a phase I. clinical trial. *Cancer Chemother. Pharmacol.* **2013**, *71*, 765–775. [CrossRef] [PubMed]

52. Berenson, J.R.; Matous, J.; Swift, R.A.; Mapes, R.; Morrison, B.; Yeh, H.S. A phase I/II study of arsenic trioxide/bortezomib/ascorbic acid combination therapy for the treatment of relapsed or refractory multiple myeloma. *Clin. Cancer Res.* **2007**, *13*, 1762–1768. [CrossRef] [PubMed]

53. Berenson, J.R.; Boccia, R.; Siegel, D.; Bozdech, M.; Bessudo, A.; Stadtmauer, E.; Talisman Pomeroy, J.; Steis, R.; Flam, M.; Lutzky, J.; et al. Efficacy and safety of melphalan, arsenic trioxide and ascorbic acid combination therapy in patients with relapsed or refractory multiple myeloma: A prospective, multicentre, phase II, single-arm study. *Br. J. Haematol.* **2006**, *135*, 174–183. [CrossRef] [PubMed]

54. Abou-Jawde, R.M.; Reed, J.; Kelly, M.; Walker, E.; Andresen, S.; Baz, R.; Karam, M.A.; Hussein, M. Efficacy and safety results with the combination therapy of arsenic trioxide, dexamethasone, and ascorbic acid in multiple myeloma patients: A phase 2 trial. *Med. Oncol.* **2006**, *23*, 263–272. [CrossRef] [PubMed]

55. Chang, J.E.; Voorhees, P.M.; Kolesar, J.M.; Ahuja, H.G.; Sanchez, F.A.; Rodriguez, G.A.; Kim, K.; Werndli, J.; Bailey, H.H.; Kahl, B.S. Phase II study of arsenic trioxide and ascorbic acid for relapsed or refractory lymphoid malignancies: A Wisconsin Oncology Network study. *Hematol. Oncol.* **2009**, *27*, 11–16. [CrossRef] [PubMed]

56. Bael, T.E.; Peterson, B.L.; Gollob, J.A. Phase II trial of arsenic trioxide and ascorbic acid with temozolomide in patients with metastatic melanoma with or without central nervous system metastases. *Melanoma Res.* **2008**, *18*, 147–151. [CrossRef] [PubMed]

57. Subbarayan, P.R.; Lima, M.; Ardalan, B. Arsenic trioxide/ascorbic acid therapy in patients with refractory metastatic colorectal carcinoma: A clinical experience. *Acta Oncol.* **2007**, *46*, 557–561. [CrossRef] [PubMed]

58. Wu, K.L.; Beksac, M.; van Droogenbroeck, J.; Amadori, S.; Zweegman, S.; Sonneveld, P. Phase II multicenter study of arsenic trioxide, ascorbic acid and dexamethasone in patients with relapsed or refractory multiple myeloma. *Haematologica* **2006**, *91*, 1722–1723. [PubMed]

59. Aldoss, I.; Mark, L.; Vrona, J.; Ramezani, L.; Weitz, I.; Mohrbacher, A.M.; Douer, D. Adding ascorbic acid to arsenic trioxide produces limited benefit in patients with acute myeloid leukemia excluding acute promyelocytic leukemia. *Ann. Hematol.* **2014**, *93*, 1839–1843. [CrossRef] [PubMed]

60. Bahlis, N.J.; McCafferty-Grad, J.; Jordan-McMurry, I.; Neil, J.; Reis, I.; Kharfan-Dabaja, M.; Eckman, J.; Goodman, M.; Fernandez, H.F.; Boise, L.H.; et al. Feasibility and correlates of arsenic trioxide combined with ascorbic acid-mediated depletion of intracellular glutathione for the treatment of relapsed/refractory multiple myeloma. *Clin. Cancer Res.* **2002**, *8*, 3658–3668. [PubMed]

61. Held, L.A.; Rizzieri, D.; Long, G.D.; Gockerman, J.P.; Diehl, L.F.; de Castro, C.M.; Moore, J.O.; Horwitz, M.E.; Chao, N.J.; Gasparetto, C. A Phase I study of arsenic trioxide (Trisenox), ascorbic acid, and bortezomib (Velcade) combination therapy in patients with relapsed/refractory multiple myeloma. *Cancer Investig.* **2013**, *31*, 172–176. [CrossRef] [PubMed]

62. Welch, J.S.; Klco, J.M.; Gao, F.; Procknow, E.; Uy, G.L.; Stockerl-Goldstein, K.E.; Abboud, C.N.; Westervelt, P.; DiPersio, J.F.; Hassan, A.; et al. Combination decitabine, arsenic trioxide, and ascorbic acid for the treatment of myelodysplastic syndrome and acute myeloid leukemia: A phase I study. *Am. J. Hematol.* **2011**, *86*, 796–800. [CrossRef] [PubMed]

63. Stephenson, C.M.; Levin, R.D.; Spector, T.; Lis, C.G. Phase I clinical trial to evaluate the safety, tolerability, and pharmacokinetics of high-dose intravenous ascorbic acid in patients with advanced cancer. *Cancer Chemother. Pharmacol.* **2013**, *72*, 139–146. [CrossRef] [PubMed]

64. Kawada, H.; Sawanobori, M.; Tsuma-Kaneko, M.; Wasada, I.; Miyamoto, M.; Murayama, H.; Toyosaki, M.; Onizuka, M.; Tsuboi, K.; Tazume, K.; et al. Phase I Clinical Trial of Intravenous L-ascorbic Acid Following Salvage Chemotherapy for Relapsed B-cell non-Hodgkin's Lymphoma. *Tokai J. Exp. Clin. Med.* **2014**, *39*, 111–115. [PubMed]

65. Polireddy, K.; Dong, R.; Reed, G.; Yu, J.; Chen, P.; Williamson, S.; Violet, P.C.; Pessetto, Z.; Godwin, A.K.; Fan, F.; et al. High Dose Parenteral Ascorbate Inhibited Pancreatic Cancer Growth and Metastasis: Mechanisms and a Phase, I./IIa study. *Sci. Rep.* **2017**, *7*, 17188. [CrossRef] [PubMed]

66. Nielsen, T.K.; Hojgaard, M.; Andersen, J.T.; Jorgensen, N.R.; Zerahn, B.; Kristensen, B.; Henriksen, T.; Lykkesfeldt, J.; Mikines, K.J.; Poulsen, H.E. Weekly ascorbic acid infusion in castration-resistant prostate cancer patients: A single-arm phase II trial. *Transl. Androl. Urol.* **2017**, *6*, 517–528. [CrossRef] [PubMed]

67. Mosteller, R.D. Simplified calculation of body-surface area. *N. Engl. J. Med.* **1987**, *317*, 1098. [CrossRef] [PubMed]

68. Vollbracht, C.; Schneider, B.; Leendert, V.; Weiss, G.; Auerbach, L.; Beuth, J. Intravenous vitamin C administration improves quality of life in breast cancer patients during chemo-/radiotherapy and aftercare: Results of a retrospective, multicentre, epidemiological cohort study in Germany. *In Vivo* **2011**, *25*, 983–990. [PubMed]

69. Riordan, H.D.; Hunninghake, R.B.; Riordan, N.H.; Jackson, J.J.; Meng, X.; Taylor, P.; Casciari, J.J.; Gonzalez, M.J.; Miranda-Massari, J.R.; Mora, E.M.; et al. Intravenous ascorbic acid: Protocol for its application and use. *P. R. Health Sci. J.* **2003**, *22*, 287–290. [PubMed]

70. Padayatty, S.J.; Riordan, H.D.; Hewitt, S.M.; Katz, A.; Hoffer, L.J.; Levine, M. Intravenously administered vitamin C as cancer therapy: Three cases. *CMAJ* **2006**, *174*, 937–942. [CrossRef] [PubMed]

14

Does Vitamin C Influence Neurodegenerative Diseases and Psychiatric Disorders?

Joanna Kocot * 🆔, Dorota Luchowska-Kocot, Małgorzata Kiełczykowska, Irena Musik and Jacek Kurzepa

Chair and Department of Medical Chemistry, Medical University of Lublin, 4A Chodźki Street, 20-093 Lublin, Poland; dorota.luchowska-kocot@umlub.pl (D.L.-K.); malgorzata.kielczykowska@umlub.pl (M.K.); irena.musik@umlub.pl (I.M.); jacek.kurzepa@umlub.pl (J.K.)

Abstract: Vitamin C (Vit C) is considered to be a vital antioxidant molecule in the brain. Intracellular Vit C helps maintain integrity and function of several processes in the central nervous system (CNS), including neuronal maturation and differentiation, myelin formation, synthesis of catecholamine, modulation of neurotransmission and antioxidant protection. The importance of Vit C for CNS function has been proven by the fact that targeted deletion of the sodium-vitamin C co-transporter in mice results in widespread cerebral hemorrhage and death on post-natal day one. Since neurological diseases are characterized by increased free radical generation and the highest concentrations of Vit C in the body are found in the brain and neuroendocrine tissues, it is suggested that Vit C may change the course of neurological diseases and display potential therapeutic roles. The aim of this review is to update the current state of knowledge of the role of vitamin C on neurodegenerative diseases including Alzheimer's disease, Parkinson's disease, Huntington's disease, multiple sclerosis and amyotrophic sclerosis, as well as psychiatric disorders including depression, anxiety and schizophrenia. The particular attention is attributed to understanding of the mechanisms underlying possible therapeutic properties of ascorbic acid in the presented disorders.

Keywords: vitamin C; Alzheimer's disease; Parkinson's disease; Huntington's disease; multiple sclerosis; amyotrophic sclerosis; depression; anxiety; schizophrenia

1. Introduction

Vitamin C (Vit C, ascorbic acid) belongs to a group of water-soluble vitamins. In organisms, Vit C can exist in two forms: reduced—the exact ascorbic acid (AA) which in physiological pH occurs in its anion form of an ascorbate—and oxidized one—dehydroascorbic acid (DHA), which is a product of two-electron oxidation of AA (Figure 1). In the course of metabolic processes an ascorbate free radical can be produced as a result of one-electron oxidation. This variety may subsequently undergo dismutation forming ascorbate and DHA [1].

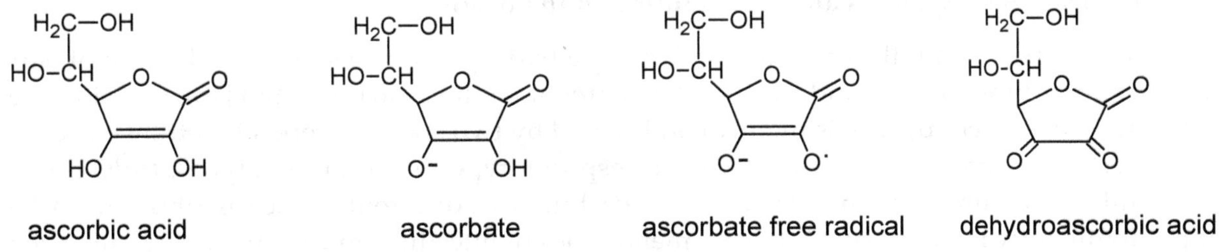

Figure 1. Forms of vitamin C occurring in organisms.

Mammalian organisms are generally capable of synthesizing Vit C themselves. However, some species like fruit bats, guinea pigs, other primates and humans are deprived of this ability due to the lack of L-gulono-1,4-lactone oxidase enzyme which is an element of the metabolic pathway responsible for synthesis of ascorbic acid from glucose [1,2]. Moreover, Vit C is not produced by intestinal microflora [3]. The above facts make these organisms strictly dependent on dietary intake. The recommended Vit C daily intake was established as 60 mg with the reservation that in smokers this value should be increased up to 140 mg [4]. According to the later recommendations, Vit C consumption should be 75 (women) and 90 (men) mg per day, whereas in smokers this value ought to be increased by 35 mg per day [3,5,6].

Vit C is a nutrient of greatest importance for proper functioning of nervous system and its main role in the brain is its participation in the antioxidant defense. Apart from this role, it is involved in numerous non-oxidant processes like biosynthesis of collagen, carnitine, tyrosine and peptide hormones as well as of myelin. It plays the crucial role in neurotransmission and neuronal maturation and functions [7]. For instance, its ability to alleviate seizure severity as well as reduction of seizure-induced damage have been proved [8,9]. On the other hand, disruption of vitamin C transport has been shown to contribute to brain damage in premature infants [10]. Furthermore, Vit C treatment has been reported to ameliorate neuropathological alterations as well as memory impairments and the neurodegenerative changes in rats exposed to neurotoxic substances like aluminum or colchicine [11,12].

Consequently, the growing interest in the issue of vitamin C deficiency, as well as vitamin C treatment in the nervous system diseases, was observed for many years. These facts made us decide to update the current state of knowledge of the role of Vit C in neurodegenerative diseases including Alzheimer's disease, Parkinson's disease, Huntington's disease, multiple sclerosis as well as amyotrophic sclerosis, as well as in psychiatric disorders including depression, anxiety disorders and schizophrenia.

2. Methods

To review the literature on brain Vit C transport/distribution and its function in central nervous system, PubMed and Scopus databases were searched using the following search terms: (vitamin C OR ascorbic acid) AND (central nervous system OR CNS) or (vitamin OR ascorbic acid) AND brain, separately.

To review the literature on the role of Vit C in neurodegenerative diseases and psychiatric disorders, PubMed and Scopus databases were searched using the following search terms: (vitamin C OR ascorbic acid) AND Alzheimer, (vitamin C OR ascorbic acid) AND Parkinson, (vitamin C OR ascorbic acid) AND Huntington, (vitamin C OR ascorbic acid) AND multiple sclerosis, (vitamin C OR ascorbic acid) AND amyotrophic sclerosis, (vitamin C OR ascorbic acid) AND depression, (vitamin C OR ascorbic acid) AND anxiety and (vitamin C OR ascorbic acid) AND schizophrenia, separately. The searching was limited to the last 10 years and human studies, but if none or a few human studies were found the criteria were expanded then to include in vitro or animal studies.

The final search was conducted in April 2017. The titles and abstracts of the articles identified through the initial search were reviewed, and the irrelevant articles were excluded. The full texts of the remaining articles were reviewed to detect studies that did were not suitable for this review.

3. Vitamin C Transport Systems and Distribution in the Brain

Two basic barriers limit the entry of Vit C (being a hydrophilic molecule) into the central nervous system: the blood-brain barrier and the blood-cerebrospinal fluid barrier (CSF) [13]. Considering the whole body, ascorbic acid uptake is mainly conditioned by two sodium-dependent transporters from the SLC23 family, the sodium-dependent Vit C transporter type 1 (SVCT1) and type 2 (SVCT2). These possess similar structure and amino acid sequence, but have different tissue distribution. SVCT1 is found predominantly in apical brush-border membranes of intestinal and renal tubular cells, whereas SVCT2 occurs in most tissue cells [14,15]. SVCT2 is especially important for the transport of Vit

C in the brain—it mediates the transport of ascorbate from plasma across choroid plexus to the cerebrospinal fluid and across the neuronal cell plasma membrane to neuronal cytosol [16]. Although dehydroascorbic acid (DHA) enters the central nervous system more rapidly than the ascorbate, the latter one readily penetrates CNS after oral administration. DHA is taken up by the omnipresent glucose transporters (GLUT), which have affinity to this form of Vit C [17,18]. GLUT1 and GLUT3 are mainly responsible for DHA uptake in the CNS [13]. Transport of DHA by GLUT transporter is bidirectional—each molecule of DHA formed inside the cells by oxidation of the ascorbate could be effluxed and lost. This phenomenon is prevented by efficient cellular mechanisms of DHA reduction and recycling in ascorbate [19]. Neurons can take up ascorbic acid using both described ways [20], whereas astrocytes acquire Vit C utilizing only GLUT transporters [21].

The brain has been found to belong to the organs of the highest ascorbate content, with neurons displaying the highest concentration of all the human organism and reaching 10 mmol/L [1,22]. Mefford et al. [23] and Milby et al. [24] showed high concentrations of Vit C in neuron-rich areas of hippocampus and neocortex in the human brain. Authors suggested that ascorbate content in above brain areas is as much as two-fold higher than in other regions. The difference in ascorbate content between neurons and glia appears to be significant [25]. It is postulated that in astrocytes and glial supported cells lacking the SVCT2, the uptake and reduction of DHA may be the only mechanism of ascorbate retention [26]. In addition to ascorbate motion in neurons and glial cells, it is also released from both types of cells. This release contributes to a certain extent to the homeostatic mechanism of extracellular ascorbate maintenance in the brain [15,19]. Moreover, the extracellular ascorbate concentration is regulated dynamically by glutamate release—increase in extracellular Vit C concentration causes heteroexchange with glutamate [27,28].

4. Vitamin C Function in Central Nervous System

It is well known that the main function of intracellular ascorbic acid in the brain is the antioxidant defense of the cells. However, vitamin C in the central nervous system (CNS) has also many non-antioxidant functions—it plays a role of an enzymatic co-factor participating in biosynthesis of such substances as collagen, carnitine, tyrosine and peptide hormones. It has also been indicated that myelin formation in Schwann cells could be stimulated by ascorbic acid [7,29].

The brain is an organ particularly exposed to oxidative stress and free radicals' activity, which is associated with high levels of unsaturated fatty acids and high cell metabolism rate [16]. Ascorbic acid, being an antioxidant, acts directly by scavenging reactive oxygen and nitrogen species produced during normal cell metabolism [30,31]. In vivo studies demonstrated that the ascorbate had the ability to inactivate superoxide radicals—the major byproduct of fast metabolism of mitochondrial neurons [32]. Moreover, the ascorbate is a key factor in the recycling of other antioxidants, e.g., alpha-tocopherol (Vitamin E). Alpha-tocopherol, found in all biological membranes, is involved in preventing lipid peroxidation by removing peroxyl radicals. During this process α-tocopherol is oxidized to the α-tocopheroxyl radical, which can result in a very harmful effect. The ascorbate could reduce the tocopheroxyl radical back to tocopherol and then its oxidized form is recycled by enzymatic systems with using NADH or NADPH [33]. Regarding these facts, vitamin C is considered to be an important neuroprotective agent.

One non-antioxidant function of vitamin C is its participation in CNS signal transduction through neurotransmitters [16]. Vit C is suggested to influence this process via modulating of binding of neurotransmitters to receptors as well as regulating their release [34–37]. In addition, ascorbic acid acts as a co-factor in the synthesis of neurotransmitters, particularly of catecholamines—dopamine and norepinephrine [26,38]. Seitz et al. [39] suggested that the modulating effect of the ascorbate could be divided into short- and long-term ones. The short-term effect refers to ascorbate role as a substrate for dopamine-β-hydroxylase. Vit C supplies electrons for this enzyme catalyzing the formation of norepinephrine from dopamine. Moreover, it may exert neuroprotective influence against ROS and quinones generated by dopamine metabolism [16]. On the other hand, the long-term effect could be connected with increased expression of the tyrosine hydroxylase gene, probably via a mechanism that entails the increase of intracellular cAMP [39]. It has been stated that the function of ascorbic acid as a neuromodulator of neural transmission may be also associated with amino acidic residues reduction [40] or scavenging of ROS generated in response to neurotransmitter receptor activation [34,41]. Moreover, some have studies showed that ascorbic acid modulates the activity of some receptors such as glutamate as well as γ-aminobutyric acid (GABA) ones [22,40,42–44]. Vit C has been shown to prevent excitotoxic damage caused by excessive extracellular glutamate leading to hyperpolarization of the N-methyl-D-aspartate (NMDA) receptor and therefore to neuronal damage [45]. Vit C inhibits the binding of glutamate to the NMDA receptor, thus demonstrating a direct effect in preventing excessive nerve stimulation exerted by the glutamate [26]. The effect of ascorbic acid on GABA receptors can be explained by a decrease in the energy barrier for GABA activation induced by this agent. Ascorbic acid could bind to or modify one or more sites capable of allosterically modulating single-channel properties. In addition, it is possible that ascorbic acid acts through supporting the conversion from the last GABA-bound closed state to the open state. Alternatively, ascorbic acid could induce the transition of channels towards additional open states in which the receptor adopts lower energy conformations with higher open probabilities [40,44].

There have also been reports concerning the effect of Vit C on cognitive processes such as learning, memory and locomotion, although the exact mechanism of this impact is still being investigated [26]. However, animal studies have shown a clear association between the ascorbate and the cholinergic and dopaminergic systems, they also suggested that the ascorbate can act as a dopamine receptor antagonist. This was also confirmed by Tolbert et al. [46], who showed that the ascorbate inhibits the binding of specific dopamine D1 and D2 receptor agonists.

Another non-antioxidant function of Vit C includes modulation of neuronal metabolism by changing the preference for lactate over glucose as an energy substrate to sustain synaptic activity. During ascorbic acid metabolic switch, this vitamin is released from glial cells and is taken up by neurons where it restraints glucose transport and its utilization. This allows lactate uptake and its usage as the primary energy source in neurons [47]. It was observed that intracellular ascorbic acid inhibited neuronal glucose usage via a mechanism involving GLUT3 [48].

Vit C is involved in collagen synthesis, which also occurs in the brain [26]. There is no doubt that collagen is needed for blood vessels and neural sheath formation. It is well recognized that vitamin C takes part in the final step of the formation of mature triple helix collagen. In this stage, ascorbic acid acts as an electron donor in the hydroxylation of procollagen propyl and lysyl residues [16]. The role of Vit C in collagen synthesis in the brain was confirmed by Sotiriou et al. [49]. According to these authors in mice deficient in SVCT2 ascorbate transporter, the concentration of ascorbate in the brain was below detection level. The animals died due to capillary hemorrhage in the penetrating vessels of the brain. Ascorbate-dependent collagen synthesis is also linked to the formation of the myelin sheath that surrounds many nerve fibers [26]. In vitro studies showed that ascorbate, added to a mixed culture of rat Schwann cells and dorsal root ganglion neurons, promoted myelin formation and differentiation of Schwann cells during formation of the basal lamina of the myelin sheath [7,29].

5. Role of Vitamin C in Neurodegenerative Diseases

Vit C is important for proper nervous system function and its abnormal concentration in nervous tissue is thought to be accompanied with neurological disorders. Studies have shown that disruption of vitamin C transport may cause brain damage in premature infants. Vit C was found to show alleviating effect on seizures severity as well as reducing influence on seizure-induced damage of hippocampus [8,9]. One of the recent studies also revealed that glutamate-induced negative changes in immature brain of rats were reduced by Vit C treatment [50]. Moreover, Vit C administration was shown to recover the colchicine-induced neuroinflammation-mediated neurodegeneration and memory impairments in rats [12] as well as ameliorate behavioral deficits and neuropathological alterations in rats exposed to aluminum chloride [11].

The fact that Vit C can neutralize superoxide radicals, which are generated in large amount during neurodegenerative processes, seems to support its role in neurodegeneration. Moreover, plasma and cellular Vit C levels decline steadily with age and neurodegenerative diseases are often associated with aging. An association of Vit C release with motor activity in central nervous system regions, glutamate-uptake-dependent release of Vit C, its possible role in modulation of N-methyl-D-aspartate receptor activity as well as ability to prevent peroxynitrite anion formation constitute further evidence pointing to the role of Vit C in neurodegenerative processes.

5.1. Alzheimer's Disease

Alzheimer's disease (AD) is the most common form of dementia, an incurable and progressive neurodegenerative disease, leading to far-reaching memory loss, cognitive decline and eventually death. There are two major forms of the AD disease: early onset (familial) and late onset (sporadic). Early-onset one is rare, accounting for less than 5% of all AD cases. Mutations in three genes, mainly amyloid precursor protein (21q21.3), presenilin-1 (14q24.3) and presenilin-2 (1q42.13), have been identified to be involved in the development of this form. Late-onset AD (LOAD) is common among individuals over 65 years of age. Although heritability of LOAD is high (79%), its etiology is considered to be polygenic and multifactorial. The apolipoprotein E ε4 allele (19q13.2) is the major known genetic risk factor for this form of AD. The E4/E4 genotype does not determine the occurrence of LOAD, but is a factor that increases susceptibility to this disease and lowers the age of disease onset. Moreover, a large number of genes have been suggested to be implicated in risk of late-onset Alzheimer's, e.g., clusterin (8p21), complement receptor 1 (1q32), phosphatidylinositol binding clathrin assembly protein (11q14.2), myc box-dependent-interacting protein 1 (2q14.3), ATP binding cassette transporter 7 (19p13.3), membrane-spanning 4-domains, subfamily A (11q12.2), ephrin type-A receptor 1 (7q34), CD33 antigen (19q13.3), CD2 associated protein (6p12.3), sortilin-related receptor 1 (11q24.1), GRB2 associated-binding protein 2 (11q13.4–13.5), insulin-degrading enzyme (10q24), death-associated protein kinase 1 (DAPK1) or gene encoding ubiquilin-1 (UBQLN1) [51,52]. The list of genes associated with AD is still growing. For instance, in the recent study, Lee et al. revealed that single-nucleotide polymorphisms in six genes, including 3-hydroxybutyrate dehydrogenase, type 1 (BDH1), ST6 beta-galactosamide alpha-2,6-sialyltranferase 1 (ST6GAL1), RAB20, member RAS oncogene family (RAB20), PDS5 cohesin associated factor B (PDS5B), adenosine deaminase, RNA-specific, B2 (ADARB2), and SplA/ryanodine receptor domain and SOCS box containing 1 (SPSB1), were directly or indirectly related to conversion of mild cognitive impairment to AD [53].

A neuropathological lesions characteristic of AD include neurofibrillary tangles (composed of hyperphosphorylated and aggregated tau protein) accumulated in the neuronal cytosol as well as the extracellular plaque deposits of the β-amyloid peptide (Aβ), with their frequency correlating with declining cognitive measures [54]. Proteolytic cleavage of amyloid precursor polypeptide chain by secretases (mainly β- and γ-secretase) produces Aβ40 and Aβ42 peptides, which consist of 40 and 42 amino acids, respectively. The latter one, due to its hydrophobicity, is characterized by a greater tendency to form fibrils and is believed to be the main factor responsible for the formation of amyloid deposits [55]. However, Nagababu et al. suggested that the enhanced toxic effect observed for Aβ42 could be attributed to a greater toxicity of the 1–42 aggregates than the 1–40 ones of a comparable size distribution and not to the formation of larger fibrils [56]. According to Ott et al. [54] pre-aggregated Aβ42 peptide induces hyperphosphorylation and pathological structural changes of tau protein and thereby directly links the "amyloid hypothesis" to tau pathology observed in AD [54]. Although the pathogenesis of AD has not been fully understood yet, many studies have demonstrated that ROS and oxidative stress are implicated in disease progression. Aβ peptide was found to enhance the neuronal vulnerability to oxidative stress and cause an impairment of electron transport chain, whereas oxidative stress was shown to induce accumulation of Aβ peptide which subsequently promotes ROS production [16,22,57]. Bartzokis et al. in turn [58] suggested that myelin breakdown in vulnerable late-myelinating regions released oligodendrocyte- and myelin-associated iron that promoted the development of the toxic amyloid oligomers and plaques. There is also the "amyloid cascade-inflammatory hypothesis" which assumes that AD probably results from the inflammatory response induced by extracellular β-amyloid protein deposits, which subsequently become enhanced by aggregates of tau protein [59]. Moreover, recent research has suggested that AD might be a prion-like disease [60,61].

The role of Vit C in AD disease was studied in APP/PSEN1 mice carrying human AD mutations in the amyloid precursor protein (APP) and presenilin (PSEN1) genes (transgenic mouse model of Alzheimer's disease) with partial ablation of vitamin C transport in the brain [9,62,63].

Warner et al. [9] demonstrated that decreased brain Vit C level in the 6-month-old SVCT2+/− APP/PSEN1 mice (obtained by crossing APP/PSEN1 bigenic mice with SVCT2+/− heterozygous knockout mice, which have the lower number of the sodium-dependent Vit C transporter) was associated with enhanced oxidative stress in brain, increased mortality, a shorter latency to seizure onset after kainic acid administration (10 mg/kg i.p.), and more ictal events following treatment with pentylenetetrazol (50 mg/kg i.p.). Furthermore, the authors reported that Vit C deficiency alone in SVCT2+/− mice increased the severity of kainic acid- and pentylenetetrazol-induced seizures [62]. According to another study even moderate intracellular Vit C deficiency displayed an important role in accelerating amyloid aggregation and brain oxidative stress formation, particularly during early stages of disease development. In 6-month-old SVCT2+/− APP/PSEN1 mice increased brain cortex oxidative stress (enhanced malondialdehyde, protein carbonyls, F2-isoprostanes) and decreased level of total glutathione as compared to wild-type controls were observed. Moreover, SVCT2+/− mice had elevated levels of both soluble and insoluble Aβ1-42 and a higher Aβ1-42/Aβ1-40 ratio. In 14-month old mice there were more amyloid-β plaque deposits in both hippocampus and cortex of SVCT2+/−APP/PSEN1+ mice as compared to APP/PSEN+ mice with normal brain Vit C level, whereas oxidative stress levels were similar between groups [62]. Ward et al. [63], in turn, showed that severe Vit C deficiency in Gulo−/− mice (lacking L-gulono-1,4-lactone oxidase (Gulo) responsible for the last step in Vit C synthesis) resulted in decreased blood glucose levels, oxidative damage to lipids and proteins in the cortex, and reduction in dopamine and serotonin metabolites in both the cortex and striatum. Moreover, Gulo−/− mice displayed a significant decrease in voluntary locomotor activity, reduced physical strength and elevated sucrose preference. All the above-mentioned behaviors were restored to control levels after treatment with Vit C (250 mg/kg, i.p.). The role of Vit C in preventing the brain against oxidative stress damage seems to be also proved by the recent study performed by Sarkar et al. [64]. The researchers share a view that cerebral ischemia-reperfusion-induced oxidative stress may initiate the pathogenic cascade leading eventually to neuronal loss, especially in hippocampus, with amyloid accumulation, tau protein pathology and irreversible Alzheimer's dementia. Being the prime source of ROS generation, neuronal mitochondria are the most susceptible to damage caused by oxidative stress. The study proved it that L-ascorbic acid loaded polylactide nanocapsules exerted a protective effect on brain mitochondria against cerebral ischemia-reperfusion-induced oxidative injury [64]. Kennard and Harrison, in turn, evaluated the effects of a single intravenous dose of Vit C on spatial memory (using the modified Y-maze test) in APP/PSEN1 mice. The study was performed on APP/PSEN1 and wild-type (WT) mice of three age spans (3, 9 or 20 months). It was shown that APP/PSEN1 mice displayed no behavioral impairment as compared to WT controls, but memory impairment along with aging was observed in both groups. Vit C treatment (125 mg/kg, i.v.) improved performance in 9-month old APP/PSEN1 and WT mice, but improvements in short-term spatial memory did not result from changes in the neuropathological features of AD or monoamine signaling, as acute Vit C administration did not alter monoamine levels in the nucleus accumbens [65]. Cognitive-enhancing effects of acute intraperitoneal (i.p.) Vit C treatment in APP/PSEN1 mice (12- and 24-month-old) were investigated by Harrison et al. Vit C treatment (125 mg/kg i.p.) improved Y-maze alternation rates and swim accuracy in the water maze in both APP/PSEN1 and wild-type mice; but like in the previous study had no significant effect on the age-associated increase in Aβ deposits and oxidative stress, and did not also affect acetylcholinesterase

(AChE) activity either, which was significantly reduced in APP/PSEN1 mice [66]. Murakami et al. [67] in turn reported that 6-month-treatment with Vit C resulted in reduced Aβ oligomer formation without affecting plaque formation, a significant decrease in brain oxidative damage and Aβ42/Aβ40 ratio as well as behavioral decline in an AD mouse model. Furthermore, this restored the declined synaptophysin and reduced the phosphorylation of tau protein at Ser396.

Besides the presented roles, Vit C has also been suggested to prevent neurodegenerative changes and cognitive decline by protecting blood–brain barrier (BBB) integrity [68].

Kook et al., in the study performed on KO-Tg mice (generating by crossing 5 familial Alzheimer's disease mutation (5XFAD) mice with mice lacking *Gulo*), found that oral Vit C supplementation (3.3 g/L of drinking water) reduced amyloid plaque burden in the cortex and hippocampus by ameliorating BBB disruption (via preventing tight junction structural changes) and morphological changes in the mitochondria [69]. This seems to be confirmed by other studies that proved that Vit C might affect levels of proteins responsible for the tightness of BBB, like tight junction-specific integral membrane proteins (occludin and claudin-5) as well as matrix metalloproteinase 9 (MMP-9). Allahtavakoli et al. demonstrated that in a rat stroke model Vit C administration (500 mg/kg; 5 h after stroke) significantly reduced BBB permeability by reducing serum levels of matrix metalloproteinase 9 [70]. Song et al. reported that Vit C (100 mg/kg i.p.) protected cerebral ischemia-induced BBB disruption by preserving the expression of claudin 5 [71], whereas Lin et al. observed that Vit C (500 mg/kg i.p.) prevented compression-induced BBB disruption and sensory deficit by upregulating the expression of both occludin and claudin-5 [72].

In the available literature, there were only few studies investigating the role of Vit C in AD disease in human and the existing ones have yielded equivocal results.

Some studies have shown significantly lower plasma/serum Vit C level in AD patients as compared to healthy individuals, whereas others have found no difference [73,74]. However, meta-analysis performed by Lopes da Silva et al. proved significantly lower plasma levels of Vit C in AD patients [75]. It seems that the above discrepancies may result from the fact that not plasma but rather intracellular Vit C may be associated with AD.

Generally, studies involving human participants are limited to assessing the effect of Vit C supplementation administered with other antioxidants on AD course.

Arlt et al. [76] found that 1-month and 1-year co-supplementation of Vit C (1000 mg/day) with vitamin E (400 IU/day) increased their concentrations not only in plasma but also in cerebrospinal fluid (which reflects the Vit C status of the brain), while cerebrospinal fluid lipid oxidation was significantly reduced only after 1 year. However, vitamins' supplementation did not have a significant effect on the course of AD [76]. These findings were aslo confirmed by the randomized clinical trial of Galasko et al. [77], which showed that treatment of AD patients for 16 weeks with vitamin E (800 IU/day) plus Vit C (500 mg/day) plus α-lipoic acid (900 mg/day) did not influence cerebrospinal fluid levels of Aβ42, tau and p181tau (widely accepted biomarkers related to amyloid or tau pathology), but decreased F2-isoprostane level (a validated biomarker of oxidative stress). Moreover, is should be emphasized that the above treatment increased risk of faster cognitive decline. This seems to be consistent with results of the recent study which revealed it that Vit C was a potent antioxidant within the AD brain, but it was not able to ameliorate other factors linked to AD pathogenesis as it was proved to be a poor metal chelator and did not inhibit Aβ42 fibrillation [78]. In the study considering an association between nutrient patterns and three brain AD-biomarkers, namely Aβ load, glucose metabolism and gray matter volumes (a marker of brain atrophy) in AD-vulnerable regions, it was found that the higher intake of carotenoids, vitamin A, vitamin C and dietary fibers was positively associated only with glucose metabolism [79].

On the other hand, a randomized control trial involving 276 elderly participants demonstrated that 16-week-co-supplementation of vitamin E and C with β-carotene significantly improved cognitive function (particularly with higher doses of β-carotene). Furthermore, the authors suggested that such a treatment markedly reduced plasma Aβ levels and elevated plasma estradiol levels [80]. Vit C and E co-supplementation for more than 3 years was also shown to be associated with a reduced prevalence and incidence of AD [81]. Moreover, an adequate Vit C plasma level seems to be associated with less progression in carotid intima-media thickness (C-IMT)—the greater C-IMT is suggested to be a risk factor in predicting cognitive decline in the general population, in the elderly population and in patients with Alzheimer's disease. Polidori et al. showed significant decrease (with a linear slope) in Vit C level among old individuals with no or very mild cognitive impairment from the first to the fourth C-IMT quartile [82].

5.2. Parkinson's Disease

Parkinson's disease (PD) is a common long-term neurodegenerative movement disorder characterized by the progressive loss of substantia nigra dopaminergic neurons and consequent depletion of dopamine in the striatum. Dementia, depression and behavioral deficiencies are common symptoms in the advanced stages of the disease [22]. PD is pathologically heterogeneous, but abnormal aggregation of α-synuclein (α-syn) within neuronal perikarya (Lewy bodies) and neurites (Lewy neurites) are neuropathological (but not pathognomonic) hallmarks of this disease [83]. The primary cause of the neurodegenerative process underlying PD is still unknown. Only about 10% of PD cases have shown to be hereditary, whereas the rest are sporadic and result from complex interactions between environmental and common genetic risk factors. Monogenic PD with autosomal-dominant inheritance is caused by mutation in α-synuclein gene (SNCA) or leucine-rich repeat kinase 2 gene (LRRK2), whereas the form with autosomal recessive inheritance by mutations in the genes encoding Parkin 2 (PARK2), PTEN-induced putative kinase 1 (PINK1), protein deglycase DJ-1 (PARK7), and protein ATP13A2 (PARK9). However, many diverse genetic defects in other loci have been suggested to be associated with PD. Candidate genes which have been reported to be associated with PD include e.g., β-glucocerebrosidase (GBA), diacylglycerol kinase θ, 110kD (GAK-DGKQ), SNCA, human leukocyte antigen (HLA), RAD51B, DYRK1A, CHCHD2, VPS35, RAB39B or TMEM230 [84,85]. Different mechanisms, including genomic factors, epigenetic changes, toxic factors, mitochondrial dysfunction, oxidative stress, neuroimmune/neuroinflammatory reactions, hypoxic-ischemic conditions, metabolic deficiencies and ubiquitin–proteasome system dysfunction, seem to be involved in PD pathogenesis [84,86–92]. Mitochondrial dysfunction has been shown to be linked to mutations in PINK1 and DJ1 genes [87,88]. Moreover, it is known that dopamine metabolism produces oxidant species, whereas oxidative stress participates in protein aggregation in PD [22,90,93]. Glutamate-mediated excitotoxicity has been proposed to be a further PD factor. It is also suggested that, like in the case of AD, PD might be a prion-like disease [94–96]. Olanow et al. [94] proposed the hypothesis that α-synuclein is a prion-like protein that can adopt a self-propagating conformation and thereby cause neurodegeneration. Scheffold et al. [97], in turn, reported that telomere shortening (one of the hallmarks of ageing) led to an acceleration of synucleinopathy and impaired microglia response and thereby might contribute to PD pathology. It is likely that not the above factors per se, but rather their synergistic interactions result in the development of the nigrostriatal damage in PD.

Vit C is believed to play a role in dopaminergic neuron differentiation. He et al. [98] in in vitro study found that Vit C enhanced the differentiation of midbrain derived neural stem cell towards dopaminergic neurons by increasing 5-hydroxymethylcytosine (5hmC) and decreasing histone H3 lysine 27 tri-methylation (H3K27m3) generation in dopamine phenotype gene promoters, which are catalyzed by ten-eleven-translocation 1 methylcytosine dioxygenase 1 (Tet1) and histone H3K27 demethylase (Jmjd3), respectively [98,99]. It seems that Vit C acts through regulation of Tet1 and Jmjd3 activities (it acts as a co-factor), since Tet1 and Jmjd3 knockdown/inhibition resulted in no effect of Vit C on either 5hmC or H3K27m3 in the progenitor cells [98]. In another in vitro study, it was shown that mouse embryonic fibroblasts cultured in Vit C-free medium displayed extremely low content of 5hmC, whereas treatment with Vit C resulted in a dose- and time-dependent increase in 5-hmC generation, which was not associated with any change in Tet genes expression. Additionally, it was found that treatment with another reducing agent as glutathione did not affect 5-hmC, whereas blocking Vit C entry into cells or knocking down *Tet* expression significantly reduced the effect of Vit C on 5-hmC [100].

Vit C is also believed to play an indirect role in α-syn oligomerization. Posttranslational α-syn modifications caused by oxidative stress, including modification by 4-hydroxy-2-nonenal, nitration and oxidation, have been implicated to promote oligomerization of α-syn, whereas Vit C as an antioxidant prevents this effect [22,101]. Jinsmaa et al. [102] found that treatment with Vit C attenuated Cu^{2+}-mediated augmentation of 3,4-dihydroxyphenylacetaldehyde (DOPAL)-induced α-syn oligomerization in rat pheochromocytoma PC12 cells, but alone (without Cu^{2+}) did not exert such an effect. Khan et al. showed, in turn, that Vit C supplementation (227.1 μM, 454.2 μM or 681.3 μM in diet, 21 days) caused a significant dose-dependent delay in the loss of climbing ability of PD Drosophila model expressing normal human α-syn in the neurons [103].

Moreover, Vit C is thought to be involved in neuroprotection against glutamate-mediated excitotoxicity occurring in PD. Ballaz et al. [104] in in vitro study performed on dopaminergic neurons of human origin showed that Vit C prevented cell death following prolonged exposure to glutamate. Glutamate induced toxicity in a dose-dependent way via the stimulation of α-amino-3-hydroxy-5-methyl-4-isoxazole propionic acid (AMPA) and metabotropic receptors and to a lesser degree by N-methyl-D-aspartate (NMDA) and kainate receptors, whereas Vit C (25–300 μM) administration protected cells against glutamate excitotoxity. The authors emphasized the fact that such a neuroprotection effect was dependent on the inhibition of oxidative stress, as Vit C prevented the pro-oxidant action of quercetin occurred over the course of prolonged exposure [104]. Vit C neuroprotection effect against dose-dependent glutamate-induced neurodegeneration in the postnatal brain was also confirmed by Shah et al. [50].

The effect of Vit C on dopamine system has also been observed. Izumi et al. [105] showed that PC12 cells treated with paraquat (50 μM, 24 h) displayed increased levels of cytosolic and vesicular dopamine, whereas pretreatment with Vit C (0.3–10 μM, 24 h) suppressed the elevations of intracellular dopamine and almost completely prevented paraquat toxicity.

Human studies have shown that Vit C deficiency among PD patients is widespread [106,107]. However, similarly like in the case of AD, not plasma but rather intracellular Vit C seems to be associated with PD. This could to be confirmed by the study performed by Ide et al. [108] who investigated the association between both lymphocyte and plasma Vit C levels in various stages of PD. Lymphocyte Vit C levels in patients with severe PD was significantly lower compared to those at less severe stages, whereas plasma Vit C levels showed a decreasing tendency; however that effect was not significant [108].

Although in the newest literature data, there are only a few human studies considering the role of Vit C treatment in PD, the existing ones give some evidences that Vit C treatment may have beneficial effect in PD course. A cohort study involving 1036 PD patients showed that dietary Vit C intake was significantly associated with reduced PD risk. However, it was not significant in a 4-year lagged analysis [109]. Quiroga et al., in turn, reported a case of a 66-year-old man with PD, pleural effusion and bipolar disorder who was found to have low serum Vit C and zinc levels. Intravenous replacement of both Vit C and zinc resulted in resolution of the movement disorder in less than 24 h [107]. The other case report concerned 83-year-old men with dementia, diabetes mellitus, hypertension, benign prostatic hypertension, paroxysmal atrial fibrillation, congestive heart failure and suspected PD. The man was treated with Vit C (200 mg) and zinc (4 mg), which resulted in complete resolution of periungual and gingival bleeding as well as palatal petechiae. Moreover, the man's orientation and mental status were found to be markedly improved and no further delusions or agitations were observed [110].

Vit C was shown to increase L-dopa (3,4-dihydroxy-L-phenylalanine, one of the main drugs used in PD therapy) absorption in elderly PD patients. However, this effect was not observed in all patients but only in those with poor baseline L-dopa bioavailability [111]. Moreover, in vitro study performed by Mariam et al. revealed that Vit C is a strong inducer of L-dopa production from pre-grown mycelia of Aspergillus oryzae NRRL-1560 [112].

5.3. Huntington's Disease

Huntington's disease (HD) is a genetic, autosomal dominant disorder characterized by general neurodegeneration in brain with marked deterioration of medium-sized spiny neurons (MSNs) in the striatum [17,113]. HD is caused by a mutation (a CAG expansion) in the huntingtin gene (*HTT*), which results in an abnormal polyglutamine expansion in the huntingtin (HTT) protein and consequently HTT aggregation [113]. The mutant HTT alters intracellular Ca^{2+} homeostasis, induces mitochondrial dysfunction, disrupts intracellular trafficking and impairs gene transcription [114].

Clinically, HD is characterized by tripartite clinical features, namely progressive motor dysfunction (so-called choreic movements), neuropsychiatric symptoms and a variety of cognitive deficits [115,116]. Neuropathologically, HD is associated with a progressive, selective neuronal dysfunction and degeneration, especially in the both part of striatum (caudate and putamen) [117,118].

HD is known to be associated with a failure in energy metabolism, impaired mitochondrial ATP production and oxidative damage [113,119–121]. Other mechanisms, such as excitotoxicity, aberrant glutamatergic, dopaminergic and Ca^{2+} signaling mechanisms, metabolic damage, immune response, apoptosis as well as autophagy are also suggested to be involved in HD pathology [119,121–124].

Vit C flux from astrocytes to neurons during synaptic activity is regarded to be essential for protecting neurons against oxidative damage and modulation of neuronal metabolism, thus permitting optimal ATP production [119]. Under physiological conditions, Vit C is released from astrocytes to striatal extracellular fluid during increased synaptic activity. The enhancement of Vit C concentration in striatal extracellular fluid results in SVCT2 translocation to the plasma membrane and consequently Vit C uptake by neurons [119]. In neurons, Vit C is able to scavenge reactive oxygen species generated during synaptic activity and neuronal metabolism. As a result, Vit C is oxidized to dihydroascorbate, which is then released into the extracellular fluid and uptaken by neighboring astrocytes, where is subsequently turned back to a reduced form, which can be used again by neurons. Vit C can interact directly with reactive oxygen species but can also act as a co-factor in the reduction of other antioxidants as glutathione and α-tocopherol. Moreover, Vit C may function as a neuronal metabolic switch, which means that it is capable to inhibit glucose consumption and permit lactate uptake/use as a substrate to sustain synaptic activity. This function is not dependent on antioxidant activity of Vit C [47] and seems to be of great importance, taking into account that decreased expression of GLUT3 in both STHdhQ cells (striatal neurons derived from knock-in mice expressing mutant huntingtin; cell model of HD) and R6/2 mice (mouse model of HD) as well as impaired GLUT3 localization at the plasma membrane in HD cells were observed [125].

Unfortunately, the mechanism mentioned above does not work properly in HD. Abnormal Vit C flux from astrocytes to neurons was found both in R6/2 mice and STHdhQ cells. Acuña et al. proved that SVCT2 failed to reach the plasma membrane in cells expressing mutant Htt, which resulted in disturbed Vit C uptake by neurons [119]. Additionally, there is some evidence that altered glutamate transporter activity (GLT1—the protein primarily found on astrocytes and responsible for removing most extracellular glutamate), observed in HD, is related to deficient striatal Vit C release into extracellular fluid [126–128]. Miller et al. performed the study on R6/2 mice receiving ceftriaxone (200 mg/kg, once daily injection per 5 days)—a β-lactam antibiotic that selectively increases the expression of GLT1. To evaluate Vit C release in vivo voltammetry combined with corticostriatal afferent stimulation was used. R6/2 mice treated with saline displayed a marked decrease in striatal extracellular Vit C level compared to control group, whereas treatment with ceftriaxone restored striatal Vit C in R6/2 mice to control level and also improved the HD behavioral phenotype. It was also shown that intra-striatal infusion of GLT1 inhibitor (dihydrokainic acid or DL-*threo*-β-benzyloxyaspartate) blocked evoked striatal Vit C release [126]. Dorner et al., in turn, observed that cortical stimulation resulted in a rapid increase in Vit C release in both R6/2 and wild-type mice, but the response had a significantly shorter duration and smaller magnitude in R6/2 group. The researchers also measured striatal Vit C release in response to treatment with d-amphetamine (5 mg/kg)—a psychomotor stimulant known to release Vit C from corticostriatal terminals independently of dopamine. Both

Vit C release and behavioral activation were diminished in R6/2 mice compared to wild-type ones. The authors concluded that the corticostriatal pathway was directly involved in behavior-related Vit C release and that this system was dysfunctional in HD [127]. It is thought that Vit C is released into striatal extracellular fluid as glutamate is uptaken—glutamate/Vit C heteroexchange. Consequently, Vit C level decreases while glutamate level increases in extracellular fluid of HD striatum owing to a downregulation of GLT1 [127,128]. Elevated glutamate level in synaptic gaps leads to abnormal signal transmission.

In addition, it is also believed that long-term oxidative stress (one of the key players in HD progression) eliminates the ability of Vit C to modulate glucose utilization [125].

The effect of Vit C treatment on behavior-related neuronal activity was studied by Rebec et al. [129]. The authors showed that in the striatum of R6/2 mice impulse activity was consistently elevated compared to wild-type mice, whereas restoring extracellular Vit C to the wild-type level by Vit C treatment (300 mg/kg, 3 days) reversed this effect. This suggests Vit C involvement in normalization of neuronal function in HD striatum. In another study, the same researchers reported that regular injections of Vit C (300 mg/kg/day, 4 days/week) restored the behavior-related release of Vit C in striatum, which was associated with improved behavioral responding. Vit C treatment significantly attenuated the neurological motor signs of HD without altering overall motor activity [130].

Although studies performed on cell and animal models of HD appear to indicate the role of Vit C in HD course, to the best of our knowledge, in the newest literature there exists a lack of studies considering the role of Vit C or the effect of its supplementation in HD human subjects.

5.4. Multiple Sclerosis

Multiple sclerosis (MS) is a progressive demyelinating process considered as an autoimmune disease of unknown etiology. MS is characterized by infiltration of immune cells (in particular T cells and macrophages), demyelination (loss of myelin sheath that surrounds and protects nerve fibers allowing them to conduct electrical impulses) and axonal pathology resulting in multiple neurological deficits, which range from motor and sensory deficits to cognitive and psychological impairment [131,132]. The etiology of MS is still unknown, but it is suggested that genetic predisposition associated with environmental factors can lead to expression of the envelope protein of MS-associated retrovirus (MSRV) and thus trigger the disease [133]. Although pathogenesis of MS has not been fully clarified yet, either destruction by the immune system or a significant extent apoptosis, particularly apoptosis of oligodendroglia cells, are believed to be underlying mechanism. Oxidative/nitrosative stress and mitochondrial dysfunction are believed to contribute to the pathophysiology of MS [131,134–137].

Having regarded the presented facts, it seems to be justified that Vit C, being a very important brain antioxidant, may affect MS course. Vit C is known to affect numerous metabolic processes directly associated with immune system. Furthermore, Vit C-dependent collagen synthesis has also been linked to formation of the myelin sheath [7].

In the literature data, there are only a few studies considering association between MS and Vit C. However, the existing ones showed that MS patients displayed significantly lower Vit C level as compared to healthy individuals [135,136,138]. Besler et al. [138], in turn, observed an inverse correlation between the serum levels of Vit C and lipid peroxidation in MS patients. The authors concluded that decreased Vit C level, observed in MS patients during relapse of the disease, might be dependent on the elevated oxidative burden as reflected by increased lipid peroxidation. Hejazi et al. [139], in turn, found no significant difference between daily intake of Vit C (recorded from a 24-h dietary recall questionnaire for 3 days) in MS patients ($n = 37$) in comparison with healthy subjects. The intake of Vit C in both groups was below dietary reference intake (DRI), however in control group it was near the DRI value.

An efficiency of antioxidant therapy in relapsing-remitting multiple sclerosis patients ($n = 14$) treated with complex of antioxidants and neuroprotectors with various mechanisms of action (α-lipoic acid, nicotinamide, acetylcysteine, triovit beta-carotine, alpha-tocopheryl acetate, ascorbic acid, selenium, pentoxifylline, cerebrolysin, amantadine hydrochloride) during 1 month, 2 times a year was investigated by Odinak et al. [140]. The treatment resulted in significant reduction of relapse frequency, decrease of required corticosteroid courses and significantly reduced content of lipid peroxide products [140]. However, it should be underlined that Vit C was only one element of multicomponent treatment. However, in another study it was shown that intrahippocampal injection of Vit C (0.2, 1, 5 mg/kg, 7 days) improved memory acquisition of passive avoidance learning (PAL) in ethidium bromide-induced MS in rats. The injection of ethidium bromide caused significant deterioration of PAL, whereas treatment with Vit C at a dose of 5 mg/kg resulted in significant improvement in PAL [141].

Summing up, the possible role of Vit C in MS course remains to be explored.

5.5. Amyotrophic Lateral Sclerosis

Amyotrophic lateral sclerosis (ALS) is an incurable, chronic progressive neurodegenerative disease characterized by the degeneration of upper motor neurons in the motor cortex and lower motor neurons in the spinal cord and the brain stem [142]; the reason why only motor neurons are targeted remains unknown. ALS results in loss of power and function of skeletal muscles, which is reflected by difficulties in walking, using the arms, speaking and swallowing. ALS occurs in two forms: hereditary one, which is called familial (5–10% of ALS cases) and not hereditary one, called sporadic. Familial ALS is indistinguishable from the much more common sporadic form, but usually it begins at a slightly younger age. It is assumed that about 2% of all cases of ALS are caused by mutations in the gene encoding copper/zinc superoxide dismutase (SOD1) on chromosome 21, but the etiology of the remaining ALS cases is not fully understood. The course of ALS is variable, but usually relatively rapid. Most patients die, usually due to respiratory failure (respiratory muscles paralysis), within 3–5 years from the onset of symptoms [143].

Although the underlying causes of motor neuron degeneration remain still unknown, researchers have suggested a contribution of oxidative stress, mitochondrial dysfunction, glutamate-mediated excitotoxicity, cytoskeletal abnormalities, and protein aggregation [144]. Because of the above-presented facts and its activity-dependent release in the brain, it seems to be possible that Vit C may be involved in ALS pathogenesis. It appears to be confirmed by Blasco et al. who compared 1 H-NMR spectra of cerebrospinal fluid (CSF) samples collected from ALS patients ($n = 44$) and patients without a neurodegenerative disease. The authors found significantly higher Vit C level in the ALS group. Vit C, apart from being free radical scavenger, was suggested to modulate neuronal metabolism by reducing glucose consumption during episodes of glutamatergic synaptic activity and stimulating lactate uptake in neurons, which is consistent with lower lactate/pyruvate ratio seen in ALS patients [144].

However, in the available literature data, there are only a few studies evaluating an association between Vit C and ALS, and the existing ones have not proved its role in the course of this disease.

Nagano et al. [145] investigated the efficacy of Vit C treatment (0.8% w/w in the diet) in familiar ALS mice, administered before or after the onset of the disease. The mice treated with Vit C before disease onset survived significantly longer by 62% than the control. However, that treatment did not affect the mean age of onset appearance and administration after disease onset did not prolong survival. Netzahualcoyotzi and Tapia [146] found that the infusion of Vit C (20 mM), alone or in combination with glutathione ethylester, did not prevent the AMPA-induced motor alterations of the rear limbs and motor neuron degradation in rats. The pooled analysis of 5 large prospective studies of about 1100 ALS patients performed by Fitzgerald et al. showed that neither supplementation (even long-term) nor high dietary intake of Vit C affected risk of ALS [147]. Okamoto et al. [148] investigated the relationship between dietary intake of vegetables, fruit and antioxidants and the risk of ALS (153 ALS patients aged 18–81 years with disease duration of 3 years) in Japan. The study showed that a higher consumption of fruits and/or vegetables was associated with a significantly reduced risk of ALS. However, no significant dose-response relationship was observed between intake of beta-carotene,

Vit C and vitamin E and the risk of ALS. Spasojević et al. [149], in turn, suggested that the use of Vit C could have an unfavorable effect in ALS patients. The researchers examined the effect of Vit C on the production of hydroxyl radicals in CSF obtained from sporadic ALS patients. Using electron paramagnetic resonance spectroscopy, the authors detected ascorbyl radicals in CSF of ALS patients, whereas in control CSF they were undetectable. Moreover, the addition of hydrogen peroxide to the CSF of ALS patients provoked further formation of ascorbyl as well as hydroxyl radicals ex vivo. Thus, it seems that herein Vit C may paradoxically induce pro-oxidative effects. This may result from the fact that Vit C is an excellent one-electron reducing agent that can reduce ferric (Fe^{3+}) ion to ferrous (Fe^{2+}) one, while being oxidized to ascorbate radical. In a Fenton reaction, Fe^{2+} reacts with H_2O_2 generating Fe^{3+} and a very strong oxidizing agent—hydroxyl radical. The presence of Vit C allows the recycling of Fe^{3+} back to Fe^{2+}, which can subsequently catalyze the successive formation of hydroxyl radicals [1,150]. Moreover, it has also been shown that high concentrations of ascorbyl radical can reduce SOD activity.

6. Role of Vitamin C in Psychiatric Disorders

Vit C is also believed to be involved in anxiety, stress, depression, fatigue and mood state in humans. It has been hypothesized that oral Vit C supplementation can elevate mood as well as reduce distress and anxiety.

6.1. Depression

Depression (DP) is a mental disorder characterized by a number of basic symptoms like low mood, biological rhythm disorders, psychomotor slowdown, anxiety, somatic disorders as well other nonspecific symptoms [151]. It has a multifactorial etiology, with biological, psychological, social and lifestyle factors of important roles [152]. Several hypotheses have been proposed to explain the mechanisms underlying depression. Firstly, it is believed that depression is associated with disturbances of serotonin, norepinephrine and dopamine neurotransmission. Moreover, many observations have supported the involvement of GABAergic system in the pathomechanism of depression [153]. GABA level in plasma and CSF of patients suffering from depression was shown to be reduced [154,155] which points to its decreased synthesis in the brain. Recent data have suggested that chronic stress, via initiating changes in the hypothalamic-pituitary-adrenal axis and the immune system, acts as a trigger for the above-mentioned disturbance. For example, glucocorticoids and proinflammatory cytokines enhance the conversion of tryptophan to kynurenine thus leading to a decrease in the synthesis of brain serotonin (because less tryptophan is available for conversion to serotonin) and an increase in the formation of neurotoxic metabolites, e.g., glutamate antagonist quinolinic acid. The activity of the dopaminergic systems was also found to be reduced in response to inflammation [156]. Secondly, some genetic factors have been suggested to be implicated in depression etiology [157]. Thirdly, apoptosis of the brain cells seems to be involved in depression development, since a numerical and morphological alterations of astrocytes in patients with major depressive disorder were observed [158–161]. This may also be dependent, at least partially, on proinflammatory cytokine actions since quinolinic acid was shown to contribute to the increase in apoptosis of astrocytes or neurons [162,163].

Basing on several animal studies [153,155,164–166], there is preliminary evidence that Vit C exerts an antidepressant-like effect via:

1. modulation of monoaminergic systems [167] (e.g., Vit C was shown to activate the serotonin 1A (5-HT1A) receptor, this activation is a mechanism of action of many antidepressant, anxiolytic and antipsychotic drugs);
2. modulation of GABAergic systems (via activation of $GABA_A$ receptors and a possible inhibition of $GABA_B$ receptors) [155];

3.   inhibition of N-methyl-D-aspartate (NMDA) receptors and L-arginine-nitric oxide (NO)-cyclic guanosine 3,5-monophosphate (cGMP) pathway—the blockade of NMDA receptor is associated with reduced levels of NO and cGMP, whereas reduction of NO levels within the hippocampus was shown to induce antidepressant-like effects [119];

4.   blocking potassium (K^+) channels—Vit C administration was shown to produce an antidepressant-like effect in the tail suspension test via K^+ channel inhibition [119]; as K^+ channels were reported to belong to the physiological targets of NO and cGMP in the brain, their inhibition plays a significant role in the treatment of depression;

5.   activation of phosphatidylinositol-3-kinase (PI3K) and inhibition of glycogen synthase kinase 3 beta (GSK-3β) activity [112,119];

6.   induction of heme oxygenase 1 expression—it is a candidate depression biomarker which may be a link factor between inflammation, oxidative stress and the biological as well functional changes in brain activity in depression; its decreased expression is associated with depressive symptoms [166,168];

7.   since depression is well known to be associated with altered anti- and prooxidant profiles, Vit C may play antidepressant function also by its antioxidant properties [118,119].

The available literature data indicate that Vit C deficiency is very common in patients with depressive disorders. Gariballa [169] in a randomized, double blind, placebo-controlled trial observed that low Vit C status was associated with increased depression symptoms following acute illness in older people. Parameters were measured at baseline as well as after 6 weeks and 6 months. Patients with Vit C depletion had significantly increased symptoms of depression as compared to those with its higher concentrations both at baseline and at 6 weeks. Significantly lower serum Vit C level in patients with depression vs. healthy controls was also shown by Bajpai et al. [170] and Gautam et al. [171]. Moreover, in the latter study dietary supplementation of Vit C (1000 mg/day) along with vitamins A and E for a period of 6 weeks resulted in a significant reduction in depression scores [171]. Furthermore, a case-control study carried out on 60 male university students showed that subjects diagnosed with depression had significantly lower intake of Vit C than the healthy ones [172]. Similarly, in another case-control study involving 116 girls identified as having depressive symptoms, depression was negatively associated with Vit C intake, even after adjusting for confounding variables [173]. Rubio-López et al. [174], in turn, examined the relationship between nutritional intake and depressive symptoms in 710 Valencian schoolchildren aged 6–9 years and also observed that nutrient intake of Vit C was significantly lower in children with depressive symptoms. Additionally, prevalence of Vit C inadequacy (below dietary recommended intakes) was significantly higher in subjects with depressive symptoms.

The efficacy of Vit C as an adjuvant agent in the treatment of pediatric major depressive disorder in a double-blind, placebo-controlled pilot trial was evaluated by Amr et al. [175]. Patients ($n = 12$) treated for six months with fluoxetine (10–20 mg/day) and Vit C (1000 mg/day) showed a significant decrease in depressive symptoms in comparison with the fluoxetine plus placebo group as measured by the Children's Depression Rating Scale and Children's Depression Inventory. No serious adverse effects were shown. Zhang et al. [176] in double-blind clinical trial investigated the effect of Vit C (500 mg twice daily) on mood in non-depressed acutely hospitalized patients. The applied therapy increased plasma and mononuclear leukocyte Vit C concentrations and was associated with a 34% reduction in mood disturbance (assessed with Profile of Mood States) [176]. Similarly, Wang et al. found that short-term Vit C (500 mg twice daily) treatment was associated with a 71% reduction in mood disturbance (assessed with Profile of Mood States) and a 51% reduction in psychological distress (assessed with Distress Thermometer) in acutely hospitalized patients with a high prevalence of hypovitaminosis C [177]. Khajehnasiri et al. [178] in a randomized, double-blind, placebo-controlled trial involving 136 depressed male shift workers observed, in turn, that Vit C administration (250 mg twice daily for 2 months) alone and in combination with omega-3 fatty acids significantly reduced the Beck Depression Inventory (BDI) score, however omega-3 fatty acid supplementation alone was more effective. Moreover, Vit C and omega-3 fatty acids supplementation alone (but not in combination) decreased significantly serum MDA levels. Fritz et al. [179] conducted a systematic review of human and observational studies assessing the efficiency of interventional Vit C as a contentious adjunctive cancer therapy and reported that it could improve quality of life, physical function, as well as prevent some side effects of chemotherapy, including fatigue, nausea, insomnia, constipation and depression.

6.2. Anxiety

Anxiety is an adaptive response to uncertain threat, but it becomes pathological when is disproportionate to the threat, persists beyond the presence of the stressor, or is triggered by innocuous stimuli or situations. Similarly like in the case of depression, neurotransmitter system disruptions (namely GABA, serotonin and noradrenalin) as well as an impaired regulation of the hypothalamic-pituitary-adrenal axis are involved in anxiety disorders [180]. Furthermore, several studies have suggested a positive correlation between oxidative stress and anxiety-like behavior.

The growing evidence, which has been recently emerged, suggests that anxiety is associated with Vit C deficit, whereas Vit C supplementation could help reduce feeling of anxiety. The underlying mechanism is not fully understood yet, but Vit C seems to play this role by: regulating neurotransmitters' activity, attenuating cortisol activity, preventing stress-induced oxidative damage and antioxidant defense in brain or some as yet undetermined effects on anxiety-related brain structures [181].

Kori et al. [182] observed that rats subjected to restrained stress (by placing in a wire mesh restrainer for 6 h per day for 21 days) displayed a significant increase in serum cortisol level with concomitant decrease in serum Vit C and E levels. Boufleur et al. [183], in turn, found decreased plasma Vit C levels in rats exposed to chronic mild stress. Interestingly, neonatal handling could prevent Vit C reduction in rats exposed to chronic mild stress in adulthood. Koizumi et al. [184] showed that Vit C status was critical for determining vulnerability to anxiety in a sex-specific manner. The study was performed on senescence marker protein–30/gluconolactones knockout mice (unable to synthesize Vit C) whose Vit C status was continuously shifted from adequate to depleted one (by providing a water with or without Vit C). It was observed that anxiety responses in the novelty-suppressed feeding paradigm were worse during Vit C depletion conditions, especially in females. Hughes et al. [181], in turn, reported that prolonged treatment with Vit C (approximately 80 mg/kg/day in drinking water, 83 days) markedly decreased anxiety-related behavior in the open field test in hooded rats. In another study, the same researchers examined the effect of Vit C treatment with three doses (61, 114 or 160 mg/kg/day in drinking water, 8 weeks) and observed that an anxiolytic effects of Vit C were displayed in higher frequencies of walking (with doses of 114 mg/kg/day and 160 mg/kg/day), higher frequencies of rearing (with dose of 61 mg/kg/day) and lower frequencies of grooming (with dose of 61 mg/kg/day) in the open field as well as more frequent occupation of the open arms in the elevated plus-maze (with dose of 61 mg/kg/day). The authors concluded that anxiolytic effects of Vit C were more typical of the lowest dose and it was to some extent dependent on anxiety intensity [185]. The effect of Vit C on adrenal gland function (an element of the stress response system) was investigated by Choi et al. [186]. An adrenalectomized (ADX) and non-ADX rats were treated with Vit C (25 or 100 m/kg, 7 days) and subsequently subjected to both Vit C treatment and electroshock stress for next 5 days. Vit C supplementation reduced corticosterone level in non-ADX rats. Stress decreased the mean value of rearing frequency in both non-ADX and ADX rats, whereas Vit C partially attenuated this effect in non-ADX group. Moreover, Vit C treatment decreased adrenocorticotropic hormone in both groups and significantly reduced freezing time increased by stress. The authors suggested that the alleviating effect of Vit C on stress-related rearing behavior was exerted via modulation of corticosterone, whereas the effect on freezing behavior via modulation of corticotropin-releasing hormone or adrenocorticotropin-releasing hormone [186]. Puty et al. [187] in turn suggested that Vit C plays anxiolytic-like effect via affecting serotonergic system. The researchers evaluated the protective effect of Vit C against methylmercury (MeHg)-induced anxiogenic-like effect in zebrafish.

MeHg produced a marked anxiogenic effects in the light/dark box test, which was accompanied by a decrease in the extracellular levels of serotonin as well an increase in its oxidized metabolite tryptamine-4,5-dione, whereas pretreatment with Vit C (2 mg/g, i.p.) prevented such alterations. Furthermore, Angrini and Leslie [188] found that pretreatment with Vit C (100 mg or 200 mg/kg) could attenuate, especially the higher dose, behavioral and anxiogenic effects of prolonged exposure to noise (100 dB for 2 months, 5 days/week, 4 h daily) on male laboratory mice.

Although there are only a few studies considering the effects of vitamin C on anxiety and stress responses in humans, the existing ones seem to provide promising results.

De Oliveira et al. [189] examined the effects of short-term oral Vit C supplementation (500 mg/day, 14 days) in high school students (n = 42) in a randomized, double-blind, placebo-controlled trial. The treatment led to higher plasma Vit C concentration that was associated with reduced anxiety levels evaluated with BIA (Beck Anxiety Inventory). Moreover, the Vit C supplementation had positive effect on the heart rate. Gautam et al. [171] observed that patients with generalized anxiety disorder had significantly lower Vit C levels in comparison with healthy controls, whereas 6-week vitamins supplementation (vitamin C accompanied with A and E) led to a significant reduction in anxiety scores [171]. Mazloom et al. [190], in turn, showed that short-term supplementation of Vit C (1000 mg/day) reduced anxiety levels (evaluated basing on Depression Anxiety Stress Scales 21-item) in diabetic patients. This effect was exerted through alleviating oxidative damage. Furthermore, recently performed a systematic review also showed that high-dose Vit C supplementation was effective in reducing anxiety as well as stress-induced blood pressure increase [191].

6.3. Schizophrenia

Schizophrenia is a severe and complex neuropsychiatric disorder that affects 1% of the population worldwide [192–194]. Symptoms of schizophrenia are described as "positive" (also so-called productive) and "negative" ones: the first include hallucinations, paranoia and delusions, while negative examples are: limited motivation, impaired speech, weakening and social withdrawal. These symptoms usually appear in early adulthood and often persist in about three-fourths of patients despite optimum treatment [192]. Some authors have suggested that insufficient dopamine level due to the loss of dopamine producing cells may lead to schizophrenia [195]. On the other hand, it has been postulated that schizophrenia has been linked to hyperactivity of brain dopaminergic systems that may reflect an underlying dysfunction of NMDA receptor-mediated neurotransmission [194]. Furthermore, there is the increasing evidence that several physiological mechanisms such as oxidative stress, altered one carbon metabolism and atypical immune-mediated responses may be involved in schizophrenia pathomechanism [192,196].

Hoffer [197] summarized in the review study the evidence showing that among others Vit C deficiency could worsen the symptoms of schizophrenia and that large doses of this vitamin could improve the core metabolic abnormalities predisposing some people to development of this disease. According to the author, it is probable that the pathologic process responsible for schizophrenia could increase ascorbic acid utilization. Sarandol et al. [198] also noted lower levels of serum Vit C as compared to control group, but this was not regarded as a statistically significant difference. Moreover, a 6-week-long antipsychotic treatment did not modify the concentration of this vitamin. The authors explained that other factors, such as nutrition, physical activity, etc., might be the reason for the discrepancy between the results of their research and other studies. Similarly, Young et al. [199] observed only a slight decrease in Vit C levels in schizophrenic group vs. control one; but interestingly, a highly significant increase in Vit C level in the control female group as compared to both control as well as schizophrenic male group was observed. The authors pointed out that this information might be relevant particularly in the light of recent reports that the risk of schizophrenia is higher in men than women. The reduced supply of Vit C with the diet in patients with schizophrenia was noted by Konarzewska et al. [200].

The review of Magalhães et al. revealed that the implementation of Vit C as a low-molecular-weight antioxidant alleviated the effects of free radicals in the treatment of schizophrenia [201]. According to Bentsen et al. [202] membrane lipid metabolism and redox regulation may be disturbed in schizophrenia. These authors conducted a study aiming at examination of the clinical effect of adding vitamins E + C to antipsychotics (D_2 receptor antagonists). Patients with schizophrenia or related psychoses received Vit C (1000 mg/day) along with vitamin E (364 mg/day) for 16 weeks. Vitamins impaired the course of psychotic symptoms, especially of persecutory delusions. The authors pointed to the usefulness of supplementation of antioxidant vitamins as agents alleviating some side effects of antipsychotic drugs. This was also confirmed by the next study involving schizophrenia patients treated with haloperidol [203]. Classical antipsychotics like haloperidol are suggested to increase oxidative stress and oxidative cell injury in brain, which may influence the course as well as treatment effects of schizophrenia. In this study, chronic haloperidol treatment connected with supplementation of a combination of ω-3 fatty acids and vitamins E and C showed a significant beneficial effect on schizophrenia treatment as measured by SANS (Simpson Angus Scale) and BPRS (Brief Psychiatric Rating Scale) scales. BPRS total score and subscale scores as well as SANS scores were significantly improved starting from the 4th week of treatment. Moreover, in patients with schizophrenia after 16 weeks of treatment, serum Vit C levels were almost twice as high as at the beginning of the study. These results supported the hypothesis of a beneficial effect of the applied supplementation both on positive and negative symptoms of schizophrenia as well as the severity of side effects induced by haloperidol [203]. Heiser et al. [204] also stated that reactive oxygen species (ROS) were involved in the pathophysiology of psychiatric disorders such as schizophrenia. Their research demonstrated that antipsychotics induced ROS formation in the whole blood of rats, which could be reduced by the application of vitamin C. The aim of their study was to demonstrate the effects of clozapine, olanzapine and haloperidol at different doses (18, 90 and 180 μg/mL) on the formation of ROS in the whole blood by using electron spin resonance spectroscopy. To demonstrate the protective capacity of Vit C the blood samples were incubated the highest concentration of each drug with Vit C (1 mM) for 30 min. Olanzapine caused significantly greater ROS formation vs. control under all treatment conditions, while in the case of haloperidol and clozapine only two higher concentrations resulted in significantly increased ROS formation. Vitamin C reduced the ROS production of all tested drugs, but for olanzapine the attenuating effect did not reach a significant level.

A relatively novel approach as for the role of Vit C in etiology and treatment of schizophrenia was presented by Sershen et al. [193]. According to the researchers, deficits in N-methyl-D-aspartate receptor (NMDAR) function are linked to persistent negative symptoms and cognitive deficits in schizophrenia. This hypothesis is supported by the fact that the flavoprotein D-amino acid oxidase (DAO) was shown to degrade the gliotransmitter D-Ser, a potent activator of N-methyl-D-aspartate-type glutamate receptors, while a lot of evidence has suggested that DAO, together with its activator, G72 protein, may play a key role in the pathophysiology of schizophrenia. Furthermore, in a postmortem study the activity of DAO was found to be two-fold higher in schizophrenia subjects [205]. Sershen et al. [193] showed that acute ascorbic acid dose (300 mg/kg i.p.) inhibited PCP-induced and amphetamine-induced locomotor activity in mouse model, which was further attenuated in the presence of D-serine (600 mg/kg). The authors suggested that this effect could result from the Vit C-depended changes in dopamine carrier-membrane translocation and/or altered redox mechanisms that modulate NMDARs. However, this issue needs to be further investigated.

7. Conclusions

The crucial role of Vit C in neuronal maturation and functions, neurotransmitter action as well as responses to oxidative stress is well supported by the evidences presented in this review (Figure 2).

The aforementioned animal studies confirmed the usefulness of using of Vit C in the treatment of neurological diseases, both neurodegenerative and psychiatric ones. Only in the case of ALS, the possible unfavorable effects were suggested. However, studies on the role of Vit C in the course of neurological disorders in human are limited and the existing ones have aimed mostly at evaluating the effect of Vit C supplementation (often co-supplementation with other agents). Recently, a tendency toward using administration of large doses of Vit C as an adjuvant in curing of many diseases was observed. Unfortunately, in the available literature there is a lack of studies considering this issue in the context of neurological disorders.

NEURODEGENERATIVE DISEASES

Alzheimer's disease
- ↑ Oxidative stres
- ↑ Acceleration of amyloid aggregation
- ↑ Neuronal loss
- Influence on the blood-brain barrier integrity
- Influence on the phosphorylation of tau protein at Ser396

Parkinson's disease
- Oligomerization: ↑ posttranslational αSyn modifications
- ↓ Dopaminergic neuron differentiation
- ↓ Neuroprotection against glutamate-mediated excitotoxicity
- Effect on dopamine system

Huntington's disease
- ↑ Oxidative stres
- Disorders in glucose transport and metabolism
- Disorders in glutamine metabolism

Multiple sclerosis
- Disorders in collagen synthesis (demyelination)
- ↑ Oxidative stres

Amyotrophic lateral sclerosis
- ↑ Oxidative stres
- Disorders in glucose and lactate metabolism

PSYCHIATRIC DISORDERS

Depression
- Modulation of monoaminergic and GABAergic systems
- Inhibition of N-methyl-D-aspartatereceptors and L-arginine-nitric oxide-(NO)-cyclic guanosine 3,5-monophosphate (cGMP) pathway
- Blocking potassium (K⁺) channels
- Activation of phosphatidylinositol-3-kinase (PI3K) and inhibition of glycogen synthase kinase 3 beta (GSK-3β) activity
- Induction of heme oxygenase 1 expression
- ↑ Oxidative stres

Anxiety
- ↑ Oxidative stres
- Disturbances in neurotransmitters' activities
- ↓ Cortisol activity

Schizophrenia
- Changes in dopamine carrier-membrane translocation
- Alteration of redox mechanisms modulating NMDARs
- ↑ Oxidative stres

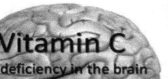

Figure 2. The main potential consequences of brain Vit C deficiency in the course and pathogenesis of neurological disorders.

In conclusion, the future studies concerning the question if Vit C could be a promising adjuvant in therapy of neurodegenerative and/or psychiatric disorders in humans, seem to be advisable.

References

1. Du, J.; Cullen, J.J.; Buettner, G.R. Ascorbic acid: Chemistry, biology and the treatment of cancer. *Biochim. Biophys. Acta* **2012**, *1826*, 443–457. [CrossRef] [PubMed]
2. Traber, M.G.; Stevens, J.F. Vitamins C and E: Beneficial effects from a mechanistic perspective. *Free Radic. Biol. Med.* **2011**, *51*, 1000–1013. [CrossRef] [PubMed]
3. Said, H.M. Intestinal absorption of water-soluble vitamins in health and disease. *Biochem. J.* **2011**, *437*, 357–372. [CrossRef] [PubMed]
4. Berger, M.M. Vitamin C requirements in parenteral nutrition. *Gastroenterology* **2009**, *137*, 70–78. [CrossRef] [PubMed]
5. Hart, A.; Cota, A.; Makhdom, A.; Harvey, E.J. The Role of Vitamin C in Orthopedic Trauma and Bone Health. *Am. J. Orthop.* **2015**, *44*, 306–311. [PubMed]
6. Waly, M.I.; Al-Attabi, Z.; Guizani, N. Low Nourishment of Vitamin C Induces Glutathione Depletion and Oxidative Stress in Healthy Young Adults. *Prev. Nutr. Food Sci.* **2015**, *20*, 198–203. [CrossRef] [PubMed]
7. Eldridge, C.F.; Bunge, M.B.; Bunge, R.P.; Wood, P.M. Differentiation of axon-related Schwann cells in vitro. I. Ascorbic acid regulates basal lamina assembly and myelin formation. *J. Cell. Biol.* **1987**, *105*, 1023–1034. [CrossRef] [PubMed]
8. Sawicka-Glazer, E.; Czuczwar, S.J. Vitamin C: A new auxiliary treatment of epilepsy? *Pharmacol. Rep.* **2014**, *66*, 529–533. [CrossRef] [PubMed]

9. Warner, T.A.; Kang, J.Q.; Kennard, J.K.; Harrison, F.E. Low brain ascorbic acid increases susceptibility to seizures in mouse models of decreased brain ascorbic acid transport and Alzheimer's disease. *Epilepsy Res.* **2015**, *110*, 20–25. [CrossRef] [PubMed]

10. Tveden-Nyborg, P.; Vogt, L.; Schjoldager, J.G.; Jeannet, N.; Hasselholt, S.; Paidi, M.D.; Christen, S.; Lykkesfeldt, J. Maternal vitamin C deficiency during pregnancy persistently impairs hippocampal neurogenesis in offspring of guinea pigs. *PLoS ONE* **2012**, *7*, e48488. [CrossRef] [PubMed]

11. Olajide, O.J.; Yawson, E.O.; Gbadamosi, I.T.; Arogundade, T.T.; Lambe, E.; Obasi, K.; Lawal, I.T.; Ibrahim, A.; Ogunrinola, K.Y. Ascorbic acid ameliorates behavioural deficits and neuropathological alterations in rat model of Alzheimer's disease. *Environ. Toxicol. Pharmacol.* **2017**, *50*, 200–211. [CrossRef] [PubMed]

12. Sil, S.; Ghosh, T.; Gupta, P.; Ghosh, R.; Kabir, S.N.; Roy, A. Dual Role of Vitamin C on the Neuroinflammation Mediated Neurodegeneration and Memory Impairments in Colchicine Induced Rat Model of Alzheimer Disease. *J. Mol. Neurosci.* **2016**, *60*, 421–435. [CrossRef] [PubMed]

13. Nualart, F.; Mack, L.; García, A.; Cisternas, P.; Bongarzone, E.R.; Heitzer, M.; Jara, N.; Martínez, F.; Ferrada, L.; Espinoza, F.; et al. Vitamin C Transporters, Recycling and the Bystander Effect in the Nervous System: SVCT2 versus Gluts. *J. Stem Cell Res. Ther.* **2014**, *4*, 209. [CrossRef] [PubMed]

14. Corpe, C.P.; Tu, H.; Eck, P.; Wang, J.; Faulhaber-Walter, R.; Schnermann, J.; Margolis, S.; Padayatty, S.; Sun, H.; Wang, Y.; et al. Vitamin C transporter Slc23a1 links renal reabsorption, vitamin C tissue accumulation and perinatal survival in mice. *J. Clin. Investig.* **2010**, *120*, 1069–1083. [CrossRef] [PubMed]

15. Tsukaguchi, H.; Tokui, T.; Mackenzie, B.; Berger, U.V.; Chen, X.Z.; Wang, Y.; Brubaker, R.F.; Hediger, M.A. A family of mammalian Na1-dependent L-ascorbic acid transporters. *Nature* **1999**, *399*, 70–75. [CrossRef] [PubMed]

16. Hansen, S.N.; Tveden-Nyborg, P.; Lykkesfeldt, J. Does vitamin C deficiency affect cognitive development and function? *Nutrients* **2014**, *6*, 3818–3846. [CrossRef] [PubMed]

17. Hosoya, K.; Nakamura, G.; Akanuma, S.; Tomi, M.; Tachikawa, M. Dehydroascorbic acid uptake and intracellular ascorbic acid accumulation in cultured Müller glial cells (TR-MUL). *Neurochem. Int.* **2008**, *52*, 1351–1357. [CrossRef] [PubMed]

18. Parker, W.H.; Qu, Z.; May, J.M. Ascorbic Acid Transport in Brain Microvascular Pericytes. *Biochem. Biophys. Res. Commun.* **2015**, *458*, 262–267. [CrossRef] [PubMed]

19. May, J.M. Vitamin C transport and its role in the central nervous system. *Subcell. Biochem.* **2012**, *56*, 85–103. [CrossRef] [PubMed]

20. Castro, M.; Caprile, T.; Astuya, A.; Millán, C.; Reinicke, K.; Vera, J.C.; Vásquez, O.; Aguayo, L.G.; Nualart, F. High-affinity sodium-vitamin C co-transporters (SVCT) expression in embryonic mouse neurons. *J. Neurochem.* **2001**, *78*, 815–823. [CrossRef] [PubMed]

21. García-Krauss, A.; Ferrada, L.; Astuya, A.; Salazar, K.; Cisternas, P.; Martínez, F.; Ramírez, E.; Nualart, F. Dehydroascorbic Acid Promotes Cell Death in Neurons Under Oxidative Stress: A Protective Role for Astrocytes. *Mol. Neurobiol.* **2016**, *53*, 5847–5863. [CrossRef]

22. Covarrubias-Pinto, A.; Acuña, A.I.; Beltrán, F.A.; Torres-Díaz, L.; Castro, M.A. Old Things New View: Ascorbic Acid Protects the Brain in Neurodegenerative Disorders. *Int. J. Mol. Sci.* **2015**, *16*, 28194–28217.

23. Mefford, I.N.; Oke, A.F.; Adams, R.N. Regional distribution of ascorbate in human brain. *Brain Res.* **1981**, *212*, 223–226. [CrossRef]

24. Milby, K.; Oke, A.; Adams, R.N. Detailed mapping of ascorbate distribution in rat brain. *Neurosci. Lett.* **1982**, *28*, 169–174. [CrossRef]

25. Rice, M.E.; Russo-Menna, I. Differential compartmentalization of brain ascorbate and glutathione between neurons and glia. *Neuroscience* **1998**, *82*, 1213–1223. [CrossRef]

26. Harrison, F.E.; May, J.M. Vitamin C function in the brain: Vital role of the ascorbate transporter SVCT2. *Free Radic. Biol. Med.* **2009**, *46*, 719–730. [CrossRef] [PubMed]

27. Miele, M.; Boutelle, M.G.; Fillenz, M. The physiologically induced release of ascorbate in rat brain is dependent on impulse traffic, calcium influx and glutamate uptake. *Neuroscience* **1994**, *62*, 87–91. [CrossRef]

28. Rice, M.E. Ascorbate regulation and its neuroprotective role in the brain. *Trends Neurosci.* **2000**, *23*, 209–216. [CrossRef]

29. Olsen, C.L.; Bunge, R.P. Requisites for growth and myelination of urodele sensory neurons in tissue culture. *J. Exp. Zool.* **1986**, *238*, 373–384. [CrossRef] [PubMed]

30. May, J.M.; Qu, Z.C. Ascorbic acid prevents oxidant-induced increases in endothelial permeability. *Biofactors* **2011**, *37*, 46–50. [CrossRef] [PubMed]

31. Hu, T.M.; Chen, Y.J. Nitrosation-modulating effect of ascorbate in a model dynamic system of coexisting nitric oxide and superoxide. *Free Radic. Res.* **2010**, *44*, 552–562. [CrossRef] [PubMed]

32. Jackson, T.S.; Xu, A.; Vita, J.A.; Keaney, J.F., Jr. Ascorbate prevents the interaction of superoxide and nitric oxide only at very high physiological concentrations. *Circ. Res.* **1998**, *83*, 916–922. [CrossRef] [PubMed]

33. Mock, J.T.; Chaudhari, K.; Sidhu, A.; Sumien, N. The influence of vitamins E and C and exercise on brain aging. *Exp. Gerontol.* **2016**. [CrossRef] [PubMed]

34. Majewska, M.D.; Bell, J.A.; London, E.D. Regulation of the NMDA receptor by redox phenomena: Inhibitory role of ascorbate. *Brain Res.* **1990**, *537*, 328–332. [CrossRef]

35. Rebec, G.V.; Pierce, R.C. A vitamin as neuromodulator: Ascorbate release into the extracellular fluid of the brain regulates dopaminergic and glutamatergic transmission. *Prog. Neurobiol.* **1994**, *43*, 537–565. [CrossRef]

36. Serra, P.A.; Esposito, G.; Delogu, M.R.; Migheli, R.; Rocchitta, G.; Grella, G.; Miele, E.; Miele, M.; Desole, M.S. Analysis of 3-morpholinosydnonimine and sodium nitroprusside effects on dopamine release in the striatum of freely moving rats: Role of nitric oxide, iron and ascorbic acid. *Br. J. Pharmacol.* **2000**, *131*, 836–842. [CrossRef] [PubMed]

37. Todd, R.D.; Bauer, P.A. Ascorbate modulates 5-[3*H*]hydroxytryptamine binding to central 5-HT3 sites in bovine frontal cortex. *J. Neurochem.* **1988**, *50*, 1505–1512. [CrossRef] [PubMed]

38. Figueroa-Méndez, R.; Rivas-Arancibia, S. Vitamin C in Health and Disease: Its Role in the Metabolism of Cells and Redox State in the Brain. *Front. Physiol.* **2015**, *23*, 397. [CrossRef] [PubMed]

39. Seitz, G.; Gebhardt, S.; Beck, J.F.; Böhm, W.; Lode, H.N.; Niethammer, D.; Bruchelt, G. Ascorbic acid stimulates DOPA synthesis and tyrosine hydroxylase gene expression in the human neuroblastoma cell line SK-N-SH. *Neurosci. Lett.* **1998**, *244*, 33–36. [CrossRef]

40. Calero, C.I.; Vickers, E.; Cid, G.M.; Aguayo, L.G.; von Gersdorff, H.; Calvo, D.J. Allosteric modulation of retinal GABA receptors by ascorbic acid. *J. Neurosci.* **2011**, *31*, 9672–9682. [CrossRef] [PubMed]

41. Majewska, M.D.; Bell, J.A. Ascorbic acid protects neurons from injury induced by glutamate and NMDA. *Neuroreport* **1990**, *1*, 194–196. [CrossRef] [PubMed]

42. Fan, S.F.; Yazulla, S. Modulation of voltage-dependent k+ currents (Ik(v)) in retinal bipolar cells by ascorbate is mediated by dopamine d1 receptors. *Vis. Neurosci.* **1999**, *16*, 923–931. [CrossRef] [PubMed]

43. Nelson, M.T.; Joksovic, P.M.; Su, P.; Kang, H.W.; Van Deusen, A.; Baumgart, J.P.; David, L.S.; Snutch, T.P.; Barrett, P.Q.; Lee, J.H.; et al. Molecular mechanisms of subtype-specific inhibition of neuronal t-type calcium channels by ascorbate. *J. Neurosci.* **2007**, *27*, 12577–12583. [CrossRef] [PubMed]

44. Kara, Y.; Doguc, D.K.; Kulac, E.; Gultekin, F. Acetylsalicylic acid and ascorbic acid combination improves cognition; via antioxidant effect or increased expression of NMDARs and nAChRs? *Environ. Toxicol. Pharmacol.* **2014**, *37*, 916–927. [CrossRef] [PubMed]

45. Sandstrom, M.I.; Rebec, G.V. Extracellular ascorbate modulates glutamate dynamics: Role of behavioral activation. *BMC Neurosci.* **2007**, *8*, 32. [CrossRef] [PubMed]

46. Tolbert, L.C.; Morris, P.E., Jr.; Spollen, J.J.; Ashe, S.C. Stereospecific effects of ascorbic acid and analogues on D1 and D2 agonist binding. *Life Sci.* **1992**, *51*, 921–930. [CrossRef]

47. Castro, M.A.; Angulo, C.; Brauchi, S.; Nualart, F.; Concha, I.I. Ascorbic acid participates in a general mechanism for concerted glucose transport inhibition and lactate transport stimulation. *Pflugers Arch.* **2008**, *457*, 519–528. [CrossRef] [PubMed]

48. Beltrán, F.A.; Acuña, A.I.; Miro, M.P.; Anulo, C.; Concha, I.I.; Castro, M.A. Ascorbic acid-dependent GLUT3 inhibition is a critical step for switching neuronal metabolism. *J. Cell. Physiol.* **2011**, *226*, 3286–3294. [CrossRef] [PubMed]

49. Sotiriou, S.; Gispert, S.; Cheng, J.; Wang, Y.H.; Chen, A.; Hoogstraten-Miller, S.; Miller, G.F.; Kwon, O.; Levine, M.; Guttentag, S.H.; et al. Ascorbic-acid transporter Slc23a1 is essential for vitamin C transport into the brain and for perinatal survival. *Nat. Med.* **2002**, *8*, 514–517. [CrossRef] [PubMed]

50. Shah, S.A.; Yoon, G.H.; Kim, H.O.; Kim, M.O. Vitamin C neuroprotection against dose-dependent glutamate-induced neurodegeneration in the postnatal brain. *Neurochem. Res.* **2015**, *40*, 875–884. [CrossRef] [PubMed]

51. Bekris, L.M.; Yu, C.E.; Bird, T.D.; Tsuang, D.W. Genetics of Alzheimer Disease. *J. Geriatr. Psychiatry Neurol.* **2010**, *23*, 213–227. [CrossRef] [PubMed]

52. Barber, R.C. The Genetics of Alzheimer's Disease. *Scientifica (Cairo)* **2012**, *2012*, 46210. [CrossRef] [PubMed]

53. Lee, E.; Giovanello, K.S.; Saykin, A.J.; Xie, F.; Kong, D.; Wang, Y.; Yang, L.; Ibrahim, J.G.; Doraiswamy, P.M.; Zhu, H. Single-nucleotide polymorphisms are associated with cognitive decline at Alzheimer's disease conversion within mild cognitive impairment patients. *Alzheimers Dement.* **2017**, *8*, 86–95. [CrossRef] [PubMed]

54. Ott, S.; Henkel, A.W.; Henkel, M.K.; Redzic, Z.B.; Kornhuber, J.; Wiltfang, J. Pre-aggregated Aβ1 42 peptide increases tau aggregation and hyperphosphorylation after short-term application. *Mol. Cell. Biochem.* **2011**, *349*, 169–177. [CrossRef] [PubMed]

55. Marszałek, M. Alzheimer's disease against peptides products of enzymatic cleavage of APP protein. Forming and variety of fibrillating peptides—Some aspects. *Postepy Hig. Med. Dosw.* **2016**, *70*, 787–796. [CrossRef] [PubMed]

56. Nagababu, E.; UsatyuK, P.V.; Enika, D.; Natarajan, V.; Rifkind, J.M. Vascular Endothelial Barrier Dysfunction Mediated by Amyloid-β Proteins. *J. Alzheimers Dis.* **2009**, *17*, 845–854. [CrossRef] [PubMed]

57. Li, Q.; Cui, J.; Fang, C.; Liu, M.; Min, G.; Li, L. S-Adenosylmethionine Attenuates Oxidative Stress and Neuroinflammation Induced by Amyloid-β Through Modulation of Glutathione Metabolism. *J. Alzheimers Dis.* **2017**, *58*, 549–558. [CrossRef] [PubMed]

58. Bartzokis, G.; Lu, P.H.; Mintzd, J. Human brain myelination and amyloid beta deposition in Alzheimer's disease. *Alzheimers Dement.* **2007**, *3*, 122–125. [CrossRef] [PubMed]

59. McGeer, P.L.; McGeer, E.G. The amyloid cascade-inflammatory hypothesis of Alzheimer disease: Implications for therapy. *Acta Neuropathol.* **2013**, *126*, 479. [CrossRef] [PubMed]

60. Dinkins, M.B.; Dasgupta, S.; Wang, G.; Zhu, G.; Bieberich, E. Exosome reduction in vivo is associated with lower amyloid plaque load in the 5XFAD mouse model of Alzheimer's disease. *Neurobiol. Aging* **2014**, *35*, 1792–1800. [CrossRef] [PubMed]

61. Málaga-Trillo, E.; Ochs, K. Uncontrolled SFK-mediated protein trafficking in prion and Alzheimer's disease. *Prion* **2016**, *10*, 352–361. [CrossRef] [PubMed]

62. Dixit, S.; Bernardo, A.; Walker, J.M.; Kennard, J.A.; Kim, G.Y.; Kessler, E.S.; Harrison, F.E. Vitamin C deficiency in the brain impairs cognition, increases amyloid accumulation and deposition, and oxidative stress in APP/PSEN1 and normally aging mice. *ACS Chem. Neurosci.* **2015**, *6*, 570–581. [CrossRef] [PubMed]

63. Ward, M.S.; Lamb, J.; May, J.M.; Harrison, F.E. Behavioral and monoamine changes following severe vitamin C deficiency. *J. Neurochem.* **2013**, *124*, 363–375. [CrossRef] [PubMed]

64. Sarkar, S.; Mukherjee, A.; Swarnakar, S.; Das, N. Nanocapsulated Ascorbic Acid in Combating Cerebral Ischemia Reperfusion—Induced Oxidative Injury in Rat Brain. *Curr. Alzheimer. Res.* **2016**, *13*, 1363–1373. [CrossRef] [PubMed]

65. Kennard, J.A.; Harrison, F.E. Intravenous ascorbate improves spatial memory in middle-aged APP/PSEN1 and wild type mice. *Behav. Brain Res.* **2014**, *264*, 34–42. [CrossRef] [PubMed]

66. Harrison, F.E.; Hosseini, A.H.; McDonald, M.P.; May, J.M. Vitamin C reduces spatial learning deficits in middle-aged and very old APP/PSEN1 transgenic and wild-type mice. *Pharmacol. Biochem. Behav.* **2009**, *93*, 113 150. [CrossRef] [PubMed]

67. Murakami, K.; Murata, N.; Ozawa, Y.; Kinoshita, N.; Irie, K.; Shirasawa, T.; Shimizu, T. Vitamin C restores behavioral deficits and amyloid-β oligomerization without affecting plaque formation in a mouse model of Alzheimer's disease. *J. Alzheimers Dis.* **2011**, *26*, 7–18. [CrossRef] [PubMed]

68. Lam, V.; Hackett, M.; Takechi, R. Antioxidants and Dementia Risk: Consideration through a Cerebrovascular Perspective. *Nutrients* **2016**, *8*, 828. [CrossRef] [PubMed]

69. Kook, S.Y.; Lee, K.M.; Kim, Y.; Cha, M.Y.; Kang, S.; Baik, S.H.; Lee, H.; Park, R.; Mook-Jung, I. High-dose of vitamin C supplementation reduces amyloid plaque burden and ameliorates pathological changes in the brain of 5XFAD mice. *Cell Death Dis.* **2014**, *5*, 1083. [CrossRef] [PubMed]

70. Allahtavakoli, M.; Amin, F.; Esmaeeli-Nadimi, A.; Shamsizadeh, A.; Kazemi-Arababadi, M.; Kennedy, D. Ascorbic Acid Reduces the Adverse Effects of Delayed Administration of Tissue Plasminogen Activator in a Rat Stroke Model. *Basic Clin. Pharmacol. Toxicol.* **2015**, *117*, 335–339. [CrossRef] [PubMed]

71. Song, J.; Park, J.; Kim, J.H.; Choi, J.Y.; Kim, J.Y.; Lee, K.M.; Lee, J.E. Dehydroascorbic Acid Attenuates Ischemic Brain Edema and Neurotoxicity in Cerebral Ischemia: An in vivo Study. *Exp. Neurobiol.* **2015**, *24*, 41–54. [CrossRef] [PubMed]

72. Lin, J.L.; Huang, Y.H.; Shen, Y.C.; Huang, H.C.; Liu, pH. Ascorbic acid prevents blood-brain barrier disruption and sensory deficit caused by sustained compression of primary somatosensory cortex. *J. Cereb. Blood Flow. Metab.* **2010**, *30*, 1121–1136. [CrossRef] [PubMed]

73. Polidori, M.C.; Mattioli, P.; Aldred, S.; Cecchetti, R.; Stahl, W.; Griffiths, H.; Senin, U.; Sies, H.; Mecocci, P. Plasma antioxidant status, immunoglobulin g oxidation and lipid peroxidation in demented patients: Relevance to Alzheimer disease and vascular dementia. *Dement. Geriatr. Cogn. Disord.* **2004**, *18*, 265–270. [CrossRef] [PubMed]

74. Schippling, S.; Kontush, A.; Arlt, S.; Buhmann, C.; Sturenburg, H.J.; Mann, U.; Griffiths, H.; Senin, U.; Sies, H.; Mecocci, P. Increased lipoprotein oxidation in Alzheimer's disease. *Free Radic. Biol. Med.* **2000**, *28*, 351–360. [CrossRef]

75. Lopes da Silva, S.; Vellas, B.; Elemans, S.; Luchsinger, J.; Kamphuis, P.; Yaffe, K.; Sijben, J.; Groenendijk, M.; Stijnen, T. Plasma nutrient status of patients with Alzheimer's disease: Systematic review and meta-analysis. *Alzheimers Dement.* **2014**, *10*, 485–502. [CrossRef] [PubMed]

76. Arlt, S.; Müller-Thomsen, T.; Beisiegel, U.; Kontush, A. Effect of one-year vitamin C- and E-supplementation on cerebrospinal fluid oxidation parameters and clinical course in Alzheimer's disease. *Neurochem. Res.* **2012**, *37*, 2706–2714. [CrossRef] [PubMed]

77. Galasko, D.R.; Peskind, E.; Clark, C.M.; Quinn, J.F.; Ringman, J.M.; Jicha, G.A.; Cotman, C.; Cottrell, B.; Montine, T.J.; Thomas, R.G.; et al. Alzheimer's Disease Cooperative Study. Antioxidants for Alzheimer disease: A randomized clinical trial with cerebrospinal fluid biomarker measures. *Arch. Neurol.* **2012**, *69*, 836–841. [CrossRef] [PubMed]

78. Chan, S.; Kantham, S.; Rao, V.M.; Palanivelu, M.K.; Pham, H.L.; Shaw, P.N.; McGeary, R.P.; Ross, B.P. Metal chelation, radical scavenging and inhibition of Aβ_{42} fibrillation by food constituents in relation to Alzheimer's disease. *Food Chem.* **2016**, *199*, 185–194. [CrossRef] [PubMed]

79. Berti, V.; Murray, J.; Davies, M.; Spector, N.; Tsui, W.H.; Li, Y.; Williams, S.; Pirraglia, E.; Vallabhajosula, S.; McHugh, P.; et al. Nutrient patterns and brain biomarkers of Alzheimer's disease in cognitively normal individuals. *J. Nutr. Health Aging* **2015**, *19*, 413–423. [CrossRef] [PubMed]

80. Li, Y.; Liu, S.; Man, Y.; Li, N.; Zhou, Y. Effects of vitamins E and C combined with β-carotene on cognitive function in the elderly. *Exp. Ther. Med.* **2015**, *9*, 1489–1493. [CrossRef] [PubMed]

81. Zandi, P.P.; Anthony, J.C.; Khachaturian, A.S.; Stone, S.V.; Gustafson, D.; Tschanz, J.T.; Norton, M.C.; Welsh-Bohmer, K.A.; Breitner, J.C. Cache County Study Group. Reduced risk of Alzheimer disease in users of antioxidant vitamin supplements: The Cache County Study. *Arch. Neurol.* **2004**, *61*, 82–88. [CrossRef] [PubMed]

82. Polidori, M.C.; Ruggiero, C.; Croce, M.F.; Raichi, T.; Mangialasche, F.; Cecchetti, R.; Pelini, L.; Paolacci, L.; Ercolani, S.; Mecocci, P. Association of increased carotid intima-media thickness and lower plasma levels of vitamin C and vitamin E in old age subjects: Implications for Alzheimer's disease. *J. Neural Transm.* **2015**, *122*, 523–530. [CrossRef] [PubMed]

83. Su, B.; Liu, H.; Wang, X.; Chen, S.G.; Siedlak, S.L.; Kondo, E.; Choi, R.; Takeda, A.; Castellani, R.J.; Perry, G.; et al. Ectopic localization of FOXO3a protein in Lewy bodies in Lewy body dementia and Parkinson's disease. *Mol. Neurodegener.* **2009**, *4*, 32. [CrossRef] [PubMed]

84. Cacabelos, R. Parkinson's Disease: From Pathogenesis to Pharmacogenomics. *Int. J. Mol. Sci.* **2017**, *18*, 551. [CrossRef] [PubMed]

85. Nalls, M.A.; Pankratz, N.; Lill, C.M.; Do, C.B.; Hernandez, D.G.; Saad, M.; DeStefano, A.L.; Kara, E.; Bras, J.; Sharma, M.; et al. Large-scale meta-analysis of genome-wide association data identifies six new risk loci for Parkinson's disease. *Nat. Genet.* **2014**, *46*, 989–993. [CrossRef] [PubMed]

86. Tanner, C.M.; Kamel, F.; Ross, G.W.; Hoppin, J.A.; Goldman, S.M.; Korell, M.; Marras, C.; Bhudhikanok, G.S.; Kasten, M.; Chade, A.R.; et al. Rotenone, paraquat, and Parkinson's disease. *Environ. Health. Perspect.* **2011**, *119*, 866–872. [CrossRef] [PubMed]

87. Hao, L.Y.; Giasson, B.L.; Bonini, N.M. DJ-1 is critical for mitochondrial function and rescues PINK1 loss of function. *Proc. Natl. Acad. Sci. USA* **2010**, *107*, 9747–9752. [CrossRef] [PubMed]

88. Gautier, C.A.; Kitada, T.; Shen, J. Loss of PINK1 causes mitochondrial functional defects and increased sensitivity to oxidative stress. *Proc. Natl. Acad. Sci. USA* **2008**, *105*, 11364–11369. [CrossRef] [PubMed]

89. Elkon, H.; Melamed, E.; Offen, D. Oxidative stress, induced by 6-hydroxydopamine, reduces proteasome activities in PC12 cells: Implications for the pathogenesis of Parkinson's disease. *J. Mol. Neurosci.* **2004**, *24*, 387–400. [CrossRef]

90. Belluzzi, E.; Bisaglia, M.; Lazzarini, E.; Tabares, L.C.; Beltramini, M.; Bubacco, L. Human SOD2 modification by dopamine quinones affects enzymatic activity by promoting its aggregation: Possible implications for Parkinson's disease. *PLoS ONE* **2012**, *7*, e38026. [CrossRef] [PubMed]

91. Rokad, D.; Ghaisas, S.; Harischandra, D.S.; Jin, H.; Anantharam, V.; Kanthasamy, A.; Kanthasamy, A.G. Role of neurotoxicants and traumatic brain injury in α-synuclein protein misfolding and aggregation. *Brain Res. Bull.* **2016**. [CrossRef] [PubMed]

92. Irwin, D.J.; Grossman, M.; Weintraub, D.; Hurtig, H.I.; Duda, J.E.; Xie, S.X.; Lee, E.B.; Van Deerlin, V.M.; Lopez, O.L.; Kofler, J.K.; et al. Neuropathological and genetic correlates of survival and dementia onset in synucleinopathies: A retrospective analysis. *Lancet. Neurol.* **2017**, *16*, 55–65. [CrossRef]

93. Rieder, C.R.; Williams, A.C.; Ramsden, D.B. Selegiline increases heme oxygenase-1 expression and the cytotoxicity produced by dopaminetreatment of neuroblastoma SK-N-SH cells. *Braz. J. Med. Biol. Res.* **2004**, *37*, 1055–1062. [CrossRef] [PubMed]

94. Olanow, C.W.; Brundin, P. Parkinson's disease and alpha synuclein: Is Parkinson's disease a prion-like disorder? *Mov. Disord.* **2013**, *28*, 31–40. [CrossRef] [PubMed]

95. Seidel, K.; Bouzrou, M.; Heidemann, N.; Krüger, R.; Schöls, L.; den Dunnen, W.F.A.; Korf, H.W.; Rüb, U. Involvement of the cerebellum in Parkinson disease and dementia with Lewy bodies. *Ann. Neurol.* **2017**. [CrossRef] [PubMed]

96. Armstrong, R.A. Evidence from spatial pattern analysis for the anatomical spread of α-synuclein pathology in Parkinson's disease dementia. *Folia Neuropathol.* **2017**, *55*, 23–30. [CrossRef] [PubMed]

97. Scheffold, A.; Holtman, I.R.; Dieni, S.; Brouwer, N.; Katz, S.F.; Jebaraj, B.M.; Kahle, P.J.; Hengerer, B.; Lechel, A.; Stilgenbauer, S.; et al. Telomere shortening leads to an acceleration of synucleinopathy and impaired microglia response in a genetic mouse model. *Acta Neuropathol. Commun.* **2016**, *4*, 87. [CrossRef] [PubMed]

98. He, X.B.; Kim, M.; Kim, S.Y.; Yi, S.H.; Rhee, Y.H.; Kim, T.; Lee, E.H.; Park, C.H.; Dixit, S.; Harrison, F.E.; et al. Vitamin C facilitates dopamine neuron differentiation in fetal midbrain through TET1- and JMJD3-dependent epigenetic control manner. *Stem Cells* **2015**, *33*, 1320–1332. [CrossRef] [PubMed]

99. Camarena, V.; Wang, G. The epigenetic role of vitamin C in health and disease. *Cell. Mol. Life Sci.* **2016**, *73*, 1645–1658. [CrossRef] [PubMed]

100. Minor, E.A.; Court, B.L.; Young, J.I.; Wang, G. Ascorbate Induces Ten-Eleven Translocation (Tet) Methylcytosine Dioxygenase-mediated Generation of 5-Hydroxymethylcytosine. *J. Biol. Chem.* **2013**, *288*, 13669–13674. [CrossRef] [PubMed]

101. Xiang, W.; Schlachetzki, J.C.; Helling, S.; Bussmann, J.C.; Berlinghof, M.; Schaffer, T.E.; Marcus, K.; Winkler, J.; Klucken, J.; Becker, C.M. Oxidative stress-induced posttranslational modifications of α-synuclein: Specific modification of α-synuclein by 4-hydroxy-2-nonenal increases dopaminergic toxicity. *Mol. Cell. Neurosci.* **2013**, *54*, 71–83. [CrossRef] [PubMed]

102. Jinsmaa, Y.; Sullivan, P.; Sharabi, Y.; Goldstein, D.S. DOPAL is transmissible to and oligomerizes alpha-synuclein in human glial cells. *Auton. Neurosci.* **2016**, *194*, 46–51. [CrossRef] [PubMed]

103. Khan, S.; Jyoti, S.; Naz, F.; Shakya, B.; Rahul, A.M.; Siddique, Y.H. Effect of L-ascorbic Acid on the climbing ability and protein levels in the brain of Drosophila model of Parkinson's disease. *J. Neurosci.* **2012**, *122*, 704–709. [CrossRef]

104. Ballaz, S.; Morales, I.; Rodríguez, M.; Obeso, J.A. Ascorbate prevents cell death from prolonged exposure to glutamate in an in vitro model of human dopaminergic neurons. *J. Neurosci. Res.* **2013**, *91*, 1609–1617. [CrossRef] [PubMed]

105. Izumi, Y.; Ezumi, M.; Takada-Takatori, Y.; Akaike, A.; Kume, T. Endogenous dopamine is involved in the herbicide paraquat-induced dopaminergic cell death. *Toxicol. Sci.* **2014**, *139*, 466–478. [CrossRef] [PubMed]

106. Medeiros, M.S.; Schumacher-Schuh, A.; Cardoso, A.M.; Bochi, G.V.; Baldissarelli, J.; Kegler, A.; Santana, D.; Chaves, C.M.; Schetinger, M.R.; Moresco, R.N.; et al. Iron and Oxidative Stress in Parkinson's Disease: An Observational Study of Injury Biomarkers. *PLoS ONE* **2016**, *11*, e0146129. [CrossRef] [PubMed]

107. Quiroga, M.J.; Carroll, D.W.; Brown, T.M. Ascorbate- and zinc-responsive parkinsonism. *Ann. Pharmacother.* **2014**, *48*, 1515–1520. [CrossRef] [PubMed]

108. Ide, K.; Yamada, H.; Umegaki, K.; Mizuno, K.; Kawakami, N.; Hagiwara, Y.; Matsumoto, M.; Yoshida, H.; Kim, K.; Shiosaki, E.; et al. Lymphocyte vitamin C levels as potential biomarker for progression of Parkinson's disease. *Nutrition* **2015**, *31*, 406–408. [CrossRef] [PubMed]

109. Hughes, K.C.; Gao, X.; Kim, I.Y.; Rimm, E.B.; Wang, M.; Weisskopf, M.G.; Schwarzschild, M.A.; Ascherio, A. Intake of antioxidant vitamins and risk of Parkinson's disease. *Mov. Disord.* **2016**, *31*. [CrossRef] [PubMed]

110. Noble, M.; Healey, C.S.; McDougal-Chukwumah, L.D.; Brown, T.M. Old disease, new look? A first report of parkinsonism due to scurvy, and of refeeding-induced worsening of scurvy. *Psychosomatics* **2013**, *54*, 277–283. [CrossRef] [PubMed]

111. Nagayama, H.; Hamamoto, M.; Ueda, M.; Nito, C.; Yamaguchi, H.; Katayama, Y. The effect of ascorbic acid on the pharmacokinetics of levodopa in elderly patients with Parkinson disease. *Clin. Neuropharmacol.* **2004**, *27*, 270–273. [CrossRef] [PubMed]

112. Mariam, I.; Ali, S.; Rehman, A. Ikram-Ul-Haq. L-Ascorbate, a strong inducer of L-dopa (3,4-dihydroxy-L-phenylalanine) production from pre-grown mycelia of Aspergillus oryzae NRRL-1560. *Biotechnol. Appl. Biochem.* **2010**, *55*, 131–137. [CrossRef] [PubMed]

113. Peña-Sánchez, M.; Riverón-Forment, G.; Zaldívar-Vaillant, T.; Soto-Lavastida, A.; Borrero-Sánchez, J.; Lara-Fernández, G.; Esteban-Hernández, E.M.; Hernández-Díaz, Z.; González-Quevedo, A.; Fernández-Almirall, I.; et al. Association of status redox with demographic, clinical and imaging parameters in patients with Huntington's disease. *Clin. Biochem.* **2015**, *48*, 1258–1263. [CrossRef] [PubMed]

114. Sari, Y. Huntington's Disease: From Mutant Huntingtin Protein to Neurotrophic Factor Therapy. *Int. J. Biomed. Sci.* **2011**, *7*, 89–100. [PubMed]

115. Paulsen, J.S. Cognitive Impairment in Huntington Disease: Diagnosis and Treatment. *Curr. Neurol. Neurosci. Rep.* **2011**, *11*, 474–483. [CrossRef] [PubMed]

116. Long, J.D.; Paulsen, J.S.; Marder, K.; Zhang, Y.; Kim, J.I.; Mills, J.A. Researchers of the PREDICT-HD Huntington's Study Group. Tracking motor impairments in the progression of Huntington's disease. *Mov. Disord.* **2014**, *29*, 311–319. [CrossRef] [PubMed]

117. Vonsattel, J.P.; Myers, R.H.; Stevens, T.J.; Ferrante, R.J.; Bird, E.D.; Richardson, E.P., Jr. Neuropathological classification of Huntington's disease. *J. Neuropathol. Exp. Neurol.* **1985**, *44*, 559–577. [CrossRef] [PubMed]

118. Postert, T.; Lack, B.; Kuhn, W.; Jergas, M.; Andrich, J.; Braun, B.; Przuntek, H.; Sprengelmeyer, R.; Agelink, M.; Büttner, T. Basal ganglia alterations and brain atrophy in Huntington's disease depicted by transcranial realtime sonography. *J. Neurol. Neurosurg. Psychiatry* **1999**, *67*, 457–462. [CrossRef] [PubMed]

119. Acuña, A.I.; Esparza, M.; Kramm, C.; Beltrán, F.A.; Parra, A.V.; Cepeda, C.; Toro, C.A.; Vidal, R.L.; Hetz, C.; Concha, I.I.; et al. A failure in energy metabolism and antioxidant uptake precede symptoms of Huntington's disease in mice. *Nat. Commun.* **2013**, *4*, 2917. [CrossRef] [PubMed]

120. Weydt, P.; Pineda, V.V.; Torrence, A.E.; Libby, R.T.; Satterfield, T.F.; Lazarowski, E.R.; Gilbert, M.L.; Morton, G.J.; Bammler, T.K.; Strand, A.D.; et al. Thermoregulatory and metabolic defects in Huntington's disease transgenic mice implicate PGC-1alpha in Huntington's disease neurodegeneration. *Cell. Metab.* **2006**, *4*, 349–362. [CrossRef] [PubMed]

121. Tereshchenko, A.; McHugh, M.; Lee, J.K.; Gonzalez-Alegre, P.; Crane, K.; Dawson, J.; Nopoulos, P. Abnormal Weight and Body Mass Index in Children with Juvenile Huntington's Disease. *J. Huntingtons. Dis.* **2015**, *4*, 231–238. [CrossRef] [PubMed]

122. Ross, C.A.; Tabrizi, S.J. Huntington's disease: From molecular pathogenesis to clinical treatment. *Lancet Neurol.* **2011**, *10*, 83–98. [CrossRef]

123. Labbadia, J.; Morimoto, R.I. Huntington's disease: Underlying molecular mechanisms and emerging concepts. *Trends Biochem. Sci.* **2013**, *38*, 378–385. [CrossRef] [PubMed]

124. Tang, T.S.; Chen, X.; Liu, J.; Bezprozvanny, I. Dopaminergic Signaling and Striatal Neurodegeneration in Huntington's Disease. *J. Neurosci.* **2007**, *27*, 7899–7910. [CrossRef] [PubMed]

125. Covarrubias-Pinto, A.; Moll, P.; Solís-Maldonado, M.; Acuña, A.I.; Riveros, A.; Miró, M.P.; Papic, E.; Beltrán, F.A.; Cepeda, C.; Concha, I.I.; et al. Beyond the redox imbalance: Oxidative stress contributes to an impaired GLUT3 modulation in Huntington's disease. *Free Radic. Biol. Med.* **2015**, *89*, 1085–1096. [CrossRef] [PubMed]

126. Miller, B.R.; Dorner, J.L.; Bunner, K.D.; Gaither, T.W.; Klein, E.L.; Barton, S.J.; Rebec, G.V. Up-regulation of GLT1 reverses the deficit in cortically evoked striatal ascorbate efflux in the R6/2 mouse model of Huntington's disease. *J. Neurochem.* **2012**, *121*, 629–638. [CrossRef] [PubMed]

127. Dorner, J.L.; Miller, B.R.; Klein, E.L.; Murphy-Nakhnikian, A.; Andrews, R.L.; Barton, S.J.; Rebec, G.V. Corticostriatal dysfunction underlies diminished striatal ascorbate release in the R6/2 mouse model of Huntington's disease. *Brain Res.* **2009**, *1290*, 111–120. [CrossRef] [PubMed]

128. Rebec, G.V. Dysregulation of corticostriatal ascorbate release and glutamate uptake in transgenic models of Huntington's disease. *Antioxid. Redox Signal.* **2013**, *19*, 2115–2128. [CrossRef] [PubMed]

129. Rebec, G.V.; Conroy, S.K.; Barton, S.J. Hyperactive striatal neurons in symptomatic Huntington R6/2 mice: Variations with behavioral state and repeated ascorbate treatment. *Neuroscience* **2006**, *137*, 327–336. [CrossRef] [PubMed]

130. Rebec, G.V.; Barton, S.J.; Marseilles, A.M.; Collins, K. Ascorbate treatment attenuates the Huntington behavioral phenotype in mice. *Neuroreport* **2003**, *14*, 1263–1265. [CrossRef] [PubMed]

131. Hadžović-Džuvo, A.; Lepara, O.; Valjevac, A.; Avdagić, N.; Hasić, S.; Kiseljaković, E.; Ibragić, S.; Alajbegović, A. Serum total antioxidant capacity in patients with multiple sclerosis. *Bosn. J. Basic Med. Sci.* **2011**, *11*, 33–36. [PubMed]

132. Rottlaender, A.; Kuerten, S. Stepchild or Prodigy? Neuroprotection in Multiple Sclerosis (MS) Research. *Int. J. Mol. Sci.* **2015**, *16*, 14850–14865. [CrossRef] [PubMed]

133. Morandi, E.; Tarlinton, R.E.; Gran, B. Multiple Sclerosis between Genetics and Infections: Human Endogenous Retroviruses in Monocytes and Macrophages. *Front. Immunol.* **2015**, *6*, 647. [CrossRef] [PubMed]

134. Pagano, G.; Talamanca, A.A.; Castello, G.; Cordero, M.D.; d'Ischia, M.; Gadaleta, M.N.; Pallardó, F.V.; Petrović, S.; Tiano, L.; Zatterale, A. Oxidative stress and mitochondrial dysfunction across broad-ranging pathologies: Toward mitochondria-targeted clinical strategies. *Oxid. Med. Cell. Longev.* **2014**, *2014*, 541230. [CrossRef] [PubMed]

135. Polachini, C.R.; Spanevello, R.M.; Zanini, D.; Baldissarelli, J.; Pereira, L.B.; Schetinger, M.R.; da Cruz, I.B.; Assmann, C.E.; Bagatini, M.D.; Morsch, V.M. Evaluation of Delta Aminolevulinic Dehydratase Activity, Oxidative Stress Biomarkers, and Vitamin D Levels in Patients with Multiple Sclerosis. *Neurotox. Res.* **2016**, *29*, 230–242. [CrossRef] [PubMed]

136. Tavazzi, B.; Batocchi, A.P.; Amorini, A.M.; Nociti, V.; D'Urso, S.; Longo, S.; Gullotta, S.; Picardi, M.; Lazzarino, G. Serum metabolic profile in multiple sclerosis patients. *Epub Mult. Scler. Int.* **2011**, *2011*, 167156. [CrossRef] [PubMed]

137. Patel, J.; Balabanov, R. Molecular mechanisms of oligodendrocyte injury in multiple sclerosis and experimental autoimmune encephalomyelitis. *Int. J. Mol. Sci.* **2012**, *13*, 10647–10659. [CrossRef] [PubMed]

138. Besler, H.T.; Comoğlu, S.; Okçu, Z. Serum levels of antioxidant vitamins and lipid peroxidation in multiple sclerosis. *Nutr. Neurosci.* **2002**, *5*, 215–220. [CrossRef] [PubMed]

139. Hejazi, E.; Amani, R.; SharafodinZadeh, N.; Cheraghian, B. Comparison of Antioxidant Status and Vitamin D Levels between Multiple Sclerosis Patients and Healthy Matched Subjects. *Mult. Scler. Int.* **2014**, *2014*, 539854. [CrossRef] [PubMed]

140. Odinak, M.M.; Bisaga, G.N.; Zarubina, I.V. New Approaches to Antioxidant Therapy in Multiple Sclerosis. Available online: http://www.ncbi.nlm.nih.gov/pubmed/12418396 (accessed on 26 June 2017).

141. Babri, S.; Mehrvash, F.; Mohaddes, G.; Hatami, H.; Mirzaie, F. Effect of intrahippocampal administration of vitamin C and progesterone on learning in a model of multiple sclerosis in rats. *Adv. Pharm. Bull.* **2015**, *5*, 83–87. [CrossRef] [PubMed]

142. Matic, I.; Strobbe, D.; Frison, M.; Campanella, M. Controlled and Impaired Mitochondrial Quality in Neurons: Molecular Physiology and Prospective Pharmacology. *Pharmacol. Res.* **2015**, *99*, 410–424. [CrossRef] [PubMed]

143. Orrell, R.W.; Lane, R.J.; Ross, M. A systematic review of antioxidant treatment for amyotrophic lateral sclerosis/motor neuron disease. *Amyotroph. Lateral Scler.* **2008**, *9*, 195–211. [CrossRef] [PubMed]

144. Blasco, H.; Corcia, P.; Moreau, C.; Veau, S.; Fournier, C.; Vourc'h, P.; Emond, P.; Gordon, P.; Pradat, P.F.; Praline, J.; et al. 1H-NMR-based metabolomic profiling of CSF in early amyotrophic lateral sclerosis. *PLoS ONE* **2010**, *5*, e13223. [CrossRef]

145. Nagano, S.; Fujii, Y.; Yamamoto, T.; Taniyama, M.; Fukada, K.; Yanagihara, T.; Sakoda, S. The efficacy of trientine or ascorbate alone compared to that of the combined treatment with these two agents in familial amyotrophic lateral sclerosis model mice. *Exp. Neurol.* **2003**, *179*, 176–180. [CrossRef]

146. Netzahualcoyotzi, C.; Tapia, R. Degeneration of spinal motor neurons by chronic AMPA-induced excitotoxicity in vivo and protection by energy substrates. *Acta Neuropathol. Commun.* **2015**, *3*, 27. [CrossRef] [PubMed]

147. Fitzgerald, K.C.; O'Reilly, É.J.; Fondell, E.; Falcone, G.J.; McCullough, M.L.; Park, Y.; Kolonel, L.N.; Ascherio, A. Intakes of vitamin C and carotenoids and risk of amyotrophic lateral sclerosis: Pooled results from 5 cohort studies. *Ann. Neurol.* **2013**, *73*, 236–245. [CrossRef] [PubMed]

148. Okamoto, K.; Kihira, T.; Kobashi, G.; Washio, M.; Sasaki, S.; Yokoyama, T.; Miyake, Y.; Sakamoto, N.; Inaba, Y.; Nagai, M. Fruit and vegetable intake and risk of amyotrophic lateral sclerosis in Japan. *Neuroepidemiology* **2009**, *32*, 251–256. [CrossRef] [PubMed]

149. Spasojević, I.; Stević, Z.; Nikolić-Kokić, A.; Jones, D.R.; Blagojević, D.; Spasić, M.B. Different roles of radical scavengers—Ascorbate and urate in the cerebrospinal fluid of amyotrophic lateral sclerosis patients. *Redox Rep.* **2010**, *15*, 81–86. [CrossRef] [PubMed]

150. Liu, Y.; Hu, N. Electrochemical detection of natural DNA damage induced by ferritin/ascorbic acid/H2O2 system and amplification of DNA damage by endonuclease Fpg. *Biosens. Bioelectron.* **2009**, *25*, 185–190. [CrossRef] [PubMed]

151. Bembnowska, M.; Jośko, J. Depressive behaviours among adolescents as a Public Health problem. *Zdr. Publ.* **2011**, *121*, 4260430.

152. Lopresti, A.L. A review of nutrient treatments for paediatric depression. *J. Affect. Disord.* **2015**, *181*, 24–32. [CrossRef] [PubMed]

153. Moretti, M.; Budni, J.; Ribeiro, C.M.; Rieger, D.; Leal, R.B.; Rodrigues, A.L. Subchronic administration of ascorbic acid elicits antidepressant-like effect and modulates cell survival signaling pathways in mice. *J. Nutr. Biochem.* **2016**, *38*, 50–56. [CrossRef] [PubMed]

154. Luscher, B.; Shen, Q.; Sahir, N. The GABAergic Deficit Hypothesis of Major Depressive Disorder. *Mol. Psychiatry* **2011**, *16*, 383–406. [CrossRef] [PubMed]

155. Rosa, P.B.; Neis, V.B.; Ribeiro, C.M.; Moretti, M.; Rodrigues, A.L.S. Antidepressant-like effects of ascorbic acid and ketamine involve modulation of GABAA and GABAB receptors. *Pharmacol. Rep.* **2016**, *68*, 996–1001. [CrossRef]

156. Capuron, L.; Pagnoni, G.; Drake, D.F.; Woolwine, B.J.; Spivey, J.R.; Crowe, R.J.; Votaw, J.R.; Goodman, M.M.; Miller, A.H. Dopaminergic mechanisms of reduced basal ganglia responses to hedonic reward during interferon alfa administration. *Arch. Gen. Psychiatry* **2012**, *69*, 1044–1053. [CrossRef] [PubMed]

157. Bigdeli, T.B.; Ripke, S.; Peterson, R.E.; Trzaskowski, M.; Bacanu, S.A.; Abdellaoui, A.; Andlauer, T.F.; Beekman, A.T.; Berger, K.; Blackwood, D.H.; et al. Genetic effects influencing risk for major depressive disorder in China and Europe. *Transl. Psychiatry* **2017**, *7*, e1074. [CrossRef] [PubMed]

158. Altshuler, L.L.; Abulseoud, O.A.; Foland-Ross, L.; Bartzokis, G.; Chang, S.; Mintz, J.; Hellemann, G.; Vinters, H.V. Amygdala astrocyte reduction in subjects with major depressive disorder but not bipolar disorder. *Bipolar Disord.* **2010**, *12*, 541–549. [CrossRef] [PubMed]

159. Cobb, J.A.; O'Neill, K.; Milner, J.; Mahajan, G.J.; Lawrence, T.J.; May, W.T.; Miguel-Hidalgo, J.; Rajkowska, G.; Stockmeiera, C.A. Density of GFAP-immunoreactive astrocytes is decreased in left hippocampi in major depressive disorder. *Neuroscience* **2016**, *316*, 209–220. [CrossRef] [PubMed]

160. Rajkowska, G.; Hughes, J.; Stockmeier, C.A.; Javier Miguel-Hidalgo, J.; Maciag, D. Coverage of blood vessels by astrocytic endfeet is reduced in major depressive disorder. *Biol. Psychiatry* **2013**, *73*, 613–621. [CrossRef] [PubMed]

161. Rubinow, M.J.; Mahajan, G.; May, W.; Overholser, J.C.; Jurjus, G.J.; Dieter, L.; Herbst, N.; Steffens, D.C.; Miguel-Hidalgo, J.J.; Rajkowska, G.; et al. Basolateral amygdala volume and cell numbers in major depressive disorder: A postmortem stereological study. *Brain Struct. Funct.* **2016**, *21*, 171–184. [CrossRef] [PubMed]

162. Guillemin, G.J.; Wang, L.; Brew, B.J. Quinolinic acid selectively induces apoptosis of human astrocytes: Potential role in AIDS dementia complex. *J. Neuroinflammation* **2005**, *2*, 16. [CrossRef] [PubMed]

163. Braidy, N.; Grant, R.; Adams, S.; Brew, B.J.; Guillemin, G.J. Mechanism for quinolinic acid cytotoxicity in human astrocytes and neurons. *Neurotox. Res.* **2009**, *16*, 77–86. [CrossRef] [PubMed]

164. Moretti, M.; Budni, J.; Ribeiro, C.M.; Rodrigues, A.L. Involvement of different types of potassium channels in the antidepressant-like effect of ascorbic acid in the mouse tail suspension test. *Eur. J. Pharmacol.* **2012**, *687*, 21–27. [CrossRef] [PubMed]

165. Moretti, M.; Budni, J.; Freitas, A.E.; Neis, V.B.; Ribeiro, C.M.; de Oliveira Balen, G.; Rieger, D.K.; Leal, R.B.; Rodrigues, A.L. TNF-α-induced depressive-like phenotype and p38(MAPK) activation are abolished by ascorbic acid treatment. *Eur. Neuropsychopharmacol.* **2015**, *25*, 902–912. [CrossRef] [PubMed]

166. Zhao, B.; Fei, J.; Chen, Y.; Ying, Y.L.; Ma, L.; Song, X.Q.; Wang, L.; Chen, E.Z.; Mao, E.Q. Pharmacological preconditioning with vitamin C attenuates intestinal injury via the induction of heme oxygenase-1 after hemorrhagic shock in rats. *PLoS ONE* **2014**, *9*, 99134. [CrossRef]

167. Binfaré, R.W.; Rosa, A.O.; Lobato, K.R.; Santos, A.R.; Rodrigues, A.L.S. Ascorbic acid administration produces an antidepressant-like effect: Evidence for the involvement of monoaminergic neurotransmission. *Prog. Neuropsychopharmacol. Biol. Psychiatry* **2009**, *33*, 530–540. [CrossRef] [PubMed]

168. Robaczewska, J.; Kędziora-Kornatowska, K.; Kucharski, R.; Nowak, M.; Muszalik, M.; Kornatowski, M.; Kędziora, J. Decreased expression of heme oxygenase is associated with depressive symptoms and may contribute to depressive and hypertensive comorbidity. *Redox Rep.* **2016**, *21*, 209–218. [CrossRef] [PubMed]

169. Gariballa, S. Poor vitamin C status is associated with increased depression symptoms following acute illness in older people. *Int. J. Vitam. Nutr. Res.* **2014**, *84*, 12–17. [CrossRef] [PubMed]

170. Bajpai, A.; Verma, A.K.; Srivastava, M.; Srivastava, R. Oxidative stress and major depression. *J. Clin. Diagn. Res.* **2014**, *8*, 4–7. [CrossRef] [PubMed]

171. Gautam, M.; Agrawal, M.; Gautam, M.; Sharma, P.; Gautam, A.S.; Gautam, S. Role of antioxidants in generalised anxiety disorder and depression. *Indian J. Psychiatry* **2012**, *54*, 244–247. [CrossRef] [PubMed]

172. Prohan, M.; Amani, R.; Nematpour, S.; Jomehzadeh, N.; Haghighizadeh, M.H. Total antioxidant capacity of diet and serum, dietary antioxidant vitamins intake, and serum hs-CRP levels in relation to depression scales in university male students. *Redox Rep.* **2014**, *19*, 133–139. [CrossRef] [PubMed]

173. Kim, T.H.; Choi, J.Y.; Lee, H.H.; Park, Y. Associations between Dietary Pattern and Depression in Korean Adolescent Girls. *J. Pediatr. Adolesc. Gynecol.* **2015**, *28*, 533–537. [CrossRef] [PubMed]

174. Rubio-López, N.; Morales-Suárez-Varela, M.; Pico, Y.; Livianos-Aldana, L.; Llopis-González, A. Nutrient Intake and Depression Symptoms in Spanish Children: The ANIVA Study. *Int. J. Environ. Res. Public Health* **2016**, *13*, 352. [CrossRef] [PubMed]

175. Amr, M.; El-Mogy, A.; Shams, T.; Vieira, K.; Lakhan, S.E. Efficacy of vitamin C as an adjunct to fluoxetine therapy in pediatric major depressive disorder: A randomized, double-blind, placebo-controlled pilot study. *Nutr. J.* **2013**, *12*, 31. [CrossRef] [PubMed]

176. Zhang, M.; Robitaille, L.; Eintracht, S.; Hoffer, L.J. Vitamin C provision improves mood in acutely hospitalized patients. *Nutrition* **2011**, *27*, 530–533. [CrossRef] [PubMed]

177. Wang, Y.; Liu, X.J.; Robitaille, L.; Eintracht, S.; MacNamara, E.; Hoffer, L.J. Effects of vitamin C and vitamin D administration on mood and distress in acutely hospitalizedpatients. *Am. J. Clin. Nutr.* **2013**, *98*, 705–711. [CrossRef] [PubMed]

178. Khajehnasiri, F.; Akhondzadeh, S.; Mortazavi, S.B.; Allameh, A.; Sotoudeh, G.; Khavanin, A.; Zamanian, Z. Are Supplementation of Omega-3 and Ascorbic Acid Effective in Reducing Oxidative Stress and Depression among Depressed Shift Workers? *Int. J. Vitam. Nutr. Res.* **2016**, *10*, 1–12. [CrossRef] [PubMed]

179. Fritz, H.; Flower, G.; Weeks, L.; Cooley, K.; Callachan, M.; McGowan, J.; Skidmore, B.; Kirchner, L.; Seely, D. Intravenous Vitamin C and Cancer: A Systematic Review. *Integr. Cancer Ther.* **2014**, *13*, 280–300. [CrossRef] [PubMed]

180. Grillon, C.H. Models and mechanisms of anxiety: Evidence from startle studies. *Psychopharmacology* **2008**, *199*, 421–437. [CrossRef] [PubMed]

181. Hughes, R.N.; Lowther, C.L.; van Nobelen, M. Prolonged treatment with vitamins C and E separately and together decreases anxiety-related open-field behavior and acoustic startle in hooded rats. *Pharmacol. Biochem. Behav.* **2011**, *97*, 494–499. [CrossRef] [PubMed]

182. Kori, R.S.; Aladakatti, R.H.; Desai, S.D.; Das, K.K. Effect of Drug Alprazolam on Restrained Stress Induced Alteration of Serum Cortisol and Antioxidant Vitamins (Vitamin C and E) in Male Albino Rats. *J. Clin. Diagn. Res.* **2016**, *10*, AF07–AF09. [CrossRef] [PubMed]

183. Boufleur, N.; Antoniazzi, C.T.; Pase, C.S.; Benvegnú, D.M.; Dias, V.T.; Segat, H.J.; Roversi, K.; Roversi, K.; Nora, M.D.; Koakoskia, G.; et al. Neonatal handling prevents anxiety-like symptoms in rats exposed to chronic mild stress: Behavioral and oxidative parameters. *Stress* **2013**, *16*, 321–330. [CrossRef] [PubMed]

184. Koizumi, M.; Kondob, Y.; Isakaa, A.; Ishigamib, A.; Suzukia, E. Vitamin C impacts anxiety-like behavior and stress-induced anorexia relative to social environment in SMP30/GNL knockout mice. *Nutr. Res.* **2016**, *36*, 1379–1391. [CrossRef] [PubMed]

185. Hughes, N.R.; Hancock, J.N.; Thompson, R.M. Anxiolysis and recognition memory enhancement with long-term supplemental ascorbic acid (vitamin C) in normal rats: Possible dose dependency and sex differences. *Ann. Neurosci. Psychol.* **2015**, *2*, 2. Available online: http://www.vipoa.org/neuropsychol (accessed on 26 June 2017).

186. Choi, J.Y.; dela Peña, I.C.; Yoon, S.Y.; Woo, T.E.; Choi, Y.J.; Shin, C.Y.; Ryu, J.H.; Lee, Y.S.; Yu, G.Y.; Cheong, J.H. Is the anti-stress effect of vitamin C related to adrenal gland function in rat? *Food Sci. Biotechnol.* **2011**, *20*, 429–435. [CrossRef]

187. Puty, B.; Maximino, C.; Brasil, A.; da Silva, W.L.; Gouveia, A., Jr.; Oliveira, K.R.; Batista Ede, J.; Crespo-Lopez, M.E.; Rocha, F.A.; Herculano, A.M. Ascorbic acid protects against anxiogenic-like effect induced by methylmercury in zebrafish: Action on the serotonergic system. *Zebrafish* **2014**, *11*, 365–370. [CrossRef] [PubMed]

188. Angrini, M.A.; Leslie, J.C. Vitamin C attenuates the physiological and behavioural changes induced by long-term exposure to noise. *Behav. Pharmacol.* **2012**, *23*, 119–125. [CrossRef] [PubMed]

189. De Oliveira, I.J.; de Souza, V.V.; Motta, V.; Da-Silva, S.L. Effects of Oral Vitamin C Supplementation on Anxiety in Students: A Double-Blind, Randomized, Placebo-Controlled Trial. *Pak. J. Biol. Sci.* **2015**, *18*, 11–18. [CrossRef] [PubMed]

190. Mazloom, Z.; Ekramzadeh, M.; Hejazi, N. Efficacy of supplementary vitamins C and E on anxiety, depression and stress in type 2 diabetic patients: A randomized, single-blind, placebo-controlled trial. *Pak. J. Biol. Sci.* **2013**, *16*, 1597–1600. [PubMed]

191. McCabe, D.; Lisy, K.; Lockwood, C.; Colbeck, M. The impact of essential fatty acid, B vitamins, vitamin C, magnesium and zinc supplementation on stress levels in women: A systematic review. *JBI Database Syst. Rev. Implement. Rep.* **2017**, *15*, 402–453. [CrossRef]

192. Arroll, M.A.; Wilder, L.; Neil, J. Nutritional interventions for the adjunctive treatment of schizophrenia: A brief review. *Nutr. J.* **2014**, *13*, 91. [CrossRef] [PubMed]

193. Sershen, H.; Hashim, A.; Dunlop, D.S.; Suckow, R.F.; Cooper, T.B.; Javitt, D.C. Modulating NMDA Receptor Function with D-Amino Acid Oxidase Inhibitors: Understanding Functional Activity in PCP-Treated Mouse Model. *Neurochem. Res.* **2016**, *41*, 398–408. [CrossRef] [PubMed]

194. Javitt, D.C. Twenty-five years of glutamate in schizophrenia: Are we there yet? *Schizophr. Bull.* **2012**, *38*, 911–913. [CrossRef] [PubMed]

195. Wabaidur, S.M.; Alothman, Z.A.; Naushad, M. Determination of dopamine in pharmaceutical formulation using enhanced luminescence from europium complex. *Spectrochim. Acta A Mol. Biomol. Spectrosc.* **2012**, *93*, 331–334. [CrossRef] [PubMed]

196. Morera-Fumero, A.L.; Díaz-Mesa, E.; Abreu-Gonzalez, P.; Fernandez-Lopez, L.; Cejas-Mendez, M.D. Low levels of serum total antioxidant capacity and presence at admission and absence at discharge of a day/night change as a marker of acute paranoid schizophrenia relapse. *Psychiatry Res.* **2017**, *249*, 200–205. [CrossRef] [PubMed]

197. Hoffer, L.J. Vitamin Therapy in Schizophrenia. *Isr. J. Psychiatry Relat. Sci.* **2008**, *45*, 3–10. [PubMed]

198. Sarandol, A.; Kirli, S.; Akkaya, C.; Altin, A.; Demirci, M.; Sarandol, E. Oxidative-antioxidative systems and their relation with serum S100 B levels in patients with schizophrenia: Effects of short term antipsychotic treatment. *Prog. Neuropsychopharmacol. Biol. Psychiatry* **2007**, *31*, 1164–1169. [CrossRef] [PubMed]

199. Young, J.; McKinney, S.B.; Ross, B.M.; Wahle, K.W.; Boyle, S.P. Biomarkers of oxidative stress in schizophrenic and control subjects. *Prostaglandins Leukot. Essent. Fatty Acids* **2007**, *76*, 73–85. [CrossRef] [PubMed]

200. Konarzewska, B.; Stefańska, E.; Wendołowicz, A.; Cwalina, U.; Golonko, A.; Małus, A.; Kowzan, U.; Szulc, A.; Rudzki, L.; Ostrowska, L. Visceral obesity in normal-weight patients suffering from chronic schizophrenia. *BMC Psychiatry* **2014**, *14*, 35. [CrossRef] [PubMed]

201. Magalhães, P.V.; Dean, O.; Andreazza, A.C.; Berk, M.; Kapczinski, F. Antioxidant treatments for schizophrenia. *Cochrane Database Syst. Rev.* **2016**, *2*, CD008919. [CrossRef] [PubMed]

202. Bentsen, H.; Osnes, K.; Refsum, H.; Solberg, D.K.; Bøhmer, T. A randomized placebo-controlled trial of an omega-3 fatty acid and vitamins E + C in schizophrenia. *Transl. Psychiatry* **2013**, *3*, e335. [CrossRef] [PubMed]

203. Sivrioglu, E.Y.; Kirli, S.; Sipahioglu, D.; Gursoy, B.; Sarandöl, E. The impact of omega-3 fatty acids, vitamins E and C supplementation on treatment outcome and side effects in schizophrenia patients treated with haloperidol: An open-label pilot study. *Prog. Neuropsychopharmacol. Biol. Psychiatry* **2007**, *31*, 1493–1499. [CrossRef] [PubMed]

204. Heiser, P.; Sommer, O.; Schmidt, A.J.; Clement, H.W.; Hoinkes, A.; Hopt, U.T.; Schulz, E.; Krieg, J.C.; Dobschütz, E. Effects of antipsychotics and vitamin C on the formation of reactive oxygen species. *J. Psychopharmacol.* **2010**, *24*, 1499–1504. [CrossRef] [PubMed]

205. Kawazoe, T.; Park, H.K.; Iwana, S.; Tsuge, H.; Fukui, K. Human D-amino acid oxidase: An update and review. *Chem. Rec.* **2007**, *7*, 305–315. [CrossRef] [PubMed]

Permissions

List of Contributors

Kinga Linowiecka and Anna A. Brożyna
Department of Human Biology, Faculty of Biological and Veterinary Sciences, Nicolaus Copernicus University, 87-100 Toruń, Poland

Marek Foksinski
Department of Clinical Biochemistry, Faculty of Pharmacy, Collegium Medicum, Nicolaus Copernicus University, 85-092 Bydgoszcz, Poland

Gry Freja Skovsted, Pernille Tveden-Nyborg, Maiken Marie Lindblad and Stine Normann Hansen
Department of Veterinary and Animal Sciences, Faculty of Health and Medical Sciences, University of Copenhagen, Ridebanevej 9, 1870 Frederiksberg C, Denmark

Jens Lykkesfeldt
Faculty of Health and Medical Sciences, University of Copenhagen, Ridebanevej 9, Frederiksberg C, 1870 Copenhagen, Denmark
Department of Veterinary and Animal Sciences, Faculty of Health and Medical Sciences, University of Copenhagen, Ridebanevej 9, 1870 Frederiksberg C, Denmark

Maria Leticia Castro and Georgia M. Carson
School of Biological Sciences, Victoria University, Wellington 6140, New Zealand

Melanie J. McConnell
School of Biological Sciences, Victoria University, Wellington 6140, New Zealand
Malaghan Institute of Medical Research, Wellington 6242, New Zealand

Patries M. Herst
Malaghan Institute of Medical Research, Wellington 6242, New Zealand
Department of Radiation Therapy, University of Otago, Wellington 6242, New Zealand

John F. Pearson
Biostatistics and Computational Biology Unit, University of Otago, Christchurch 8140, New Zealand

Juliet M. Pullar and Margreet C. M. Vissers
Department of Pathology, University of Otago, Christchurch 8140, New Zealand

Renee Wilson and Vicky A. Cameron
Department of Medicine, University of Otago, Christchurch 8140, New Zealand

Janet K. Spittlehouse
Department of Psychological Medicine, University of Otago, Christchurch 8140, New Zealand

Paula M. L. Skidmore
Department of Human Nutrition, University of Otago, Dunedin 9054, New Zealand

Bente Juhl
Medical Department, Aarhus University Hospital, Nørrebrogade 44, 8000 Aarhus C, Denmark

Finn Friis Lauszus
Gynecology & Obstetrics Department, Herning Hospital, Gl. Landevej 61, 7400 Herning, Denmark

Gwendolyn N. Y. van Gorkom, Roel G. J. Klein Wolterink, Catharina H. M. J. Van Elssen, Wilfred T. V. Germeraad and Gerard M. J. Bos
Division of Hematology, Department of Internal Medicine, GROW-School for Oncology and Developmental Biology, Maastricht University Medical Center, 6202AZ Maastricht, The Netherlands

Lotte Wieten
Department of Transplantation Immunology, Maastricht University Medical Center, 6202 AZ Maastricht, The Netherlands

Nerea Martín-Calvo
Department of Preventive Medicine and Public Health, University of Navarra, 31008 Pamplona, Navarra, Spain
IdiSNA, Navarra Institute for Health Research, 31008 Pamplona, Navarra, Spain
CIBER Physiopathology of Obesity and Nutrition (CIBERobn), Carlos III Institute of Health, 28029 Madrid, Spain

Miguel Ángel Martínez-González
Department of Preventive Medicine and Public Health, University of Navarra, 31008 Pamplona, Navarra, Spain
IdiSNA, Navarra Institute for Health Research, 31008 Pamplona, Navarra, Spain
CIBER Physiopathology of Obesity and Nutrition (CIBERobn), Carlos III Institute of Health, 28029 Madrid, Spain
Department of Nutrition, Harvard T.H. Chan School of Public Health, Boston, MA 02115, USA

Renée Wilson, Richard Gearry and Chris Frampton
Department of Medicine, University of Otago, Christchurch 8011, New Zealand

Jinny Willis
Lipid and Diabetes Research Group, Canterbury District Health Board, Christchurch 8011, New Zealand
Lipid & Diabetes Research Group, Canterbury District Health Board, Christchurch 8140, New Zealand

Paula Skidmore and Elizabeth Fleming
Department of Human Nutrition, University of Otago, Dunedin 9016, New Zealand

Anitra Carr
Department of Pathology, University of Otago, Christchurch 8011, New Zealand

Karel Tyml
Centre for Critical Illness Research, Lawson Health Research Institute, London, ON N6A 5W9, Canada
Department of Medical Biophysics, University of Western Ontario, London, ON N6A 5C1, Canada

Harri Hemilä
Department of Public Health, University of Helsinki, Helsinki FI-00014, Finland

Nicola Baillie
Integrated Health Options Ltd., Auckland 1050, New Zealand

Anitra C. Carr
Department of Pathology & Biomedical Science, University of Otago, Christchurch 8140, New Zealand

Selene Peng
Feedback Research Ltd., Auckland 1050, New Zealand

Silvia Maggini
Bayer Consumer Care Ltd., Peter-Merian-Strasse 84, 4002 Basel, Switzerland

Gina Nauman and Mark Levine
National Institutes of Health, National Institute of Diabetes and Digestive and Kidney Diseases, Clinical Nutrition Section, Bethesda, MD 20892, USA

Javaughn Corey Gray, Rose Parkinson and Channing J. Paller
Sidney Kimmel Comprehensive Cancer Center, Johns Hopkins Medical Institutions, Baltimore, MD 21287, USA

Joanna Kocot, Dorota Luchowska-Kocot, Małgorzata Kiełczykowska, Irena Musik and Jacek Kurzepa
Chair and Department of Medical Chemistry, Medical University of Lublin, 4A Chodźki Street, 20-093 Lublin, Poland

Index

Printed in the USA
CPSIA information can be obtained
at www.ICGtesting.com
JSHW051405091023
49903JS00006B/292